CRANIOFACIAL
DYSMORPHOLOGY
Studies
In Honor of Samuel Pruzansky

CRANIOFACIAL DYSMORPHOLOGY
Studies
In Honor of Samuel Pruzansky

EDITORS
M. Michael Cohen, Jr.
Dalhousie University
Halifax, Nova Scotia
Canada

Beverly R. Rollnick
Center for Craniofacial Anomalies
University of Illinois
College of Medicine
Chicago, Illinois

These papers are being printed both as the Journal of Craniofacial Genetics and Developmental Biology, Supplement 1, 1985, Michael Melnick and Harold C. Slavkin, Editors, and as Craniofacial Dysmorphology: Studies in Honor of Samuel Pruzansky, edited by M. Michael Cohen, Jr. and Beverly R. Rollnick.

ALAN R. LISS, INC., NEW YORK

**Address All Inquiries to the Publisher
Alan R. Liss, Inc., 41 East 11th Street, New York, NY 10003**

Copyright © 1985 Alan R. Liss, Inc.

Printed in the United States of America.

Under the conditions stated below the owner of copyright for this book hereby grants permission to users to make photocopy reproductions of any part or all of its contents for personal or internal organizational use, or for personal or internal use of specific clients. This consent is given on the condition that the copier pay the stated per-copy fee through the Copyright Clearance Center, Incorporated, 27 Congress Street, Salem, MA 01970, as listed in the most current issue of "Permissions to Photocopy" (Publisher's Fee List, distributed by CCC, Inc.), for copying beyond that permitted by sections 107 or 108 of the US Copyright Law. This consent does not extend to other kinds of copying, such as copying for general distribution, for advertising or promotional purposes, for creating new collective works, or for resale.

Library of Congress Cataloging in Publication Data
Main entry under title:

Craniofacial dysmorphology.

    "These papers are being printed both as the Journal of craniofacial genetics and developmental biology supplement 1, 1985 . . . and as Craniofacial dysmorphology."
    "Publications of Samuel Pruzansky": p.
    Bibliography: p.
    Includes index.
    1. Otolaryngology—Addresses, essays, lectures.
2. Face—Abnormalities—Genetic aspects—Addresses, essays, lectures. 3. Skull—Abnormalities—Genetic aspects—Addresses, essays, lectures. 4. Pruzansky, Samuel, 1920–1984—Addresses, essays, lectures.
I. Pruzansky, Samuel, 1920–1984. II. Cohen, M. Michael (Meyer Michael), 1937–   . III. Rollnick, Beverly R.
RF71.C73 1985   617′.51   85-10391
ISBN 0-8451-0247-8

CONTENTS

ix	Contributors
1	Foreword

I. INTRODUCTION

5	Samuel Pruzansky, 1920–1984: Background, Achievements, and Reminiscences M. Michael Cohen, Jr. and Beverly R. Rollnick
9	Acknowledgments
10	Publications of Samuel Pruzansky

II. OVERVIEW SECTION

19	Sam Pruzansky As I Remember Him Paul Tessier
23	Congenital Anomalies of the Face and Associated Structures: An International Symposium Twenty-Five Years Ago Josef Warkany
25	Samuel Pruzansky and the Center for Craniofacial Anomalies Celia I. Kaye and Beverly R. Rollnick
31	The Application of Roentgencephalometry to the Study of Craniofacial Anomalies Sven Kreiborg
43	Dysmorphic Growth and Development and the Study of Craniofacial Syndromes M. Michael Cohen, Jr.
57	Regional Specification of Cell-Specific Gene Expression During Craniofacial Development Harold C. Slavkin

III. OROFACIAL CLEFTING

69	Timing Cleft Palate Closure—Age Should Not Be the Sole Determinant Samuel Berkowitz
85	Excess of Parental Non-Righthandedness in Children With Right-Sided Cleft Lip: A Preliminary Report F.C. Fraser and A. Rex
89	An Investigation to Relate the Overall Size of the Maxillary Arch and the Area of Palatal Mucosa in Cleft Lip and Palate Cases at Birth to the Overall Size of the Upper Dental Arch at Five Years of Age Arnold G. Huddart and Angela M. Huddart

97 Velopharyngeal Inadequacy in the Absence of Overt Cleft Palate
Sally J. Peterson-Falzone

IV. CEPHALOMETRIC STUDIES

127 Contrasting Mandibular Growth and Facial Development in Long Face Syndrome, Juvenile Rheumatoid Polyarthritis, and Mandibulofacial Dysostosis
Arne Björk and Vibeke Skieller

139 A Morphometric Analysis of the Craniofacial Configuration in Achondroplasia
M. Michael Cohen, Jr., Geoffrey F. Walker, and Ceib Phillips

167 Craniovertebral Malformations in Hemifacial Microsomia
Alvaro A. Figueroa and Hans Friede

179 The Beckwith-Wiedemann Syndrome: A Longitudinal Study of the Macroglossia and Dentofacial Complex
Hans Friede and Alvaro A. Figueroa

189 Cardiorespiratory Disease Associated With Hallermann-Streiff Syndrome: Analysis of Craniofacial Morphology by Cephalometric Roentgenograms
Hans Friede, Melvin Lopata, Elizabeth Fisher, and Ira M. Rosenthal

199 Skeletal and Functional Craniofacial Adaptations in Plagiocephaly
Sven Kreiborg, Eigild Møller, and Arne Björk

211 Craniofacial Dysmorphology in Syndromes Associated With Abnormal Physical Growth
Nobuyoshi Motohashi

227 The Degenerative, Regenerative Mandibular Condyle: Facial Asymmetry
J. Daniel Subtelny

V. OTHER CONTRIBUTIONS

241 Agnathia-Holoprosencephaly: A Developmental Field Complex Involving Face and Brain. Report of 3 Cases
David Bixler, Richard Ward, and David D. Gale

251 A Computerized Multi-Use Craniofacial Patient Record
Carla A. Evans and Richard L. Christiansen

259 Evaluation of Chromosomal Damage in Males Exposed to Agent Orange and Their Families
Celia I. Kaye, Sita Rao, Stacy J. Simpson, Flori S. Rosenthal, and Maimon M. Cohen

267 Dental Maturation in Hemifacial Microsomia
Hannelore T. Loevy and Scott W. Shore

273 Association of Duane Retraction Syndrome With Craniofacial Malformations
Marilyn T. Miller

283 The Dubowitz Syndrome: A Retrospective
Karlind T. Moller and Robert J. Gorlin

287 Hemifacial Microsomia and the Branchio-Oto-Renal Syndrome
Beverly R. Rollnick and Celia I. Kaye

VI. EXPERIMENTAL ANIMAL STUDIES

299 **The Significance of Receptor Physiology for Corticosterone-Induced Cleft Palate in A/J Mice**
Kenneth S. Brown and Robert M. Hackman

305 **Genetic Variation in Spontaneous and Diphenylhydantoin-Induced Craniofacial Malformations in Mice**
Kenneth S. Brown, Mark I. Evans, and Leslie C. Harne

313 **Blebs and Hematomas in the Lips of CL/Fr and A/J Mice**
Kenneth S. Brown, Suzanne C. Hetzel, Leslie C. Harne, and Sally Long

323 **Experimental Fusion of the Naturally Cleft, Embryonic Chick Palate**
Mark W.J. Ferguson and Lawrence S. Honig

339 **Experimental Teratological Studies With the Mouse CNS Mutations Cranioschisis and Delayed Splotch**
H. Kalter

343 **Index**

Contributors

Samuel Berkowitz, Cranio-Facial Anomalies Program, University of Miami School of Medicine, Miami, FL 33101 **[69]**

David Bixler, Department of Oral Facial Genetics, Ball Residence, Indiana University Schools of Dentistry and Medicine, 1226 W. Michigan St., Indianapolis, IN 46223 **[241]**

Arne Björk, Department of Orthodontics, Royal Dental College, Jagtveg 160, DK-2100, Copenhagen, Denmark **[127, 199]**

Kenneth S. Brown, Laboratory of Developmental Biology and Anomalies, National Institute of Dental Research, National Institutes of Health, Building 30, Room 414, Bethesda, MD 20205 **[299, 305, 313]**

Richard L. Christiansen, School of Dentistry, University of Michigan, Ann Arbor MI 48109 **[251]**

M. Michael Cohen, Jr., Department of Biology, Dalhousie University, Halifax, Nova Scotia, Canada B3H 3J5 **[5, 43, 139]**

Maimon M. Cohen, Genetics Division, Children's Memorial Hospital, 2300 Children's Plaza, Chicago, IL 60614 **[259]**

Carla A. Evans, Craniofacial Program, Children's Hospital, 300 Longwood Ave., Boston, MA 02115 **[251]**

Mark I. Evans, Department of Obstetrics and Gynecology, George Washington University Medical School, Washington, DC 20037 **[305]**

Mark W.J. Ferguson, Department of Basic Dental Sciences, Turner Dental School, University Dental Hospital of Manchester, Higher Cambridge Street, Manchester M15 6FH, England **[323]**

Alvaro A. Figueroa, The Center for Craniofacial Anomalies, University of Illinois College of Medicine, P.O. Box 6998, Chicago, IL 60680 **[167, 179]**

Elizabeth Fisher, Department of Pediatrics, University of Illinois College of Medicine, P.O. Box 6998, Chicago, IL 60680 **[189]**

F.C. Fraser, Division of Community Medicine, Memorial University, Health Sciences Center, St. John's, Newfoundland A1B 3V6 Canada **[85]**

Hans Friede, The Center for Craniofacial Anomalies, University of Illinois College of Medicine, P.O. Box 6998, Chicago, IL 60680 **[167, 179, 189]**

David D. Gale, College of Allied Health and Nursing, Eastern Kentucky University, Richmond, KY 40475 **[241]**

Robert J. Gorlin, Department of Oral Pathology and Genetics, University of Minnesota, 515 Delaware Street S.E., Minneapolis, MN 55455 **[283]**

Robert M. Hackman, Laboratory of Developmental Biology and Anomalies, National Institute of Dental Research, National Institutes of Health, Bethesda, MD 20205 **[299]**

Leslie C. Harne, Laboratory of Developmental Biology and Anomalies, National Institute of Dental Research, National Institutes of Health, Bethesda MD 20205 **[305, 313]**

Suzanne C. Hetzel, Laboratory of Developmental Biology and Anomalies, National Institute of Dental Research, National Institutes of Health, Bethesda, MD 20205 **[313]**

Lawrence S. Honig, Laboratory for Developmental Biology, Andrus Gerontology Center, University of Southern California, University Park MC0191, Los Angeles, CA 90089-0191 **[323]**

Arnold G. Huddart, West Midlands Regional Plastic Unit, Wordsley Hospital, Wordsley, Near Stourbridge, West Midlands DY8 4JB England **[89]**

The number in brackets is the opening page number of the contributor's article.

Contributors

Angela M. Huddart, West Midlands Regional Plastic Unit, Wordsley Hospital, Wordsley, Near Stourbridge, West Midlands DY8 4JB England **[89]**

H. Kalter, Children's Hospital Research Foundation, Elland and Bethesda Avenues, Cincinnati, OH 45229 **[339]**

Celia I. Kaye, Section of Genetics, Lutheran General Hospital, 1775 Dempster St., Park Ridge, IL 60068 **[25, 259, 287]**

Sven Kreiborg, Department of Orthodontics, The Royal Dental College, Jagtvej 160, DK-1200, Copenhagen, Denmark **[31, 199]**

Hannelore T. Loevy, Department of Pediatric Dentistry, University of Illinois College of Dentistry, P.O. Box 6998, Chicago, IL 60680 **[267]**

Sally Long, Department of Anatomy, Medical College of Wisconsin, Milwaukee, WI 53233 **[313]**

Melvin Lopata, Center for Craniofacial Anomalies, Department of Medicine, University of Illinois College of Medicine, P.O. Box 6998, Chicago, IL 60680 **[189]**

Marilyn T. Miller, Department of Ophthalmology, University of Illinois College of Medicine, Eye and Ear Infirmary, 1855 West Taylor Street, Chicago, IL 60612 **[273]**

Karlind T. Moller, Cleft Palate Maxillofacial Clinic, University of Minnesota, 515 Delaware Street S.E., Minneapolis, MN 55455 **[283]**

Eigild Møller, Department of Oral Physiology, The Royal Dental College, Jagtvej 160, DK-2100, Copenhagen, Denmark **[199]**

Nobuyoshi Motohashi, Department of Orthodontics II, School of Dentistry, Tokyo Medical and Dental University, 5-45 Yushima, 1-chome, Bunkyo-ku, Tokyo 113, Japan **[211]**

Sally J. Peterson-Falzone, Center for Craniofacial Anomalies, University of Illinois College of Medicine, P.O. Box 6998, Chicago, IL 60608 **[97]**

Ceib Phillips, School of Dentistry, The University of North Carolina, Chapel Hill, NC 27514 **[139]**

Sita Rao, Department of Pediatrics, Cook County Children's Hospital, 700 South Wood Street, Chicago, IL 60612 **[259]**

A. Rex, Department of Medical Genetics, The Montreal Children's Hospital, Montreal, Quebec, Canada **[85]**

Beverly R. Rollnick, Center for Craniofacial Anomalies, University of Illinois College of Medicine, P.O. Box 6998, Chicago, IL 60680 **[5, 25, 287]**

Ira M. Rosenthal, Department of Pediatrics, University of Illinois College of Medicine, P.O. Box 6998, Chicago, IL 60680 **[189]**

Flori S. Rosenthal, Department of Pediatrics, Cook County Children's Hospital, 700 South Wood Street, Chicago, IL 60612 **[259]**

Scott W. Shore, Department of Pediatric Dentistry, University of Illinois College of Dentistry, P.O. Box 6998, Chicago, IL 60680 **[267]**

Stacy J. Simpson, Genetics Division, Children's Memorial Hospital, 2300 Children's Plaza, Chicago, IL 60614 **[259]**

Vibeke Skieller, Institute of Orthodontics, Royal Dental College, Jagtvej 160, DK-1200, Copenhagen, Denmark **[127]**

Harold C. Slavkin, Laboratory for Developmental Biology, Department of Basic Sciences, School of Dentistry, University Park MC-0101, University of Southern California, Los Angeles, CA 90089-0191 **[57]**

J. Daniel Subtelny, Department of Orthodontics, Eastman Dental Center, 625 Elmwood Avenue, Rochester, NY 14620 **[227]**

Paul Tessier, Centre Medico-Chirurgical Foch, Paris, France **[19]**

Geoffrey F. Walker, School of Dentistry, University of Michigan, Ann Arbor, MI 48109 **[139]**

Richard Ward, Department of Oral Facial Genetics, Ball Residence, Indiana University Schools of Dentistry and Medicine, 1226 W. Michigan Street, Indianapolis, IN 46223 **[241]**

Josef Warkany, University of Cincinnati, The Children's Hospital Research Foundation, Elland and Bethesda Avenues, Cincinnati, OH 45229 **[23]**

Foreword

Prior to Dr. Samuel Pruzansky's recent death, some members of the Center that he started—the Center for Craniofacial Anomalies—approached him about planning a Festschrift in his honor. At that time, Dr. Pruzansky was consulted about a list of contributors. He asked us to co-edit the Festschrift volume. Sadly, a Festschrift meeting could not be convened prior to Dr. Pruzansky's death. Therefore, this volume is entitled "Craniofacial Dysmorphology: Studies in Honor of Samuel Pruzansky." We approached Drs. Harold Slavkin and Michael Melnick, the editors of the *Journal of Craniofacial Genetics and Developmental Biology*, who kindly consented to publish this volume and graciously permitted us to be the guest editors.

The response of the many contributors to this volume has been most gratifying to us because of the high quality of the research manuscripts submitted in spite of the time constraints placed on their preparation. We wish to thank all the contributors for their help, cooperation, and rapid response. We are also grateful to Hal Slavkin, Michael Melnick, and Alan R. Liss, Inc. for making this publication a reality.

M. Michael Cohen, Jr.
Dalhousie University

Beverly R. Rollnick
University of Illinois

I. INTRODUCTION

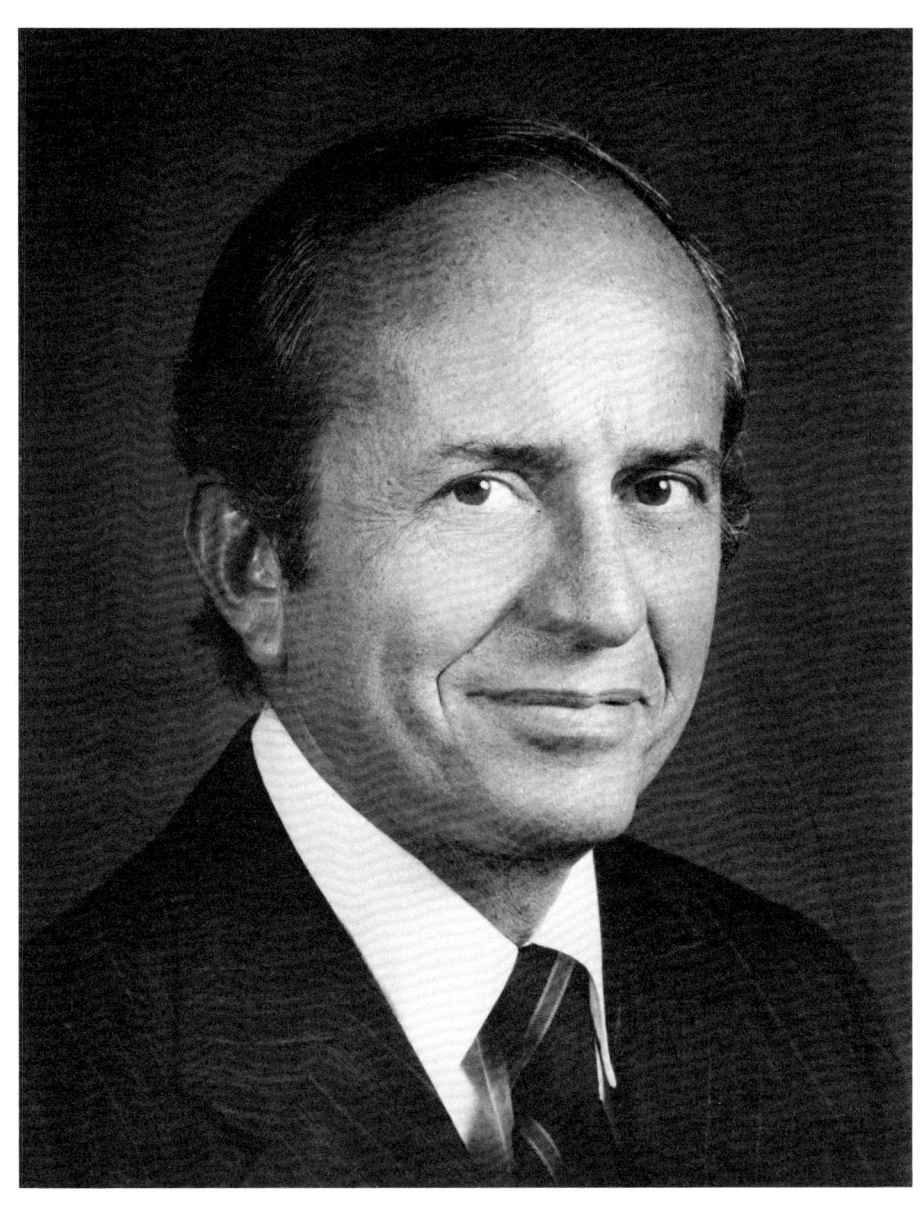

SAMUEL PRUZANSKY
1920–1984

Samuel Pruzansky 1920–1984 Background, Achievements, and Reminiscences

M. Michael Cohen, Jr. and Beverly R. Rollnick
Dalhousie University, Halifax, Nova Scotia, Canada (M.M.C.) and Center for Craniofacial Anomalies, University of Illinois College of Medicine, Chicago (B.R.R.)

Sam Pruzansky was an internationally renowned research scholar, clinician, and teacher. In a professional career that spanned 35 years, he authored more than 190 original publications, received 16 national and international awards for scientific merit, and was the founding Director of the world's first Center for Craniofacial Anomalies at the University of Illinois College of Medicine.

Sam was the first-born child of Russian Jewish immigrants. His father was a watchmaker and jeweler; his mother was a seamstress. His early Talmudic training taught him how to think and to seek knowledge and provided the foundation for what was to follow. Growing up on the lower east side of New York City, he attended Seward High School where, in addition to his studies, he was a member of the varsity soccer team. He attended night school at the City College of New York for 5 years while working during the daytime to save money for his advanced education. Although he was offered a fellowship at Columbia in physics, he pursued his chosen career of dentistry at the University of Maryland. By 1945, he held the B.S. and D.D.S. degrees.

Continuing his education at Tufts University in Boston, Sam Pruzansky was exposed to oral surgery, periodontology, and microbiology, finally earning an advanced degree in oral pathology. During this period of time, he was a part-time clinical instructor in prosthetics as well. Next, he moved on to the University of Illinois where he received his orthodontic training. When he finished, he accepted a part-time position with his mentor, Allan G. Brodie, while he devoted most of his time to pursing Ph.D. level courses in physiology for the next 3 years. His area of special interest was neuromuscular physiology.

A pivotal event that gave focus to Sam Pruzansky's professional career occurred in 1949 when he received a grant from the federal government to conduct long-term growth studies of children born with orofacial clefts. From 1953–1955, he was a Commissioned Officer in the United States Public Health Service. During this period, he served as the Acting Chief of the Clinical Investigations Branch of the National Institute for Dental Research and wrote the initial policy statements that became incorporated into the Institute's mission to study craniofacial anomalies.

In 1959, under the auspices of the National Institute for Dental Research, Sam Pruzansky chaired what was to be regarded as the seminal meeting on craniofacial anomalies. At this meeting—the first international symposium on the subject—critical questions in the field were raised that are still being studied. As Josef Warkany (1985) observes in his contribution to this volume, it was Sam Pruzansky's work and energy that made the now famous Gatlinburg Conference an epoch-making success. The

© 1985 Alan R. Liss, Inc.

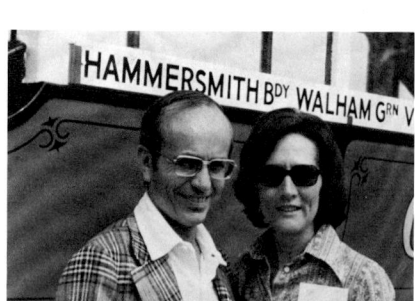
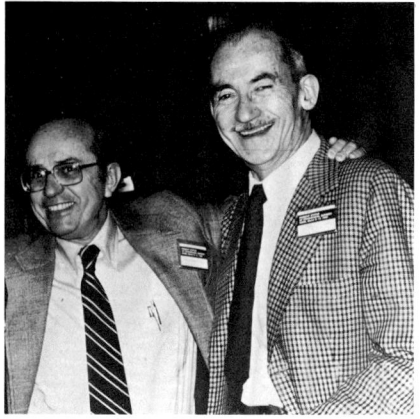
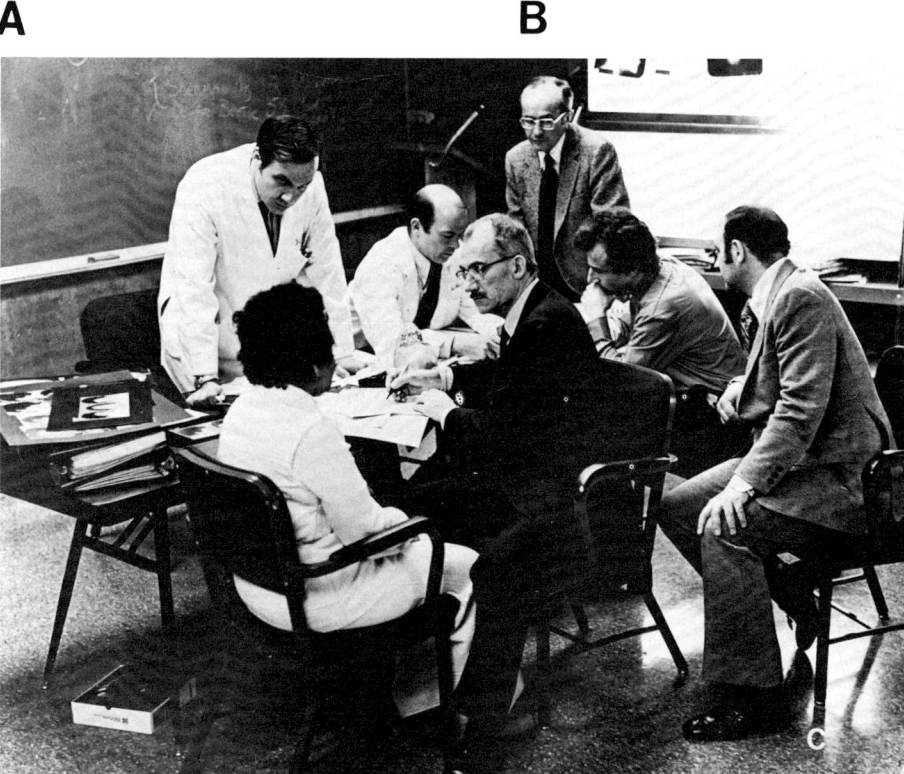

A) Sam and Donna Pruzansky at the meeting of the European Orthodontic Society, London, England, 1973. B) Sam Pruzansky and Paul Tessier at a meeting in Rome, Italy, 1982, on "The Present Status of Craniofacial Surgery." C) Sam Pruzansky with Paul Tessier, Howard Aduss, and others in a working session at the Center for Craniofacial Anomalies, Illinois.

conference proceedings are commemorated in the volume that Sam Pruzansky edited in 1961—*Congenital Anomalies of the Face and Associated Structures.*

Sam Pruzansky was destined to spend the most productive years of his academic life at the University of Illinois. In 1956, he became the Associate Director of the Cleft Palate Clinic. As patients with more complex craniofacial anomalies were referred to the Clinic, its mission was broadened in 1967 to become the first Center for Craniofacial Anomalies. Sam Pruzansky was its founding Director. By 1972, he became Professor of Orthodontics in the Pediatrics Department of the College of Medicine and, in 1980, he assumed the post of Director of Research at the Center to devote the rest of his professional life to research, teaching, and writing.

During his very active academic career, he was a visiting professor at many universities within the United States as well as abroad in Denmark, Japan, Colombia, Sweden, Australia, and Italy. He was a consultant to Crippled Children's Programs in eight different states. He served as President of the American Cleft Palate Association, the Teratology Society, and the International Society for Craniofacial Biology. He was an active member of numerous NIH advisory committees.

The many honors and awards bestowed on Sam Pruzansky are too numerous to recount in detail. Suffice it to say that he was awarded first prize for his research essay by the American Association of Orthodontists in 1957, the William John Gies Award by the American College of Dentistry in 1968, and the Honors Award by the American Cleft Palate Association in 1976. He delivered the Sheldon Friel Memorial Lecture in Copenhagen in 1977 and he was the only nonsurgeon ever invited to deliver the V.H. Kazanjian Lecture in Plastic Surgery at New York University in 1972.

During his career at the Center, Sam Pruzansky was the principal investigator of numerous, major, broad-based, NIH research grants. He initiated longitudinal growth studies of patients with craniofacial anomalies and continued to pursue these studies and to expand their scope. Extensive records were available for every specialist claiming an interest in the head and neck. The extraordinarily rich data base of the Center continues to be unique in the world today.

Sam Pruzansky's professional focus centered around three basic issues: 1) his concern with proper interdisciplinary care for patients with craniofacial anomalies and hence his interest in developing a craniofacial center, 2) his interest in understanding dysmorphic craniofacial growth and development, and 3) his adaptation of cephalometric techniques and modifications of them to document dysmorphic growth, to plan treatment properly, and to evaluate the long-term results of various surgical procedures.

Three articles in the Overview Section of this volume address these topics. Of the three remaining articles that appear in the Overview Section, two are personal reminiscences of Paul Tessier and Josef Warkany about Sam Pruzansky. The other paper reviews the emerging research activities that utilize recombinant DNA technology to investigate the problem of regional specification of cell specific gene expression. Sam Pruzansky was fascinated by the subject of genetics and attended many genetics meetings and lectures to keep abreast of the latest developments in the field.

Sam Pruzansky was an eloquent speaker and was much sought after to deliver keynote addresses around the world. He also had a way of expressing himself in his writings that was almost poetic. The following excerpt is taken from his paper "Clinical Investigation of the Experiments of Nature" [Pruzansky, 1973]:

> The skull is a community of bones and organ systems of diverse phylogenetic origin and variable patterns of development, altogether relating to several functions vital to the life and well-being of the organism. If in the course of development one member of this community is affected adversely, inevitably other parts will suffer.

He was capable of being just as poetic in his correspondence, as in the following paragraph from a letter to a colleague:

> Craniosynostosis intrigues as a drama of nature in which the Sturm und Drang of a growing brain and its hydrodynamic forces compete against the rigidities and sometimes yielding barriers of a brain case derived from dermal placodes and primitive cartilage. In the second act, the drama is intensified by the surgeon's knife that unlocks nature's barriers, stills the storm and brings tranquility in form and size. Now, the third act is to be written. How will it turn out over the long term?

Two sensitively written In Memoriam articles have already appeared in the scientific literature—one by Dan Subtelny [1984], the other by Celia Kaye [1984]. Both review Sam Pruzansky's life's work and capture the essence of his character—his intense enthusiasm, his boundless energy, his capacity for hard work, his strong sense of personal integrity, his intellectual honesty, his zeal for scientific accuracy, his dedication to excellence and his impatience with those of lesser commitment, his inspired teaching, his support and encouragement of those who were willing to learn and willing to work hard, his sensitivity to the problems of patients and their families, and, finally, his charm, his wit, and his humor.

We asked contributors to this volume to send us any personal reminiscences or anecdotes involving Sam Pruzansky. Only a few of these can be reproduced here. Various colleagues spoke of Sam Pruzansky's influence on their choice of a career or about his unfailing support for a project of theirs or his ability to discuss various problems of craniofacial biology with remarkable insight. For example, one professor observes:

> I can honestly say that his encouragement was instrumental in my ultimately pursuing a career in craniofacial developmental anomalies. . . . Because Sam Pruzansky was a true missionary in this area, he never hesitated to give all his support to those of us who were coming along behind him.

Another colleague relates an incident that took place at a scientific meeting. He described to Sam Pruzansky a new project that he was anxious to carry out: "Sam's excitement soon matched mine and before we returned to the hotel, I was promised the necessary research material and financial support as well!" A physician colleague observes:

> I shall miss the important intellectual input he provided to my academic life but mostly I shall miss the person I so often sought when I wanted to share a new observation or conclusion. . . . He could be an interested listener, a devil's advocate, or an enthusiastic supporter.

Sam's beloved wife Donna, a coworker at the Center for Craniofacial Anomalies, predeceased him. Around the anniversary of her death, a close colleague shares the following paragraph from a letter written by Sam Pruzansky:

> It is fortunate that I enjoy what I do and I am grateful for the highs I experience in scholastic endeavors. When I become depressed and lonely and think of my profound loss, especially at this time of year, I find comfort in my studies and I become the son of my forefathers bent over the Talmud in some candle-lit synagogue in east Europe. These are the long-term rewards of a tradition dedicated to education and study.

In a light vein, two colleagues relate a humorous anecdote that occurred at a time when Sam Pruzansky was deeply involved with electromyography in studying the muscles of mastication. At dinner, a rib roast was served and it was rare. With a twinkle in his eye, Sam said, "If I had a spare electrode, I bet I could get a twitch."

Sam Pruzansky will be affectionately remembered and missed by the many colleagues whose lives he touched. In the words of Joe Warkany (1985), "In the change of dentistry from a service occupation to a scientific profession, Sam Pruzansky was a pioneer and leader who left permanent imprints in the field of craniofacial biology."

ACKNOWLEDGMENTS

Numerous people have been particularly generous in their support of this volume. The following merit our special acknowledgment: K.R. Allen, Kenneth W. Bell, Lynn and Samuel Berkowitz, Georgia Lloyd Berndt, James F. Bosma, Ernesto Caronni, Peter J. Coccaro, Sr., Nancy Davidson, Fred L. DeMarco, Nicholas and Sally Peterson-Falzone, Alvaro Figueroa, Jack D. Fisher, Hans Friede, T.M. Garber, Celia Kaye, Elbert W. King, L. Klapper, Takayuki Kuroda, Fujio Miura, Nobuyoshi Motohashi, Kimie and Takashi Ohyama, H.T. Perry, Robert Ricketts, Ethel and Ira Rosenthal, Mamoru Sakuda, Harold Slavkin, Tod Sloan, Thomas P. Sperry, Joanne and Daniel Subtelny, Dan Watkins, and S. Anthony Wolfe.

REFERENCES

Kaye CI: In Memoriam: Samuel Pruzansky, September 10, 1920–February 3, 1984. Am J Med Genet 18:377–378, 1984.
Pruzansky S: Clinical investigation of the experiments of nature. ASHA Report 8:62–94, 1973.
Subtelny JD: Samuel Pruzansky (1920–1984) Am J Orthod 84:529–530, 1984.
Warkany J: Congenital anomalies of the face and associated structures: An international symposium twenty-five years ago. J Craniofac Genet Dev Biol (Suppl 1): 23–24, 1985.

Publications of Samuel Pruzansky

Glickman I, Trafidlo EJ, Pruzansky S: Calcified epithelial cyst in the subcutaneous buccal tissues. Am J Orthod Oral Surg 32:187–190, 1946.
Pruzansky S: A method of storing and spruing wax patterns. Dent. Digest 53:501, October 1947.
Glickman I, Pruzansky S, Ostrach M: The healing of extraction wounds in the presence of retained root remnants and bone frangments. Am J Orthod Oral Surg 33:263–283, 1947.
Pruzansky S: The application of electromyography to dental research. J Am Dent Assoc 44:49–68, January 1952.
Pruzansky S: Serial growth studies of newborns with cleft lip and palate at the University of Illinois. Newslett Am Assoc Cleft Palate Rehab 3:24, January 1953.
Pruzansky S: Electromyographic measurement of the function of muscles of mastication in man. Proc. Inst Med Chicago 19:316–19, June 1953.
Pruzansky S: Description, classification and analysis of unoperated clefts of the lip and palate. Am J Orthod 39:590–611, 1953.
Slaughter WB, Pruzansky S: The rationale for velar closure as a primary procedure in the repair of cleft palate defects. Plast Reconstr Surg 13:341–357, 1954.
Pruzansky S, Richmond JB: Growth of mandible in infants with micrognathia. Am J Dis Child 88:29–42, 1954.
Pruzansky S: The role of the orthodontist in the cleft palate team. Plast Reconstr Surg 14:10–29, 1954.
Bronstein IP, Rosenthal IM, Pruzansky S, Sandord HN: Pseudosenilism of progeria. Am J Dis Child 90:564–565, 1955.
Grossman HJ, Pruzansky S, Rosenthal IM: Progeroid syndrome. Report of a case of Pseudo-senilism. Pediatrics 15:413–423, April 1955.
Pruzansky S: The contributions of recent research in total management of the cleft palate child. The Therapist, April 1955. A publication of the Department of Speech, State University of Iowa.
Pruzansky S: The multi-discipline approach to the treatment of cleft palate in children: Integration of multi-professional resources through a program of basic research. J Int College Surg 24:370–379, 1955.
Pruzansky S: Factors determining arch form in clefts of the lip and palate. Am Jour Orthod 41:827–851, 1955.
Beers MD, Pruzansky S: The growth of the head of an infant with mandibular micrognathia, glossoptosis and cleft palate following the Beverly Douglas operation. Plast Reconstr Surg 16:189–193, 1955.
Pruzansky S: Dentistry's contribution to the treatment of cleft lip and palate. Alpha Omegan, 50:102, September 1956.
Rosenthal IM, Bronstein IP, Dallenbach FD, Pruzansky S, Rosenwald AK: Progeria. A case report with cephalometric roentgenograms and abnormally high concentration of lipoproteins in the serum. Pediatrics 18:565–577, October 1956.
Lis EF, Pruzansky S, Koepp-Baker H, Kobes HR: Cleft lip and palate: Perspectives in management. Pediatr Clin North Am 3:955–1028, November 1956.
Slaughter WB, Pruzansky S, Harris HL: Cleft lip and cleft palate, surgical considerations. Pediatr Clin North Am 3:1029–1047, November 1956.
Pruzansky S: Role of team approach in caring for the handicapped child. J Dent Educ 21:70–75, January 1957.
Lloyd RS, Pruzansky S, Subtelny JD: Prosthetic rehabilitation of cleft palate patient subsequent to multiple surgical and prosthetic failures. J Prosthet Dent 7:216–230, March 1957.
Pruzansky S: Foundations of the Cleft Palate Center and Training Program at the University of Illinois. Angle Orthod 27:69–82, April 1957.
Subtelny JD, Pruzansky S, Subtelny J: Application of roentgenography in the study of speech. In: Kaiser L (ed): "Manual of Phonetics." Amsterdam: North Holland Publishing Co., 1957.

Pruzansky S, Lis EF: Roentgenography of infants: Sedation, instrumentation and research. Am J Orthod 44:159–186, 1958.

Joram PR, Grogan HT, Pruzansky S: Flexible rubber molds for accurate multiple reproductions of plaster casts. J Prosthet Dent 8:100–106, 1958.

Poulton DR, Pruzansky S: Report of a case with super-numerary teeth and treatment. J Dent Child Third Quarter:212–214, 1958.

Pruzansky S: Congenital malformations. J Am Dent Assoc 56:633–637, 1958.

Slaughter WB, Pruzansky S, Harris H, Berger JC: A new surgical concept for repair of congenital clefts of lip and palate. Surg Clin North Am 945–958, August 1958.

Pruzansky S: Orthodontics in other health services, orthodontics in mid-century. In: Moyers RE (ed): "Transactions of Workshops in Orthodontics." St. Louis: C.V. Mosby Co., 1959.

Curtin JW, Greeley PW: Osteochondroma of the mandibular condyle (with EMG and cephalometric analysis by S. Pruzansky). Plast Reconstr Surg 24:511–521, 1959.

Kobes HM, Pruzansky S: The cleft palate team: A historical review. Am J Public Health 50:200–205, 1960.

Pruzansky S: Applicability of electromyographic procedures as a clinical aid in the detection of occlusal disharmony. Dent Clin North Am pp 117–130, March 1960.

Barber TK, Pruzansky S, Lauterstein A, Kindelsperger R: Application of roentgenographic cephalometry to pedodontic research. J Dent Child 27:97–106, 1960.

Pruzansky S: Contributions of roentgenographic cephalometry to the study of congenital and acquired malformations of the face. Dent Clin North Am 395–417, 1960.

Pruzansky S (ed): "Congenital Malformations of the Face and Associated Structures." Springfield, Illinois: Charles C. Thomas Co., 1960.

Barber TK, Pruzansky S, Kindelsperger R: An evaluation of the oblique cephalometric film. J Dent Child Second Quarter:94–105, 1961.

Pruzansky S: Panel discussion of essays presented at the scientific sessions of the American Association of Orthodontists, 1961. Am J Orthod 48:290–293, April 1962.

Pruzansky S: Annotated bibliography for panel discussion on oral pharyngeal physiology and its relation to orthodontic problems. Am J Orthod 48:290–293, April 1962.

Ruess AL, Pruzansky S, Lis EF, Pateau L: The oro-facial digital syndrome: A multiple congenital condition of females with associated chromosomal abnormalities. Pediatrics 29:985–995, June 1962.

Coccaro PJ, Subtelny JD, Pruzansky S: Growth of soft palate in cleft palate children: A serial cephalometric study. Plast Reconstr Surg 30:43–55, July 1962.

Lauterstein A, Pruzansky S, Barber TK: Effect of deciduous mandibular molar pulpotomy on the eruption of succedaneous premolar. J Dent Res 41:1367–1372, 1962.

Pruzansky S: Pre-surgical orthopedics and bone grafting for infants with cleft lip and palate: A dissent. Cleft Palate J 1:164–182, April 1964.

Aduss H, Pruzansky S: Postnatal craniofacial development in children with the oral-facial digital syndrome. Arch Oral Biol 9:193–203, 1964.

Pruzansky S, Aduss H: Arch form and the deciduous occlusion in complete unilateral clefts. Cleft Palate J 1:411–418, October 1964.

Lauterstein A, Pruzansky S: A roentgencephalometric study of the inflated labial vestibule. Angle Orthod 34:314–325, October 1964.

Coccaro PJ, Pruzansky S: Longitudinal study of skeletal and soft tissue profile in children with unilateral cleft lip and cleft palate. Cleft Palate J 2:1–12, January 1965.

Pruzansky S (Chairman): Report of the planning conference on Maxillofacial Prosthetics: National Institute of Dental Research, February 18, 1965.

Ruess AL, Pruzansky S, Lis EF: Intellectual development and the OFD syndrome: A review. Cleft Palate J 2:350–356, October 1965.

Pruzansky S: Is roentgencephalometry being fully exploited as an instrument for clinical investigation? Dent Clin North Am pp 211–217, March 1966.

Pruzansky S, Ruess AL, Buzdygan D: Oral-facial-digital syndrome in a Negro female. Plast Reconstr Surg 37:221–226, March 1966.

Pruzansky S: Book review of "Treatment of Cleft Lip and Palate" (Proceedings of an International Symposium held in Zurich, April 9–11, 1964, Hans Huber Published, 1964, pp. 224 Fr/Dms 8.50), Rudolf H (ed). Cleft Palate J 3:301–309, 1966.

Kraus BS, Jordan RE, Pruzansky S: Dental abnormalities in the deciduous and permanent dentition of individuals with cleft lip and palate. J Dent Res 45:1736–1746, 1966.

Pruzansky S: Letter to the editor. Cleft Palate J 4:184–186, 1967.

Aduss H, Pruzansky S: The nasal cavity in complete unilateral cleft lip and palate. Arch Otolaryngol 85:53–61, January 1967.

Lauterstein A, Pruzansky S, Levine NL: Bilateral asymmetry in mandibular tooth development. J Dent Res 46:279–285, 1967.

Pruzansky S, Elliott CR, Curtin JW, Gold HO: Somatic and psychological rehabilitation of facially deformed young adult. J Am Dent Assoc 74:1474–1479, June 1967.

Coccaro PJ, Pruzansky S, Subtelny, JD: Nasopharyngeal growth. Cleft Palate J 4:214–226, July 1967.

Meskin LH, Pruzansky S: Validity of the birth certificate in the epidemiologic assessment of facial clefts. J Dent Res 46:1456–1459, 1967.

Pruzansky S, Aduss H: Prevalence of arch collapse and malocclusion in complete unilateral cleft lip and palate. Trans Eur Orthod Soc pp 365–382, 1967.

Pruzansky S: Discussion of early treatment of cleft lip and palate including feeding of infants. Trans Eur Orthod Soc pp 410–414, 1967.

Meskin LH, Pruzansky S, Gullen WH: An epidemiologic investigation of factors related to the extent of facial clefts. I. Sex of patient. Cleft Palate J 5:23–29, 1968.

Aduss H, Pruzansky S: The width of the cleft at level of tuberosities in complete unilateral cleft lip and palate. Plast Reconstr Surg 41:113–123, February 1968.

Berkowitz S, Pruzansky S: Stereophotogrammetry of serial casts of cleft palate. Angle Orthod 38:136–149, April 1968.

Handelman CS, Pruzansky S: Occlusion and dental profile with complete bilateral cleft lip and palate. Angle Orthod 38:185–198, July 1968.

Lauterstein A, Pruzansky S: Bilateral symmetry in mandibular apical tooth growth. Arch Oral Biol 13:1047–1055, September 1968.

Pruzansky S: What is craniofacial biology? J Dent Res 47:931–933, 1968.

Meskin LH, Pruzansky S: Epidemiologic relationship of age of parents to type and extent of facial clefts. Acta Chir Plast 10:249–259, 1968.

Pruzansky S: Kinesiologic studies in craniofacial malformations. Proceedings of the 1st International Congress of Electromyographic Kinesiology, Montreal, August 1968. Electromyography [Suppl 1] 8:77–87, 1968.

Pruzansky S: Postnatal development of craniofacial malformations. J Dent Res 47:936–940, 1968.

Pruzansky S: Not all dwarfed mandibles are alike. Birth Defects IV:120–129, February 1969.

Lauterstein A, Pruzansky S: Tooth anomalies in the oral-facial-digital syndrome. Teratology 2:137–145, May 1969.

Meskin LH, Pruzansky S: A malformation profile of facial cleft patients and their siblings. Cleft Palate J 6:309–315, July 1969.

Pruzansky S, Mason RM: The "stretch-factor" in soft palate function. J Dent Res 40(5):972, 1969.

Pruzansky S: Discussion. Early treatment of cleft lip and palate. Proceedings of Second International Symposium, April 19–20, 1969, Northwestern University Dental School, pp 163–173, 1969.

Shah CV, Pruzansky S, Harris WS: Cardiac malformations with facial clefts, with observations of the Pierre Robin syndrome. Am J Dis Child 119:238–244, March 1970.

Solomon LM, Fretzin D, Pruzansky S: Pilosebaceous abnormalities in Apert's syndrome. Arch Dermatol 102:381–385, October 1970.

Solomon LM, Fretzin D, Pruzansky S: Pilosebaceous dysplasia in the oral-facial-digital syndrome. Arch Dermatol 102:598–602, December 1970.

Pruzansky S, Markovic M, Buzdygan D: Twins with clefts. Acta Genet Med Gemellol 19:224–229, 1970.

Osborne GS, Pruzansky S, Koepp-Baker H: Upper cervical spine anomalies and osseous nasopharyngeal depth. J Speech Hearing Res 14:14–22, March 1970.

Aduss H, Pruzansky S, Miller M: Interorbital distance in cleft lip and palate. Teratology 4:171–182, May 1971.

Pruzansky S: Book review of "The Uniqueness of Man," Roslansky JD (ed), Amsterdam: North Holland, 1969. Teratology, 4:214–215, May 1971.

Pruzansky S: Book review of "Advice to Parents of a Cleft Palate Child," by Wicka DK, Falk ML. Springfield, Illinois: Charles C. Thomas, 1970. J Am Dent Assoc 82:1436–1437, June 1971.

Pruzansky S: The challenge and opportunity in craniofacial anomalies. Cleft Palate J 8:239–250, July 1971.

Gorlin RJ, Cervenka J, Pruzansky S: Facial clefting and its syndromes. Birth Defects VII:3–49, June 1971.

Pruzansky S: Twins with Pierre Robin syndrome. Birth Defects VII:72–75, June 1971.

Shapiro B, Meskin LH, Cervenka J, Pruzansky S: Cleft uvula: A microform of facial clefts and its genetic basis: Birth Defects VII:80–82, June 1971.

Solomon L, Cohen MM, Pruzansky S: Pilosebaceous abnormalities in Apert type acrocephalosyndactyly. Birth Defects VII:193–195, June 1971.

Pashayan H, Pruzansky D, Pruzansky S: Are anticonvulsants teratogenic? Letter to the editor. Lancet 2:702–703, September 21, 1971.

Pruzansky S: The growth of the premaxillary-vomerine complex in complete bilateral cleft lip and palate. Tandlaegebladet 75:1157–1169, 1971.

Curtin JW, Pruzansky S: The stapling operation for complete bilateral cleft lip and palate. Trans Fifth Int Congr of Plast Reconstr Surg. Butterworths, 1971, pp 182–84.

Battle CU, Pruzansky S: Pedodontics and Dr. Bernick's articles. Letter to the editor. Clin Pediatr 11:85, February 1972.

Pruzansky S: Book review of "Cleft Lip and Palate," Grabb WC, Rosenstein SW, Bzoch KC (eds). Boston: Little-Brown Co., 1971. J Am Dent Assoc 84:649–650, March 1972.

Friede H, Pruzansky S: Longitudinal study of growth in bilateral cleft lip and palate from infancy to adolescence. Plast Reconstr Surg 49:392–403, April 1972.

Friede H, Pruzansky S: Changes in profile in complete bilateral cleft lip and palate from infancy to adolescence. Trans Eur Orthod Soc pp 1–11, July 1972.

Pruzansky S: Genetic Engineering. Letter to the editor. Am J Orthod 62:539–542, November 1972.

Kreiborg S, Pruzansky S, Pashayan H: The Saethre-Chotzen syndrome. Teratology 6:287–294, December 1972.

Horowitz SL, Berkowitz S, Broadway ES, Gorlin RJ, Harvold E, Hixon EH, Pruzansky S, Rosse RD: Cleft lip and cleft palate: Research relevant to clinical management in dentistry. An NIDR State of the Art Report. Am J Orthod 63:398–406, 1973.

Pashayan H, Pruzansky S, Putterman A: A family with blepharo-naso-facial malformation. Am J Dis Child 125:389–393, March 1973.

Pruzansky S: The temporomandibular joint. Otolaryngol Clin North Am 6:523–548, June 1973.

Aduss H, Pruzansky S: Orthodontic diagnosis. In: Cohen L (ed): "Oral Diagnosis and Treatment Planning." Springfield, Illinois: Charles C. Thomas Co., 1973, pp 219–234.

Sadowsky CL, Aduss H, Pruzansky S: The soft tissue profile in unilateral clefts. Angle Orthod 43:233–246, July 1973.

Pruzansky S: Cleft lip and palate: Therapy and prevention. J Am Dent Assoc 87:1048–1054, October 1973.

Battle CU, Pashayan H, Pruzansky S: Special management of craniofacial problems. In: Behrman RE (ed): "Neonatology: Diseases of the Fetus and Infant." St. Louis: C.V. Mosby Co., 1973.

Pruzansky S: Oral-facial clefts and other malformations. In: Carlos JP (ed): "Prevention and Oral Health." Fogarty International Center Series on Preventive Medicine, Vol. 1. Bethesda: DHEW, 1973.

Pruzansky S: Clinical investigations of the experiments of nature. ASHA Report 8:63–94, 1973.

Pashayan H, Pruzansky S: Polyostotic fibrous dysplasia (McCune-Albright syndrome). Am J Dis Child 126:618, 1973.

Solomon L, Medenica MM, Pruzansky S, Kreiborg S: Apert syndrome and palatal mucopolysaccharides. Teratology 8:287–292, December 1973.

Putterman AM, Pashayan H, Pruzansky S: Eye findings in the blepharo-naso-facial malformation syndrome. Am J Ophthalmol 76:825–831, November 1973.

Pruzansky S: Book review of "Third Symposium on Oral Sensation and Perception: The Mouth of the Infant," Bosma JF (ed). J Dent Educ 37:55–56, October 1973.

Pruzansky S: Concluding comment II. In: Bosma JF (ed): "Fourth Symposium Oral Sensation and Perception." Bethesda: DHEW Publication No. 73-546 (NIH), 1973, pp 390–408.

Pruzansky S: Monitoring growth of the infant with cleft lip and palate. Trans Eur Orthod Soc 49:538–546, 1973.

Pruzansky S, Miller M, Kammer JF: Ocular defects in craniofacial syndromes. In: Goldberg MF (ed):

"Genetics and Metabolic Eye Disease." Boston: Little-Brown & Co., 1974.

Berkowitz S, Krischer J, Pruzansky S: Quantitative analysis of cleft palate casts. Cleft Palate J 2:134–161, April 1974.

Pries C, Mittelman D, Miller M, Solomon LM, Pashayan H, Pruzansky S: The EEC syndrome. Am J Dis Child 127:840–844, June 1974.

Peterson S, Pruzansky S: Palatal anomalies in the syndromes of Apert and Crouzon. Cleft Palate J 11:394–403, October 1974.

Pashayan H, Pruzansky S, Solomon L: The EEC syndrome: Report of six patients. Birth Defects X:105–127, 1974.

Pruzansky S: Organization of an interdisciplinary unit for the study of craniofacial anomalies. In: "Symposium Dental Management of the Handicapped Child." Iowa City: University of Iowa Press, 1974.

Aduss H, Friede H, Pruzansky S: Management of the protruding premaxilla. In: Georgiade N (ed): "Proceedings of Conference on Cleft Lip and Palate," Education Foundation Society of Plastic and Reconstructive Surgery. St. Louis: C.V. Mosby Co., 1974.

Curtin JW, Pruzansky S: Unilateral mandibulomaxillary agenesis: Components of research and surgical reconstruction. In: Georgiade N (ed): "Proceedings of Conference on Cleft Lip and Palate," Education Foundation Society of Plastic and Reconstructive Surgery. St. Louis: C.V. Mosby Co., 1974.

Battle C, Pashayan H, Pruzansky S: Streeter's bands. Birth Defects X:117–120, 1974.

Pashayan H, Fraser FC, Pruzansky S: Variable limb malformations in the Brachmann-Cornelia de Lange syndrome. Birth Defects XI:147–156, 1975.

Battle C, Harris W, Pashayan H, Pruzansky S: AA-association of microtia with supravalvular aortic stenosis. Birth Defects XI:410–414, 1975.

Pruzansky S: Roentgencephalometric studies of tonsils and adenoids in normal and pathologic states. Ann Otol Rhinol Laryngol 84:55–62, 1975.

Neiman GS, Peterson SJ, Pruzansky S: Delayed pharyngeal flap success: Report of a case. Cleft Palate J 12:244–246, April 1975.

Roberts FG, Pruzansky S, Aduss H: An X-radiocephalometric study of mandibulofacial dysostosis in man. Arch Oral Biol 20:265–281, 1975.

Pruzansky S, Pashayan H, Kreiborg S, Miller M: Roentgencephalometric studies of the premature craniofacial synostoses: Report of a family with Saethre-Chotzen syndrome. Birth Defects XI:226–237, 1975.

Ohyama T, Gold H, Pruzansky S: Maxillary obturator with silicone-lined hollow extension. J Prosthet Dent 34:336–341, September 1975.

Milenkovich PM, Gold HO, Pruzansky S: Orthodontic prosthodontic collaboration in the treatment of craniofacial anomalies. Trans Eur Orthod Soc 143–154, 1975.

Pruzansky S: Anomalies of the face and brain. Birth Defects V:183–204, 1975.

Katz A, Pruzansky S: Training program in maxillofacial prosthetics for medical artists. Jour Dent Educ 39:216–221, 1975.

Pruzansky S, Friede H: Two sisters with unoperated bilateral cleft lip and palate, age 6 and 4 years. Br J Plast Surg 28:251–258, 1975.

Pruzansky S: Roentgencephalometry of infants: 1949–73. In: "Transactions of the Third International Orthodontic Congress." London: Crosby Lockwood Staples, 1975, pp 101–117.

Pruzansky S, Pashayan H: Letter to the editor. Cleft Palate J 13:76–77, 1976.

Pruzansky S: Clinical Conferences: A new feature in the Cleft Palate J 13:85–87, 1976.

Pruzansky S, Aduss H: Cleft lip and palate. J Clin Orthod 10:380–395, May 1976.

Falzone-Peterson S, Pruzansky S: Cleft palate and congenital palatopharyngeal incompetency in mandibulofacial dysostosis: Frequency and problems in treatment. Cleft Palate J 13:354–360, October 1976.

Beligere N, Caldarelli D, Pruzansky S: Bilateral congenital choanal atresia and absence of respiratory distress. Cleft Palate J 13:342–349, October 1976.

Morris AL (Chairman), Ackerman JL, Fleisch R, Kerrigan JP, Logan TP, Moore AW, Proffit WR, Pruzansky S, White RP: "Seriously Handicapping Orthodontic Conditions." Washington, DC: National Academy of Sciences, May 1976.

Hutchinson JC, Caldarelli DD, Valvassori GE, Pruzansky S, Parris P: The otologic manifestations of mandibulofacial dyostosis. Trans Am Acad Ophthalmol Otolaryngol 84:520–528, 1977.

Aduss H, Schwarz CJ, McDaniel RT, Pruzansky S: Serial extraction. J Am Dent Assoc 95:573–581, 1977.
Pruzansky S: Time: The fourth dimension in syndrome analysis applied to craniofacial malformations. Birth Defects XIII:3–28, 1977.
Pashayan H, Pruzansky S: Congenital malformations: Special management of craniofacial anomalies. In: Behrman RE (ed): "Neonatal Perinatal Medicine: Disease of the Fetus and Infant." St. Louis: C.V. Mosby, 1977, pp 879–894.
Pruzansky S: Radiocephalometric studies of the basicranium in craniofacial malformations. In: Bosma JF (ed): "Symposium on Development of the Basicranium." HEW Publications, 1977, pp 278–300.
Pruzansky S, Parris P, Laffer J: The making of a data bank for the Center for Craniofacial Anomalies. In: McCormick BH (ed): Proceedings of the Third Illinois Conference on Medical Information Systems." Chicago: University of Illinois Medical Center, 1977.
Tanaka Y, Gold HO, Pruzansky S: A simplified technique for fabricating a lightweight obturator. J Prosthet Dent 38:638–642, December 1977.
Solomon LM, Pruzansky S: Disseminate pigmented nevi and short stature. Mod Probl Paediatr 20:165–166, 1978.
Jamehdor M, Beligere N, Kaye CI, Pruzansky S, Rosenthal IM: Incomplete EEC syndrome in a patient with mosaic monosomy 21. Cleft Palate J 15:390–397, 1978.
Gold HO, Pruzansky S: Multiple abutment fixed partial dentures in maxillofacial prosthetics. J Prosthet Dent 41:424–444, 1979.
Herring SW, Rowlatt UF, Pruzansky S: Anatomical abnormalities in mandibulofacial dysostosis. Am J Med Genet 3:225–259, 1979.
Wong W, Cohen MM, Miller M, Pruzansky S, Rosenthal IM: Case report for syndrome identification. Cleft Palate J 16:286–290, 1979.
Pruzansky S, Laffer J, Parris P: Congenital palatopharyngeal incompetence: Utilization of a data bank for clinical, epidemiological and genetic studies. In: Williams BT (ed): "Proceedings of the Fourth Illinois Conference on Medical Information Systems." Urbana: University of Illinois, 1979.
Kaye CI, Rollnick BR, Pruzansky S: Malformations of the auricle: Isolated and in syndromes. IV. Cumulative pedigree data. Birth Defects XV:163–169, 1979.
Pruzansky S: Foreword. In: Slavkin HC (ed): "Developmental Craniofacial Biology." Philadelphia: Lea & Febinger, 1979.
Helmi C, Pruzansky S: Craniofacial and extracranial malformations in the Klippel-Feil syndrome. Cleft Palate J 17:65–88, 1980.
Tanaka Y, Gold H, Pruzansky S: Copperplated molds for facial prostheses. J Prosthet Dent 43:445–449, 1980.
Caldarelli DD, Hutchinson J, Pruzansky S, Valvassori G: Comparison of microtia and temporal bone anomalies in hemifacial microsomia and mandibulofacial dysostosis. Cleft Palate J 17:103–110, 1980.
Poonawalla HH, Kaye CI, Rosenthal I, Pruzansky S: Hemifacial microsomia in a patient with Klinefelter syndrome. Cleft Palate J 17:194–196, 1980.
Rowlatt U, Pruzansky S: Premaxillary agenesis, ocular hypotelorism holoprosencephaly, and extracranial anomalies in an infant with a normal karyogram. Cleft Palate J 17:197–204, 1980.
Pruzansky S: Congenital craniofacial malformations. In: Grossman H, Stubblefield R (eds): "The Physician and the Mental Health of the Child, II, Psychological Concomitants of Illness." American Medical Association, 1980, pp 103–106.
Miller M, Pruzansky S: Craniofacial anomalies. In: Peyman Sanders, and Goldberg (eds): "Principles and Practice of Ophthalmology." Philadelphia: W.B. Saunders Co., 1980.
Pruzansky S: Letter to the editor. Cleft Palate J 17:264, 1980.
Pruzansky S: Comment. Birth Defects XVI:179–180, 1980.
Pruzansky S: The Dentist on a craniofacial team. Birth Defects XVI:115–124, 1980.
Motohashi N, Pruzansky S, Day D: Roentgencephalometric analysis of craniofacial growth in the Johanson-Blizzard syndrome. J Craniofac Genet Dev Biol 1:57–72, 1981.
Motohashi N, Pruzansky S, Kawata T: Roentgencephalometric analysis of cerebral gigantism: Report of four patients. J Craniofac Genet Dev Biol 1:73–94, 1981.
Motohashi N, Pruzansky S: Long-term effects of premaxillary excision in patients with complete bilateral cleft lips and palates. Cleft Palate J 18:177–187, 1981.

Peterson-Falzone SJ, Pruzansky S, Parris P, Laffer JL: Nasopharyngeal dysmorphology in the syndromes of Apert and Crouzon. Cleft Palate J 18:237–250, 1981.

Rollnick BR Pruzansky S: Genetic services at a Center for Craniofacial Anomalies. Cleft Palate J 18:304–313, 1981.

Beligere N, Harris V, Pruzansky S: Progressive bony dysplasia in Apert syndrome. Radiology 39:593–597, 1981.

Milenkovich PM, Gold HO, Pruzansky S: Orthodontic-prosthodontic collaboration in the treatment of craniofacial anomalies. Int J Orthod 19:9–18, 1981.

Pruzansky S: Center for Craniofacial Anomalies: Spin-offs for medical education and delivery of health care. Otolaryngol Clin North Am 14:777–782, 1981.

Mafee MF, Valvassori GE, Dobben A, Kumar SE, Pruzansky S: Radiographic evaluation of the first and second branchial arch syndromes. Proc XVth Int Congress, Neuroradiology, pp 26–37, 1981.

Kreiborg S, Pruzansky S: Craniofacial growth in premature craniofacial synostosis. Scand J Plast Reconstr Surg 15:171–186, 1981.

Pruzansky S: Craniofacial surgery: The experiment on nature's experiment. II. Historical perspectives. In: McNamara JA, Jr., Carlson DS, Ribbens KA (eds): "The Effect of Surgical Intervention on Craniofacial Growth." Monograph No. 12, Craniofacial Growth Series, University of Michigan, 1981.

Pruzansky S: Premaxillary excision. Letter to the editor. Cleft Palate J 19:146–149, 1982.

Figueroa A, Pruzansky S: Terminal transverse defects with orofacial malformations (TTV-OAV): Case reports with mandibular prognathism and submucous cleft palate. Cleft Palate J 19:139–144, 1982.

Pruzansky S, Slavkin HC: Congenital and acquired craniofacial malformations. An evaluation and assessment of the State of the Science. Bethesda: NIH, 1982.

Pruzansky S: Bone grafting in clefts. Letter to the editor. Plast Reconstr Surg 70:271–272, 1982.

Beligere N, Brigham G, Pruzansky S: Perinatal intensive care in craniofacial anomalies. In: Aladjem S, Vidyasagar D (eds): "Atlas of Perinatology." Philadelphia: W.B. Saunders Co., 1982, pp 127–140.

Pruzansky S, Costaras M, Rollnick BR: Radiocephalometric findings in a family with craniofrontonasal dysplasia. Birth Defects XVIII:121–138, 1982.

Costaras M, Pruzansky S, Broadbent BH, Jr: Bony interorbital distance (BIOD), head size, and level of the cribriform plate relative to orbital height: I. Normal standards for age and sex. J Craniofac Genet Dev Biol 2:5–18, 1982.

Costaras M, Pruzansky S: Bony interorbital distance (BIOD), head size, and level of the cribriform plate relative to orbital height: II. Possible pathogenesos or orbital hypertelorism. J Craniofac Genet Dev Biol 2:19–34, 1982.

Pruzansky S: Craniofacial surgery: The experiment on nature's experiment. Review of three patients operated by Paul Tessier. Eur J Orthod 4:151–171, 1982.

Weiss E, Loevy H, Saunders A, Pruzansky S, Rosenthal IM: Monozygotic twins discordant for Ullrich-Turner syndrome. Am J Med Genet 13:389–399, 1982.

Figueroa AA, Pruzansky S: The external ear, mandible, and other components of hemifacial microsomia. J Maxillofac Surg 4:200–211, 1982.

Figueroa A, Pruzansky S, Rollnick BR: Meige Disease (familial lymphedema praecox) and cleft palate: Report of a family and review of the literature. Cleft Palate J 20:151–157, 1983.

Pruzansky S: Discussion of "The use of cranial bone grafts in the closure of alveolar and anterior palatal clefts" by Wolfe SA and Berkowitz S. Plast Reconstr Surg 72(2):669–671, 1983.

Costaras-Volarich M, Pruzansky S: Is the mandible intrinsically different in operated Crouzon syndromes? Am J Orthod 85:475–487, 1984.

Figueroa AA, Gans BJ, Pruzansky S: Long term follow-up of a mandibular costochondral graft. Oral Surg (in press), 1984.

Pruzansky S: Otocraniofacial syndromes: Clinical studies on mandibulofacial dysostosis, hemifacial microsomia and variants. In: Caronni EP (ed): "Craniofacial Surgery: Published Proceedings of an International Course on the Present Status of Craniofacial Surgery, Rome, 1982." Boston: Little Brown & Co., (in press), 1984.

Pruzansky S: Longitudinal growth studies of craniofacial anomalies 1949–1983. What have we learned? Presented at the First International Meeting of the Craniofacial Society of Great Britain, Birmingham, England, July 13–16, 1983 (in press), 1985.

Mafee MF, Corrales MM, Valvassori GE, Dobben GD, Capek V, Pruzansky S: Computed tomography in the evaluation of the orbit and the bony inter-orbital distance (B.I.O.D.). Am J Neuroradiol (in press), 1985.

II. OVERVIEW SECTION

Sam Pruzansky As I Remember Him

Paul Tessier
Centre Medico-Chirurgical Foch, Paris, France

On February 3, 1984, Sam Pruzansky died at the peak of his scientific career. We all lost a master. I lost a personal friend, and I write these pages in honor of my departed friend.

With his analytic abilities, Sam could think anatomically as an anatomist. He understood pathological conditions like a well-educated pediatrician. He understood craniofacial growth and development better than anyone, and he often understood the consequences of craniofacial surgery better than the surgeons themselves, and this irritated some of them.

Sam and I met for the first time at a workshop conducted by the late John Converse in 1968. When I presented the concepts and techniques of craniofacial surgery, the field was in its infancy. Some of the concepts and procedures were in contradiction to Sam's own beliefs, but he was open-minded. He sometimes seemed reluctant about surgical concepts and procedures and gave the impression that he did not fully realize what craniofacial surgery could offer for his own analysis.

We met again at another workshop organized by John Converse at New York University in 1971. During the three intervening years, Sam had assimilated the new ideas about Crouzon syndrome, Apert syndrome, Treacher Collins syndrome, and hypertelorbitism. Moreover, he had added his own personal visions to the field, which, after discussion, I thought correct. For example, he wanted to see whether or not, with maxillary advancement and bone grafting, I could improve the secondary deformities of a cleft palate patient he had prepared by orthodontics. The field trial was satisfactory, and the case was beautifully analyzed by Sam.

In 1972, Sam invited me to examine and operate on patients at the Center for Craniofacial Anomalies at the University of Illinois. The visits were sponsored by the Chicago surgeons. For 5 years, I went to the Center twice each year for a 2-week period to work with Sam. In November, 1974, Sam conducted a 2-day workshop on the surgery that I had performed in the United States over a 3-year period. A series of 74 cases was analyzed and criticized by my former hosts John Converse, Tom Cronin, Mike Lewin, Joe Murray, Peter Randall, and Ken Salyer. Based on the workshop, Sam wrote a paper entitled: "Craniofacial surgery: The experiment on nature's experiment" [Pruzansky, 1982]. (Dr. Pruzansky wrote a second paper in this series [Pruzansky, 1981] (*ed.*).

Sam once showed me an adult Crouzon patient in whom he had corrected the malocclusion to near perfection during an earlier 3-year period. A Le Fort III midface advancement was no longer possible for this patient. I hesitated awhile before I said,

© 1985 Alan R. Liss, Inc.

"Sam, this is a remarkable orthodontic result, but you will have to reverse the result to its original condition so that I can surgically correct all of the facial malformations together, including the severe occular proptosis and midface deficiency." Sam was silent, but after a moment he accepted that his efforts were wrong when the new craniofacial surgical concepts and procedures were considered. He reversed the result, and during the following year I operated on the patient.

Sam and I thought that in Crouzon and Apert syndromes the junction between the maxillary tuberosity and the pterygoid process was partly the cause of the retrusion of the maxilla and the midface. We both thought that following a midface advancement, the maxilla would grow posteriorly and that alveolar growth would foster the correction. Years of follow-up studies demonstrated that this was not the case, and the malocclusion reappeared. I thought it represented a relapse. Sam observed the cephalograms and demonstrated that the position of the maxilla had remained unchanged but that the mandible was growing faster and overlapped the maxilla which did not grow either posteriorly or anteriorly at the same rate as the mandible. The surgical procedure changed the position but did not change the intrinsic growth potential of the maxilla which was affected with primary hypoplasia. The cephalometric analysis confirmed what we had both already observed in nonoperated patients—that a discrepancy between the jaws, sometimes ignored in infancy, progressed with growth.

The Treacher Collins syndrome was among the disorders that intrigued Sam the most. He thought in terms of hypoplasia of the zygoma; I thought in terms of agenesis. I remember one patient in whom Sam palpated a resistant bone lateral to the orbit and thought it was the zygomatic arch. I then asked the patient to perform some mandibular movements which demonstrated that the bone was, in fact, the coronoid process. Sam wanted to observe and study for himself what the missing zygoma represented in terms of the whole craniofacial skeleton. From that moment on, he did not stop working on pictures, radiographs, and dental models for making a copy of the Treacher Collins skull. For 2 years, elbow to elbow, we worked with medical artists, explaining each aspect of the skull that would be represented in the model. We were never satisfied. Finally, a solid model of a Treacher Collins skull was made in acrylic. Today the technology exists to make such models in a few hours with spatial reconstructions from CT scans and CAD-CAM programs.

Working with Sam during the 5-year period at the Center for Craniofacial Anomalies was one of the most exciting experiences of my life. He was very spirited. He believed in treatment on the one hand and a research program on the other to analyze the results of treatment with a view towards possible modification. He would present patients and we would examine them from different standpoints. I would indicate the required surgery, which he did not often dispute. Sometimes, on the basis of discussion, I would modify my plans. Six or 12 months later, when looking at the results, Sam's critical faculties would be at work.

The surgical sponsorship for this new high-risk surgery performed by a foreigner came to an end in 1976. Sam, with loyalty to both the patients and to me, wanted all the patients who had been either examined or operated on by me during the past 5 years to be reviewed. There was a bit of sadness in this last consultation because both of us saw the end of what should have continued to be productive common work at the Center.

The last time I saw Sam was in February, 1982, at a course on craniofacial malformations held in Rome. On this occasion, he was, as usual, a precise analyst and critic. His remarks were always pertinent.

During his professional life, Sam received all the honors, awards, and recognition that it was possible to receive. Many of his publications, especially during the past 10 years, will remain as classics in the medical and scientific literature.

Sam compiled and organized a monumental number of patient medical records, cephalometric radiographs, dental casts, and drawings. I hope that such a vast accumulation of data will not fall to ashes but will resurge like the phoenix.

REFERENCES

Pruzansky S: Craniofacial surgery: The experiment on nature's experiment. Review of 3 patients operated by Paul Tessier. Eur J Orthodont 4:151–171, 1982.

Pruzansky S: Craniofacial surgery: The experiment on nature's experiment. Historical perspectives. In McNamara JA Jr, Carlson DS, Ribbens KA (eds): "The Effect of Surgical Intervention on Craniofacial Growth." Ann Arbor: University of Michigan, 1981. (Monogr No. 12, Craniofacial Growth Series.)

Congenital Anomalies of the Face and Associated Structures: An International Symposium Twenty-Five Years Ago

Josef Warkany
University of Cincinnati, The Children's Hospital Research Foundation, Cincinnati, Ohio.

It was characteristic of Dr. Samuel Pruzansky that he had the vision and the courage to organize an international symposium on dentofacial anomalies in 1959. Although Sam was supported by the Dental Study Section of the National Institutes of Health, it was his energy that made the conference held in Gatlinburg, Tennessee, on December 6–9, 1959 a success. This was the very first international symposium ever held on the subject of craniofacial anomalies. He also edited the book that commemorates the Proceedings, a volume that is still most valuable to the student of dentofacial anomalies [Pruzansky, 1961].

It was snowing when 125 scientists from the United States, Great Britain, Denmark, and Switzerland gathered in the small town of Gatlinburg—scientists working in different fields with different methods. They lived together for several days and listened to expositions of experts from many fields. The development of the facial and branchial regions was described by Drs. Bradley M. Patten and Alexander Barry, and this was followed by a talk on embryology, pathogenesis, and classification of facial clefts by Dr. Richard Boies Stark. The reader of the published Proceedings will find many of the slides used during the presentations reproduced and interpreted by the authors of these and subsequent articles. The references added to the chapters are still valuable lists of publications up to the year 1959. An article by Professor Gian Töndury on the mechanisms of cleft lip formation deals in great detail with events that take place in the development of the nasal cavity. The old theory of arrested development as the "cause" of cleft lip had been replaced by observations of epithelial bridges between the nasal cavities and the nostrils, and the disturbances of their fusion processes. Inheritance patterns of cleft lip and cleft palate were presented by Dr. P. Fogh-Andersen who had studied over 700 Danish families that contained members with facial clefts and had arrived at a series of empirical figures of genetic prognosis. This classical work is still the basis of classification of human facial clefts

---

Address reprint requests to Josef Warkany, M.D., University of Cincinnati, The Children's Hospital Research Foundation, Elland and Bethesda Avenues, Cincinnati, OH 45229.

© 1985 Alan R. Liss, Inc.

and of genetic counseling. He had found that the cleft lip complex (with or without associated cleft palate) and cleft palate alone must be distinguished, and he had recognized that, in the case of accompanying congenital fistulas of the lower lip, dominant inheritance occurred irrespective of the type of cleft. The importance of Fogh-Andersen's work was the recognition of the complex etiology of facial clefts and the futility of searches for simplistic explanations. Discussion of experimental induction of cleft palate was assigned to Dr. F. Clarke Fraser, who pointed out the role of dose, developmental stage, and genotype. He described the elevation of the palatal shelves over the tongue in mice as the embryological basis for the strain differences in cleft palate frequency. A special talk by Dr. C.W. Asling was devoted to congenital clefts produced in rats following maternal deficiency of folic acid, a method particularly useful in analyses of short-term treatments of mothers. These reports showed how far advanced the experimental work was at that time, as there were already about 20 methods available for experimental production of facial clefts. The conference turned then to problems of patients. Dr. J.D. Subtelny described the configuration of the nasopharynx and palatal segments in children with clefts and Dr. W.M. Krogman reported on the growth of the head and face revealed by cephalometry in cleft palate cases; this was supplemented by Drs. A. Björk and E. Harvold's roentgencephalometric growth analyses. Cineradiography was shown to be a fertile field for analyses of speech problems by Drs. J. Subtelny and F.A. Hofmann. Psychosocial aspects connected with cleft palate patients and educational questions were included in the Proceedings.

This incomplete summary of the symposium illustrates the breadth of Dr. Pruzansky's concept of congenital anomalies of the face. Most of the articles in the Proceedings are still timely and not surpassed by subsequent publications. The comprehensive approach was later realized in the Chicago Center for Craniofacial Anomalies, started, organized, and directed by Dr. Pruzansky for many years.

One of the subjects that was only briefly treated at the time was the field of associated anomalies, which has grown vigorously in the following decades. Syndromology, which is one of the sciences developed with great enthusiasm since the symposium of 1959, encompasses many branches of medicine besides those dealing with the face, teeth and cranium. The syndromes established since are very helpful in classification and interpretation of craniofacial anomalies, as pointed out by Fogh-Andersen, who stated that among his patients about 10% had accompanying malformations, which may help in etiologic differentiations. Anomalies of the head and neck have since become leading symptoms in the analysis of general syndromes. In the change of dentistry from a service occupation to a scientific profession, Sam Pruzansky was a pioneer and leader who left permanent imprints in the field of dental and craniofacial biology.

REFERENCE

Pruzansky S (ed): "Congenital Anomalies of the Face and Associated Structures." Charles C. Thomas, Publishers: Springfield, IL, 1961.

Samuel Pruzansky and the Center for Craniofacial Anomalies

Celia I. Kaye and Beverly R. Rollnick

The Center for Craniofacial Anomalies, University of Illinois College of Medicine, Chicago (B.R.R., C.I.K.), Section of Genetics, Lutheran General Hospital, Park Ridge (C.I.K.), Illinois

> The professional career of Samuel Pruzansky was intimately related to the development and success of the world's first Center for Craniofacial Anomalies (CCFA) at the University of Illinois-Chicago. Pruzansky conceived of the idea, officiated at the birth, and presided over the growth of this Center.

Key words: Samuel Pruzansky, Center for Craniofacial Anomalies–Chicago, cleft lip-palate, team care

INTRODUCTION

The idea of the Center for Craniofacial Anomalies (CCFA) had its genesis in the concept of the team as the basic unit most appropriate to care for the child with multiple handicaps.

"Norbert Wiener gave us the reason for the formation of multidisciplinary teams. It is to solve the problems that are too complex for the single scientist to handle and which require the correlated efforts of varied specialists for solution. . . . For our purpose, the handicapped child has been defined as one who has either a congenital or acquired organic defect which is chronic and sufficiently disabling to present an intertwined medical, dental, emotional, social, educational, and vocational problem requiring prolonged supervision for optimum rehabilitation."

"No one specialist is so omniscient and omnipotent that he can deal with all of these problems. No one doctor can go it alone for he will soon find himself at cross-purpose with the efforts of other isolationists, who seek to serve the needs of the same child. It has also become abundantly clear that these problems are not being resolved satisfactorily within the departmentalized structure of the university hospital or medical and dental schools" [Pruzansky, 1957a].

THE TEAM APPROACH

In recognizing the benefits to children of a team approach to management of complex handicapping conditions, Pruzansky was quick to recognize that the definition of the team and its interpersonal working relationships was itself a central problem.

Address reprint requests to Celia I Kaye, The Center for Craniofacial Anomalies, The University of Illinois-Chicago, P.O. Box 6998, Chicago, IL 60680.

© 1985 Alan R. Liss, Inc.

"In defining a team, it is sometimes easier to say what it is not than what it should be. Certainly, a team is a great deal more than a room full of specialists examining or discussing the same patient. First, the various disciplines represented on the team must learn to communicate with each other. This is no simple task, for there are serious semantic and emotional barriers that must be reduced in the process. . . . This does not imply that the dentist offers surgical judgments, or that the pediatrician prescribes a program of speech therapy. What does count is that the specialist in one field develops a knowledge of the sequence of therapeutic events and of the possibilities and limitations of other forms of therapy. Above all, he knows when to seek advice and from whom to seek advice" [Pruzansky, 1956].

THE CLEFT PALATE CENTER AT THE UNIVERSITY OF ILLINOIS

Recognizing the value of the team in caring for the handicapped child, Pruzansky chose to place the team in a "center." That center was the Cleft Palate Center of the Chicago Professional Colleges of the University of Illinois, later to become the University of Illinois College of Medicine. In addition to caring for the cleft palate child, "this Center was designed to provide interested specialists in the health services with additional training in their particular field; to promote knowledge of, and consideration for, all dimensions of the cleft palate person's need, and to foster research" [Pruzansky, 1954].

Research as the partner of patient care was fundamental in the development of the Center.

"In order to develop a background of fundamental information supportive to the objectives of the Cleft Palate Center, a longitudinal growth study of newborn infants with cleft lip and palate was instituted. The purpose of this research was to provide solutions to the following general problems which were held basic to the establishment of a sound rationale for the management of the various clinical problems that confront the cleft palate team:

1. How does the pattern of growth of the head of a child with a cleft lip and palate compare with that of a normal child?

2. What are the effects of surgery, in terms of kind of surgery and age at surgery, on the growth of the head of the child with a cleft?" [Pruzansky, 1954].

Although a relatively new concept in the care of the cleft palate child, Pruzansky saw the development of the Cleft Palate Center at the University of Illinois as an outgrowth of the work of others.

"When the Cleft Palate program was launched at the University of Illinois in 1949, it was not so much the planting of new seeds as it was the harvest of a crop previously prepared by many individuals working in different fields. In many ways, it all began back in the 1930s. First, there was B. Holly Broadbent and the introduction of cephalometric roentgenology—that capital investment of the orthodontic research industry. . . . While orthodontists were preoccupied with mesuring tooth eruptions and the growth of facial bones from cephalometric x-rays, experimental speech physiologists were employing precisely the same tools in the analysis of organ positions and their spatial relations within the vocal tract during sound production. . . . Speech physiologists were quick to seize the opportunity offered by the x-ray. . . . It seems that orthodontists and speech physiologists engaged in cephalometric research pursued their special interests in ignorance of each other's progress and the inter-relatedness of their separate research efforts. It was only as orthodontists and speech physiologists came to work together on problems of cleft palate that their common interest in cephalometric research was discovered. The establishment of the Cleft Palate Center (in 1949) provided the symbiotic environment in which team research could become a reality" [Pruzansky, 1957b].

At its inception in 1949, the Cleft Palate Center at the University of Illinois was not unique. The first Cleft Palate Center in the United States was established in Lancaster, Pennsylvania, in 1938. "There were many scattered throughout the country. . . . The unique attribute of the University of Illinois program was that it was primarily a training program, which was designed to provide additional training to specialists, to promote fuller knowledge about all aspects of the problem of the person with a cleft palate, and by utilizing the service cases that received care to develop a research program which would point the way toward the problems and methods of the future" [Kobes and Pruzansky, 1960].

However, Pruzansky's initial role in the Cleft Palate Center was a unique one. "I was appointed to develop a longitudinal growth study which relied mainly on photographs, study casts and cephalometric radiographs. There were no hypotheses to be tested, only the abiding conviction that it was important to study the natural history of clefts by the limited means at our dosposal. At that time, no one had developed a technique for roentgencephalometry of infants. The taking of alginate impressions of the face and palate on babies was yet to be tested, and special color cameras to provide calibrated photographs had to be designed. Although these investigations have proven their value and the methods utilized have been demonstrated to be safe in studies on humans, it is probable that a similar proposal submitted today would be rejected on the grounds that there was no hypothesis to be tested, there were no clearly delineated research protocols, and the principal investigator had no prior experience in the field" [Pruzansky, 1980].

The process of developing a longitudinal growth study had salutory outcomes in addition to research findings. Pruzansky and his colleagues amassed varied longitudinal data on the craniofacies and other bodily structures. Recognizing the need to store, retrieve, and analyze these data, Pruzansky developed a computer-based data bank. Today, the CCFA data bank stores data on over 6,500 patients and offers rich ore for craniofacial research. The third part of the CCFA triad (The Center and the Data Bank are two components) is the Maxillofacial Prosthetics Clinic. Pruzansky developed this clinic to work in close collaboration on craniofacial patients. His special contribution was to train and staff the Maxillofacial Prosthetics Clinic with medical artists who create three-dimensional models of proposed facial reconstructions.

With time, the referral patterns, and ultimately the mission, of the Cleft Palate Center changed.

"Since patients with clefts often present with other malformation syndromes affecting the head, it was inevitable that the scope of the Center's interest should become diversified especially as the core staff was competent to manage the related problems. In time, the number of referrals of other craniofacial syndromes, independent of facial clefts, began to equal or exceed cleft referrals. This occurred without any quantitative reduction in the number of clefts referred to the Center. Thus, by virtue of a progressive change in the diagnostic mix of the Center's patient inflow, we evolved into a Center for Craniofacial Anomalies" [Pruzansky, 1980]. Pruzansky had the widsom to understand this change, and the foresight to respond in a manner that would guide the future.

THE CENTER FOR CRANIOFACIAL ANOMALIES

The first Center for Craniofacial Anomalies was established in 1967 by the Chancellor of the University of Illinois Medical Center at Chicago, with Pruzansky as Director. From 1969 until his death in 1984, a major source of funding for the Center was a program project grant from the National Institute of Dental Research, with Pruzansky as principal investigator. However, the fact that support for most of the CCFA research staff was derived from grant money posed a dilemma for Pruzansky that exists to this day. Pruzansky's administrative frustrations were more than offset by his prodigious output of research, exemplified herein by his list of publications. The output of the training grant was also impressive. Pruzansky's former students and fellows staff craniofacial centers, cleft palate clinics and related facilities worldwide. Many return to mine the riches of the CCFA data bank for special research projects.

Pruzansky was sensitive to the uniqueness of the Center following its inception. "The question is sometimes asked, 'What is so unique about craniofacial anomalies that they deserve to be singled out for special attention?' The face of man is his window to the world. It contains the organs of sight, hearing and speech with which he communicates with his environment, receiving information and responding to it. The face reflects state of health, emotion and character. It is the facade by which others perceive and judge the individual. This most visible part of the body influences acceptability to society in general, and, more specifically, acceptability in human transactions" [Pruzansky, 1974].

In time, the case load of the CCFA grew and diversified. By 1984, the Center had the responsibility of storing, retrieving, and analyzing data on more than 6,500 patients. About 250 new patients were added annually, and about 1,600 patient visits were recorded each year. Within this increasingly complex patient population, over 124 syndromes were diagnosed, and 60% of the patients had multiple congenital anomalies in addition to craniofacial anomalies [Rollnick and Pruzansky, 1981]. On a given day, a single patient might undergo 12 different examinations by an equivalent number of specialists and technicians [Pruzansky et al, 1976]. Core staff of the Center consisted of pediatricians, plastic surgeons, otolaryngologists, speech pathologists, orthodontists, psychologists, audiologists, nurses, and geneticists. Pruzansky was one of the first to recognize that genetic services were essential to a center for craniofacial anomalies. Many members of the "core" staff were drawn from other medical centers and institutions in the Chicago area, forming an interhospital consortium. The geographic area of this consortium was widened when Pruzansky attracted Dr. Paul Tessier of Paris to do his first craniofacial surgery in the United States on CCFA patients. Central to the operation, then, were patient care, education, and research. As the core Center staff became larger and more diverse, so too did the research contributions.

As the Center grew, its broader significance concerned and intrigued Pruzansky. He viewed the evolution of the team as that of an academic community with shared interests. "My concern is with the academic team as differentiated from the service team. The academic team is a community of independent scholars working together in the no-man's-land between the territories claimed by traditional disciplines, not as subordinates of some great executive officer, but joined by the desire, indeed by the necessity, to understand the region as a whole and to lend one another the strength of that understanding.

"It is a team comprised of broadly trained scientists who recognize that the study of life processes like life itself is an unbroken continuum. One may enter this continuum at the level of the molecule and the cell, or by studying the organism in its ecologic setting, or at points in between. Once inside, we must be able to take excursions conceptually and operationally in any direction without encountering barriers to comprehension and logical consistency" [Pruzansky, 1980].

Pruzansky also saw the team acting as a meeting place for scientific inquiry.

"[A] by-product of the team's involvement in problems of craniofacial biology has been a gradual dissolution of the unfortunate dichotomy that has separated the clinical investigator from the laboratory scientist. By tradition it seemed that the investigator lost the cloak of scientist once he left the laboratory to work in the ward, clinic or community. It was far easier to gain prestige through investigative work in the laboratory. As a cadre of clinical investigators trained in scientific discipline emerged from federally sponsored training programs, it became possible to build bridges between clinical and laboratory science. Clues derived from clinical experience had to be tested in the laboratory. What was needed was a clinician who could recognize the problem, formulate a hypothesis and suggest the means for testing it in the laboratory. Conversely, experiments that affect man cannot be duplicated in the laboratory at will and so afford the laboratory scientist a unique opportunity to study the interrelationships of abnormal form and function" [Pruzansky, 1974].

Finally, Pruzansky was sensitive to the special role played by the dentist in the craniofacial team and in research.

"Like many other professionals, the dentist is overtrained for what he is allowed to do by law and tradition, and undertrained for what he might like to do. . . . Dentists, no less than other specialists, enrich the interdisciplinary group by the addition of their special training and experience. In the process of assimilation within the group, dentists, like all the others, become generalists. Indeed, an outsider attending staff seminars might be hard-pressed to identify representatives of specific disciplines by their contributions to the dialogue. This phenomenon is a tribute to the continuing educational forum created by the team" [Pruzansky, 1980].

Always the man of letters as well as of science, Pruzansky compared the Center to Janus.

"Janus, the ancient figure of mythology, was represented by two faces, one looking backward to the beginning of things and the other into the future. The Center for Craniofacial Anomalies may be similarly represented. In one direction, the Center seeks to understand and control the mechanisms of abnormal development. In the other direction, the Center is concerned with the growth, maturation, and treatment of the affected child" [Pruzansky].

REFERENCES

Kobes HR, Pruzansky S: The cleft palate team—A historical review. Am J Public Health 50:200–205, 1960.
Pruzansky S: The role of the orthodontist in a cleft palate team. Plast Reconstr Surg 14:10–29, 1954.
Pruzansky S: Role of the team approach in caring for the handicapped child. J Dent Educ 73–78, 1957a.

Pruzansky S: The foundations of the Cleft Palate Center and Training Program at the University of Illinois. Angle Orthod 27:69–81, 1957b.

Pruzansky S: Organization of an interdisciplinary unit for the study of craniofacial anomalies. Symposium on the Dental Management of the Handicapped Child. Iowa City, IO: Univ. Iowa Press, 1974.

Pruzansky S: The dentist on a craniofacial team. Birth defects 16:115–124, 1980.

Pruzansky S, Parris P, Laffer J: The making of a data bank for the Center for Craniofacial Anomalies. In: McCormick B (ed): Proceedings of Third Illinois Conference on Medical Information Systems. Department of Information Engineering, University of Illinois at Chicago Circle, Chicago, Illinois, 1976.

Rollnick BR, Pruzansky S: Genetic Services at a Center for Craniofacial Anomalies. Cleft Palate J 18:304–313, 1981.

The Application of Roentgencephalometry to the Study of Craniofacial Anomalies

Sven Kreiborg
Department of Orthodontics, The Royal Dental College, Copenhagen, Denmark

> Objective quantitative methods for standardized reproducible descriptions of the findings of an examination are prerequisite for the optimal care of patients with congenital or acquired craniofacial anomalies. The present report gives a brief review of the development of roentgencephalometry with special emphasis on the infant roentgencephalometric techniques pioneered by Dr. Samuel Pruzansky. In addition, some of the significant findings that have emerged from the application of these techniques to patients with craniofacial anomalies are presented, again, with emphasis on the contributions made by Dr. Pruzansky and co-workers. Finally, perspectives for future clinical and research work within the field are outlined. These perspectives include (1) improvement of cephalometric units for studies of patients with craniofacial anomalies; (2) inclusion of additional cephalometric projections, especially in patients with craniofacial asymmetry; (3) increased utilization of infant cephalometry; (4) utilization of metallic implants in selected cases; (5) greater utilization of computerized cephalometrics and multivariate statistics; and (6) combined use of longitudinal cephalometric studies and various longitudinal physiological examinations, eg, electromyography, kinesiography, and air flow studies, in the individual patient.

Key words: roentgencephalometry, craniofacial anomalies, infant cephalometry, cephalometric techniques

INTRODUCTION

The clinical management of children with congenital or acquired craniofacial anomalies poses a number of extremely complex problems. These problems relate to diagnosis, prognosis, genetics, timing and planning of various therapeutic maneuvers, and recording the patient's response to treatment. These problems require accurate assessment of the initial state and the changes in craniofacial morphology with time, both before and after treatment.

Objective quantitative methods that provide standardized reproducible descriptions of the individual are prerequisite for optimal patient care, and most of the problems listed above lend themselves to solutions with roentgencephalometric techniques.

Address reprint requests to Dr. Kreiborg, Department of Orthodontics, The Royal Dental College, Jagtvej 160, DK-1200 Copenhagen ø, Denmark.

© 1985 Alan R. Liss, Inc.

The following is a brief review of the development of general roentgencephalometric techniques and cephalometric analysis with special emphasis on infant roentgencephalometry as pioneered by Dr. Samuel Pruzansky. In addition, a review of some of the significant findings emerging from the application of these techniques to patients with craniofacial anomalies will be presented with comments on future clinical and research perspectives within the field.

ROENTGENCEPHALOMETRY
Techniques

The techniques of roentgencephalometry were originally developed more than 50 years ago by orthodontic researchers [Hofrath, 1931; Broadbent, 1931], searching for a method that would make possible the longitudinal study of growth of the jaws in children.

The method is based on utilization of a standardized, oriented apparatus in which the x-ray source is in a fixed relationship to the object. The head is positioned in a headholder, thereby controlling the desired projection. Hofrath only employed the lateral projection, whereas Broadbent's cephalometer was designed to obtain both lateral and frontal cephalograms.

Broadbent's technique has gained worldwide acceptance within the field of orthodontics as an indispensable clinical and research tool. Perspectives in the application of roentgencephalometry to clinical orthodontics have been extensively reviewed by Ricketts [1981].

Although the basic technique of Broadbent's cephalometric method has remained almost unaltered over the years, several significant technical improvements have been made, which again have led to development of refined analytical methods. Some of

TABLE I. Some of the Significant Steps in the Development of Roentgencephalometric Techniques

Source	Steps
Hofrath [1931]	Lateral projection
Broadbent [1931]	Lateral and frontal projections
Margolis [1940]	Oblique lateral projection
Ortiz and Brodie [1949]	Infant cephalometry; lateral projection
Björk [1951]	Axial projection; fixed distances from midsagittal and transmeatal planes to film; fixed enlargement
Cartright and Harvold [1954]	High-kilovoltage cephalometry
Pruzansky and Lis [1958]	Infant cephalometry; lateral and frontal projections; sedation method
Pruzansky (1966)	Infant cephalometry; axial projection
Björk [1968]	Improved orientation system with image intensifier, TV-monitor, and a light-cross projected on face
Björk [1968]	Cephalometric unit movable in vertical direction to accommodate standing subjects
Björk [1971]	Oblique frontal projection
Dahan [1974]	Infant cephalometry; axial projection
Kreiborg et al [1977]	Infant cephalometry; high-kilovoltage, fixed distances from midsagittal and transmeatal planes to film; fixed enlargement; improved orientation system with light-cross projected on face; axial projection
Solow and Kreiborg [1985]	Improved orientation system with image intensifier, TV-monitor and six laser beams projected on face and head

the significant steps in the technical development of cephalometry are listed in Table I. The technical improvements are related to the introduction of high kilovoltage [Cartright and Harvold, 1954], more projections [Margolis, 1940; Björk, 1951, 1971], fixed enlargement [Björk, 1951], and improved orientation systems [Björk, 1968; Solow and Kreiborg, 1985].

Conventional roentgencephalometry generally cannot be applied to children younger than 4 years of age, since some cooperation is required to secure an accurate and stationary position of the patient's head during the exposure.

Infant Cephalometry

Ortiz and Brodie [1949] constructed a cephalometric machine for infants utilizing the same basic design as the Broadbent-Bolton cephalometer. The infant unit differed in that it was built around a table instead of a dental chair and had only one x-ray tube for the lateral projection. The position of the infant's head had to be maintained by an assistant to avoid blurring of the image owing to movement. These problems were overcome by Pruzansky, a student of Brodie, who together with Lis in 1958 introduced an improved infant cephalometer (based on the Ortiz-Brodie design). At the same time, they described a procedure for the safe and uniform sedation of the infants to be examined. Sedation was achieved by rectal administration of secobarbital.

Pruzansky and Lis's cephalometer included both lateral and frontal projections. Since that time, an axial exposure has been added [Pruzansky, 1966; Dahan, 1974; Kreiborg et al, 1977]. Kreiborg et al. subsequently introduced the use of high kilovoltage x-ray tubes, a secondary diaphragm, and an improved orientation system [Björk, 1968] in their infant cephalometric unit (Figs. 1, 2).

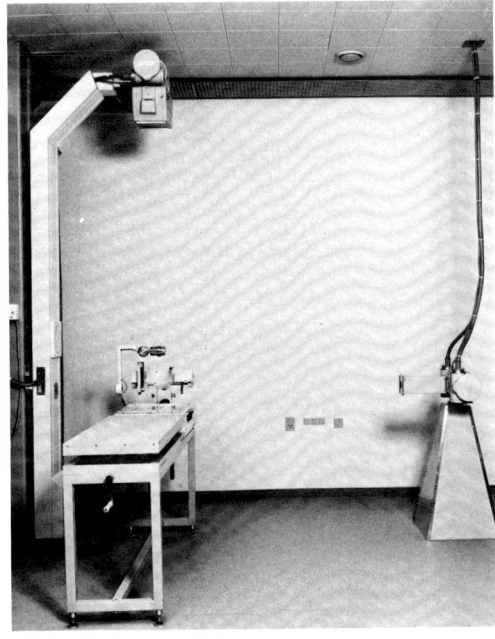

Fig. 1. Roentgencephalometric unit with two high kilovoltage x-ray tubes for infants (Kreiborg et al, 1977].

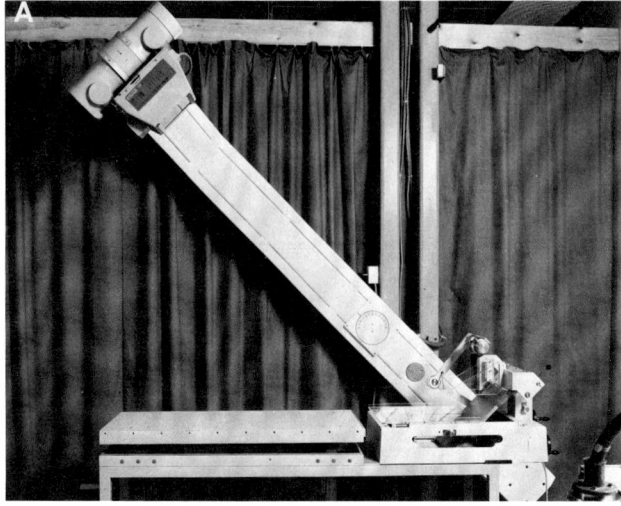

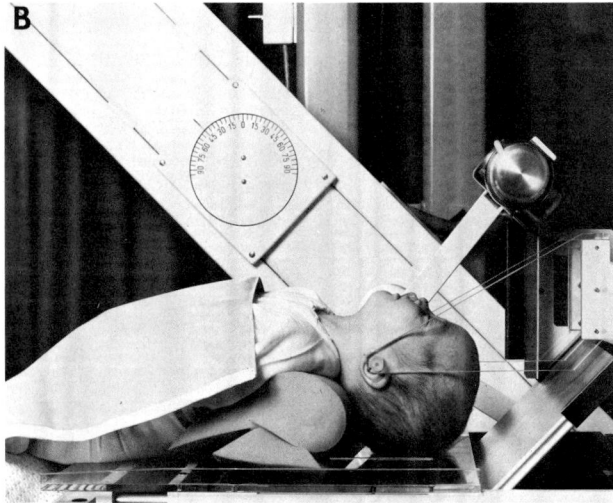

Fig. 2. A. The x-ray tube above the cephalostat is tilted 45° for the axial projection. The center of rotation is located at the axial ray of the x-ray tube for the lateral projection. B. The position of the infant's head for the axial projection. The correct orientation is secured by the ear-rods and a light-cross projected on the face. Note that the casette holder for this projection has an angulation of 45° to the vertical plane [Kreiborg et al, 1977].

Roentgencephalometric Analysis

Analytical improvements in roentgencephalometry included the combined use of roentgencephalometry and metallic implants in the jaws [Björk, 1955b, 1968] and the application of computers to cephalometric data (Table II) [Walker, 1967, 1972; Solow, 1970; Ricketts et al, 1972]. The use of metallic implants in the jaws has made it possible to distinguish between displacement and remodeling of the individual jaw in longitudinal studies of facial growth [Björk, 1968; Björk and Skieller, 1972, 1983].

TABLE II. Some Significant Steps in the Development of Cephalometric Analysis

Source	Steps
Brodie [1941]	Adjustment for enlargement for each film; growth analysis with sella-nasion as reference
Björk [1955a]	Fixed enlargement; direct growth analysis with sella-nasion as reference
Björk [1955b]	Metallic implants in the jaws to differentiate between displacement and surface remodeling of jaws
Björk [1961]	Direct growth analysis with superimposition on stable bony structures in the anterior cranial base
Brown et al [1965] Solow [1966] Harris [1972]	Multivariate statistics applied to cephalometric data
Walker [1967] Solow [1970]	Application of image processing to cephalometric films
Walker [1967] Ricketts [1969] Solow [1970] Walker [1972]	Computerized cephalometrics
Walker and Kowalski [1971] Ricketts et al, [1972] Solow [1973]	Computerized growth and treatment simulation

This method of analysis of jaw growth has been a major step forward in our understanding of normal growth of the face.

The application of computers to the field of cephalometric analysis has dramatically reduced the amount of manual work required in the statistical calculations [Walker, 1967, 1972; Ricketts, 1969; Solow, 1970]. Further, the use of computers has made it possible to handle large amounts of data and carry out multivariate analyses [Brown et al, 1965; Solow, 1966; Harris et al, 1972]. A few attempts have been made to simulate facial growth and the effect of orthodontic treatment [Walker and Kowalski, 1971; Ricketts et al, 1972; Solow, 1973].

CRANIOFACIAL ANOMALIES

The earliest roentgencephalometric investigations of patients with anomalies were carried out by Brodie and co-workers at the Department of Orthodontics, University of Illinois [Schour et al, 1934; Engel et al, 1941; Brodie and Sarnat, 1942; Engel and Brodie, 1947]. The studies dealt with analyses of craniofacial morphology and growth in patients with pituitary insufficiency, hypothyroidism, ectodermal dysplasia, and juvenile rheumatoid arthritis. During this same period, Brodie [1941] published normative data on the growth of the human head from the third month to the eighth year of life based on the Bolton records. Pruzansky had been working with improved techniques since 1949 and had systematically collected longitudinal roentgencephalometric data on infants with clefts and other craniofacial anomalies. Publication of his findings dramatically expanded our understanding of the natural history of several different syndromes [Pruzansky and Richmond, 1954; Beers and Pruzansky, 1955; Grossman et al, 1955; Pruzansky, 1955; Rosenthal et al, 1956]. In their prize-winning paper in 1958, Pruzansky and Lis presented growth analyses on infants with oxycephaly, cleft lip and palate, mandibulofacial dysostosis, ectodermal dysplasia, and progeria. For the first time, the growth pattern of the calvaria in oxycephaly could be documented both before and after linear craniectomy, and the earlier subjective discussions of the effect of linear craniectomy on skull growth could now be quantified. Later studies have had direct influence on the development of new treatment procedures for craniosynostosis. In addition, the long term effect of lip repair and palatal closure in children with clefts was now subjected to quantitative analysis. These studies and studies on the growth pattern of the mandible and the development of the airway in different syndromes with mandibular retrognathia [Pruzansky, 1969] had a direct impact on the differential diagnosis and clinical management of these patients. Since the time of these early reports, other publications dealing with the morphology and growth of the craniofacial complex in patients with craniofacial anomalies have been published from all over the world, but there has always been a continuous predominance of these from Pruzansky's group.

In 1981, Cohen attempted to compile references to all the cephalometric studies of dysmorphic syndromes. He found that, in addition to the many reports on cleft lip/palate, more than 30 different syndromes had been documented by roentgencephalometry. Today this figure has probably increased to about 40, and it should be noted that Pruzansky, alone or with co-workers, provided cephalometric data on more than 25 of these syndromes. These studies were aimed at identifying those morphologic variables that could be utilized as a basis for a numerical taxonomy that would be syndrome specific. These studies also attempted to predict growth problems and suggested modes of interceptive treatment in cases of anticipated complications.

In a publication in 1966, Pruzansky posed the rhetorical question: "Is roentgencephalometry being fully exploited as an instrument for clinical investigation?" Pruzansky pointed to the restricted utilization of roentgencephalometry in most clinical investigations and drew attention to the vast potential of the cephalometric method as a research tool. Among the suggestions he outlined was the application of roentgencephalometry to determine the significance of hypertrophic tonsils and adenoids on posture of the tongue, soft palate, mandible, head, and neck. Most of these areas have since been explored by several researchers including Pruzansky [1975], and the preliminary results have contributed significantly to our understanding of craniofacial function and growth in the normal subject as well as in the subject with a craniofacial anomaly. Interaction between facial growth and function of the masticatory muscles in patients with acquired or congenital anomalies has also been documented [Pruzansky, 1973a; Kreiborg et al, 1978].

Roentgencephalograms of patients with craniofacial anomalies can be analyzed in both a qualitative and a quantitative manner. All the qualitative signs that can be evaluated in a conventional skull radiograph can be equally, and sometimes better, observed in the cephalometric radiograph since distortion is reduced to a minimum. The quantitative analyses are not restricted to the jaws and teeth but can deal with size, shape, and relative position of all soft tissue and skeletal structures recognizable in the film, eg, soft tissue profile, eye globe, soft palate, tongue, pharynx, adenoids, tonsils, calvaria, cranial base, orbit, maxillary complex, mandible, cervical spine, and hyoid bone. The analyses then become meaningful not only to the orthodontist, but also to the radiologist, the pediatrician, the geneticist, the plastic surgeon, the neurosurgeon, the oral surgeon, the ophthalmologist, the otolaryngologist, and the speech pathologist.

Nowhere has the multidisciplinary utilization of roentgencephalometry been more clearly revealed than in the clinical and surgical management of patients with severe craniofacial anomalies, eg, Crouzon and Apert syndromes, requiring craniofacial surgery, as pioneered by Dr. Paul Tessier [1971]. Roentgencephalometry has served as a diagnostic tool for several disciplines to define the initial state, the changes with time, and to provide an individual blueprint for the osteotomies to be employed in facial reconstruction as well as to monitor the subsequent state [Pruzansky et al, 1974; Peterson and Pruzansky, 1974; Pruzansky, 1973b, 1976, 1977, 1982; Kreiborg and Pruzansky, 1981].

In dealing with patients with congenital anomalies, two central questions arise: (1) what can we do for the patient and his family? and (2) what can we learn from the patient and his family? On several occasions, Pruzansky [1973b, 1977] has drawn attention to the special value of craniofacial anomalies as experiments of nature. With the development of craniofacial surgery, Pruzansky [1982] extended this line of thought to include the phrase "the experiment on nature's experiment." Roentgencephalometric and physiological studies in such cases may add insight into the etiology of the disease and into the general developmental mechanisms involved in craniofacial morphogenesis.

PERSPECTIVES

Not all the developments possible with roentgencephalometric techniques (Table I) have, as yet, been adapted to the study of craniofacial anomalies. The basic roentgencephalometer employed in clinical and research studies of patients with craniofacial anomalies should be of the highest standards in order to secure high-quality radiographs of these rare conditions, particularly in those cases where bony structures are markedly deranged and difficult to interpret. The use of high kilovoltage x-ray tubes, rotating anodes, and a small focal spot size lead to improved resolution. Further, the risk of blurring owing to head movement during exposure is reduced. The use of primary and secondary diaphragms and fine grain intensifying screens will improve the final image and reduce the amount of radiation to the patient.

The use of fixed distances from the midsagittal plane and the plane through the ear rods to the film is recommended to allow direct superimposition of the films in a longitudinal series [Björk, 1951, 1968]. To secure as uniform an adjustment of the head as possible in longitudinal studies, various orientation systems should be employed in addition to the conventional headholding devise [Björk, 1968; Kreiborg et al, 1977; Solow and Kreiborg, 1985]. Such a need is clearly exemplified by the problems involved in the longitudinal study of patients with hemifacial microsomia or plagiocephaly. Additionally, the use of the frontal, oblique-frontal, and axial projections is advocated, especially in patients exhibiting craniofacial asymmetry [Björk, 1951, 1971; Lund, 1974; Kreiborg, 1981a; Dahl et al, 1982].

From the literature, it would appear that surprisingly few centers for craniofacial anomalies employ infant cephalometry [Pruzansky and Lis, 1958; Mazaheri and Sahni, 1969; Robertson and Hilton, 1971; Dahan, 1974; Friede et al, 1977; Kreiborg et al, 1977; Coccaro et al, 1980]. Yet, the greatest increments in postnatal growth of the craniofacial complex occur in the first few years of life. The importance of greater utilization of infant cephalometry is emphasized.

Utilization of the metallic implant technique developed by Björk [1955, 1968] has also been used in relatively few studies of facial growth in patients with anomalies [Björk, 1962; Pruzansky, 1971; Robertson and Hilton, 1971; Kreiborg and Pruzansky, 1972; Hogeman and Willmar, 1974; Friede et al, 1977; Kreiborg and Björk, 1977; Dahl, 1979; Kreiborg, 1981b; Björk and Skieller, 1983]. The combined use of metallic implants and roentgencephalometry makes it possible to distinguish between displacement and surface remodeling of bones and is a very precise tool for monitoring the functional status of sutures and the stability of craniofacial surgical results [Kreiborg, 1981b, 1985].

The application of multivariate statistics, eg, Fourier analysis and discriminant function analysis, to cephalometric data on craniofacial anomalies has only been carried out in a few studies [Ohyama et al, 1974; Walker and Kowalski, 1974; Kreiborg, 1975; Lestrel and Roche, 1976]. These methods would seem to merit greater utilization for improved taxonomy and for recognition of the heterozygote. By applying computerized cephalometrics to the study of groups of patients with craniofacial anomalies, more comprehensive analyses can be carried out which are of multidisciplinary interest [Kisling, 1966; Cohen, 1979; Kreiborg, 1981b]. Although computer technology for the simulation of craniofacial growth and the results of treatment has been available for several years (Table II), it has, as yet, barely been adapted to research and treatment planning for severe craniofacial anomalies. Not only could these techniques be helpful in planning treatment, but they could also be useful in generating and testing hypotheses related to the developmental mechanisms involved in craniofacial morphogenesis.

Some of the greatest progress in our understanding of the natural history of various types of craniofacial anomalies has, to date, emerged from the longitudinal "multidisciplinary roentgencephalometric approach" employed by Pruzansky and co-workers. Consequently, increased utilization of the combined use of longitudinal roentgencephalometric studies and relevant physiologic longitudinal examinations of the individual patients, ie, electromyography, kinesiography, air flow studies, etc, seems to be called for at the present time.

CONCLUSIONS

Clearly, the scope of the pioneering work of Dr. Samuel Pruzansky in the field of applied roentgencephalometry for the study of craniofacial anomalies beginning in infancy exemplifies the pluralistic interests of this unique investigator and reflects the many years of study required to master, comprehend, and combine the wide range of topics covered by his research. Pruzansky's scientific work will rank as key references not only with respect to the anomalies he has examined, but also as a yardstick against which future roentgencephalometric studies of other craniofacial syndromes will be measured. The value of Pruzansky's roentgencephalometric research will transcend its application to the specific disorders considered but will also serve to challenge the paradigms that explain normal growth of the craniofacial complex.

ACKNOWLEDGMENTS

The author is most grateful to Dr. Howard Aduss for valuable advice in the translation and preparation of the manuscript.

REFERENCES

Beers MD, Pruzansky S: The growth of the head of an infant with mandibular micrognathia, glossoptosis and cleft palate following the Beverly Douglas operation. Plast Reconstr Surg 16:189–193, 1955.

Björk A: Some biological aspects of prognathism and occlusion of the teeth. Angle Orthod 21:3–21, 1951.

Björk A: Cranial base development. A follow-up x-ray study of the individual variation in growth occurring between the ages of 12 and 20 years and its relation to brain case and face development. Am J Orthod 41:198–225, 1955a.

Björk A: Facial growth in man studied with the aid of metallic implants. Acta Odontol Scand 31:9–34, 1955b.

Björk A: Roentgencephalometric growth analysis. In Pruzansky S (ed): "Congenital Anomalies of the Face and Associated Structures." Springfield IL Charles C. Thomas Company, 1961, pp 237–250.

Björk A: Facial growth in bilateral hypoplasia of the mandibular condyles. A radiographic, cephalometric study of a case, using metallic implants. In Kraus and Ridel (eds): "Vistas in Orthodontics." Philadelphia: Lea and Febiger, 1962, pp 347–358.

Björk A: The use of metallic implants in the study of facial growth in children. Method and application. Am J Phys Anthropol 29:243–254, 1968.

Björk A: Kaebernes relationer til det øvrige kranium. In Lundström A (ed): "Nordisk Lärobok i Ortodonti. Uppl 3." Stockholm: Sveriges Tandläkarforbunds Förlagsförening, 1971, p 163.

Björk A, Skieller V: Facial development and tooth eruption. An implant study at the age of puberty. Am J Orthod 62:339–383, 1972.

Björk A, Skieller V: Normal and abnormal growth of the mandible. A synthesis of longitudinal cephalometric implant studies over a period of 25 years. Eur J Orthod 5:1–46, 1983.

Broadbent BH: A new x-ray technique and its application to orthodontia. Angle Orthod 1:45–66, 1931.

Brodie AG: On the growth pattern of the human head from the third month to the eighth year of life. Am J Anat 68:209–262, 1941.

Brodie AG, Sarnat BG: Ectodermal dysplasia (Anhidrotic type) with complete anodontia. Am J Dis Child 64:1046–1054, 1942.

Brown T, Barrett MJ, Darroch JN: Craniofacial factors in two ethnic groups. Growth 29:109–123, 1965.

Cartright LJ, Harvold EP: Improved radiographic results in cephalometry through the use of high kilovoltage. Can Dent Assoc J 20:260–263, 1954.

Coccaro PH, McCarthy JG, Epstein FJ, Wood-Smith D, Converse JM: Early and late surgery in craniofacial dysostosis: A longitudinal cephalometric study. Am J Orthod 77:421–436, 1980.

Cohen MM Jr: Studies in achondroplasia. Thesis, University of Minnesota, 1979.

Cohen MM Jr: A critical review of cephalometric studies of dysmorphic syndromes. Proc Finn Dent Soc 77:17–25, 1981.

Dahan J: Die dreidimensionale röntgenkephalometrische Untersuchung von Fällen mit Pierre-Robin-Syndrom. Fortschr Kieferorthop 35:240–255, 1974.

Dahl E: Transverse maxillary growth in combined cleft lip and palate. A longitudinal roentgencephalometric study by the implant method. Cleft Palate J 16:34–41, 1979.

Dahl E, Kreiborg S, Jensen BL, Fogh-Andersen P: Comparison of craniofacial morphology in infants with incomplete cleft lip and infants with isolated cleft palate. Cleft Palate J 19:258–266, 1982.

Engel MB, Brodie AG: Condylar growth and mandibular deformities. Surgery 22:976–992, 1947.

Engel MB, Bronstein IP, Brodie AG, Wesoke P: A roentgenographic cephalometric appraisal of untreated and treated hypothyroidism. Am J Dis Child 61:1193–1214, 1941.

Friede H, Johanson B, Ahlgren J, Thilander B: Metallic implants as growth markers in infants with craniofacial anomalies. Acta Odontol Scand 35:265–273, 1977.

Grossman HJ, Pruzansky S, Rosenthal IM: Progeroid syndrome. Pediatrics 15:413–423, 1955.

Harris JE, Kowalski CJ, Walker GF: Discrimination between normal and class II individuals using Steiner's analysis. Angle Orthod 42:212–220, 1972.

Hofrath H: Die Bedeutung der Röntgenfern-und Abstandsaufnahme für die Diagnostik der Kieferanomalien. Fortschr Orthod 1:232–258, 1931.

Hogeman K-E, Willmar K: On Le Fort III osteotomy for Crouzon's disease in children. Report of a four-year follow-up in one patient. Scand J Plast Reconstr Surg 8:169–172, 1974.

Kisling E: "Cranial Morphology in Down's Syndrome. A Comparative Roentgencephalometric Study in Adult Males." Copenhagen: Munksgaard, 1966.

Kreiborg S: En røntgencephalometrisk metode til analyse af kranieform. Et metodestudie appliceret på en gruppe voksne maend med Down's syndrom og en kontrolgruppe. Thesis, The Royal Dental College, Copenhagen, 1975.

Kreiborg S: Craniofacial growth in plagiocephaly and Crouzon syndrome. Scand J Plast Reconstr Surg 15:187–197, 1981a.

Kreiborg S: Crouzon syndrome. A clinical and roentgencephalometric study. Scand J Plast Reconstr Surg 15 [suppl 18], 1981b.

Kreiborg S: Postnatal growth and development of the craniofacial complex in premature craniosynostosis. In Cohen MM Jr (ed): "Handbook on Craniosynostosis." New York: Raven Press, 1985 (in press).

Kreiborg S, Björk A: Craniofacial growth in Crouzon's syndrome studied by the implant method. Third Int Cong Cleft Palate (Abstract 191), 1977.

Kreiborg S, Dahl E, Prydsoe U: A unit for infant roentgencephalometry. Dentomaxillofac Radiol 6:107–111, 1977.

Kreiborg S, Jensen BL, Møller E, Björk A: Craniofacial growth in a case of congenital muscular dystrophy. A roentgencephalometric and electromyographic investigation. Am J Orthod 74:207–215, 1978.

Kreiborg S, Pruzansky S: Roentgencephalometric and metallic implant studies in Apert's syndrome. 50th General Session IADR (Abstract 289), 1972.

Kreiborg S, Pruzansky S: Craniofacial growth in patients with premature craniosynostosis. Scand J Plast Reconstr Surg 15:171–186, 1981.

Lestrel PE, Roche AF: Fourier analysis of the cranium in trisomy 21. Growth 40:385–398, 1976.

Lund K: Mandibular growth and remodelling processes after condylar fracture. A longitudinal roentgencephalometric study. Acta Odontol Scand 32 [suppl 64], 1974.

Margolois HI: Standardized x-ray cephalographics. Am J Orthod 26:725–740, 1940.

Mazaheri M, Sahni PP: Techniques of cephalometry, photography and oral impressions of infants. J Prosth Dent 21:315–323, 1969.

Ortiz MH, Brodie AG: On the growth of the human head from birth to the third month of life. Anat Rec 103:311–333, 1949.

Ohyama K, Pruzansky S, Heinze W, Parris P: Discriminant function analysis in the diagnosis of Pierre Robin syndrome. Teratology 9:A–32, 1974.

Peterson SJ, Pruzansky S: Palatal anomalies in the syndrome of Apert and Crouzon. Cleft Palate J 11:394–403, 1974.

Pruzansky S: Factors determining arch form in clefts of the lip and palate. Am J Orthod 41:827–851, 1955.

Pruzansky S: Is roentgencephalometry being fully exploited as an instrument for clinical investigation? Dent Clin North Am. Philadelphia: WB Saunders Company, 1966, pp 211–217.

Pruzansky S: Not all dwarfed mandibles are alike. Birth Defects: Original Articles Series V(2):120–129, 1969.

Pruzansky S: The growth of the premaxillary-vomerine complex in complete bilateral cleft lip and palate. Tandlaegebladet 75:1157–1169, 1971.

Pruzansky S: Concluding comment II. In Bosma JF (ed): "Fourth Symposium on Oral Sensation and Perception." Bethesda: MD DHEW Publication No. (NIH) 73-546, 1973a, pp 390–408.

Pruzansky S: Clinical investigation of the experiments of nature. ASHA Report 8:62–94, 1973b.

Pruzansky S: Roentgencephalometric studies of tonsils and adenoids in normal and pathologic states. Ann Otol Rhinol Laryngol 84 [suppl 19], pp 1–8, 1975.

Pruzansky S: Radiocephalometric studies of the basicranium in craniofacial malformations. In Bosma JF (ed): "Development of the Basicranium." Bethesda: MD DHEW Publication No. (NIH) 76-989, 1976, pp 278–298.

Pruzansky S: Time: The fourth dimension in syndrome analysis applied to craniofacial malformations. Birth Defects: Original Articles Series XIII (3C):3–28, 1977.

Pruzansky S: Craniofacial surgery: The experiment on nature's experiment. Review of three patients operated by Paul Tessier. Eur J Orthod 4:151–171, 1982.

Pruzansky S, Lis EF: Cephalometric roentgenography of infants: Sedation, instrumentation, and research. Am J Orthod 44:159–186, 1958.

Pruzansky S, Miller M, Kammer JF: Ocular defects in craniofacial syndromes. In Goldberg MF (ed): "Genetic and Metabolic disease." Boston: Little Brown and Company, 1974, pp 487–498.

Pruzansky S, Richmond JB: Growth of the mandible in infants with micrognathia. Am J Dis Child 88:29–42, 1954.
Ricketts RM: The evolution of diagnosis to computerized cephalometrics. Am J Orthod 55:795–803, 1969.
Ricketts RM: Perspectives in the clinical application of cephalometrics. Angle Orthod 51:115–150, 1981.
Ricketts RM, Bench R, Hilgers JJ, Schulhof R: An overview of computerized cephalometrics. Am J Orthod 61:1–28, 1972.
Robertson NRE, Hilton R: The changes produced by pre-surgical orthopaedics. Br J Plast Surg 24:57–68, 1971.
Rosenthal IM, Bronstein IP, Dallenback FM, Pruzansky S, Rosenwald AK: Progeria. Pediatrics 18:565–577, 1956.
Schour BSE, Brodie AG, King EQ: The hypophysis and the teeth. Angle Orthod 4:285–304, 1934.
Solow B: The pattern of craniofacial associations. A morphological and methodological correlation and factor analysis study on young male adults. Acta Odontol Scand 24 [suppl 46], 1966.
Solow B: Computers in cephalometric research. Comput Biol Med 1:41–49, 1970.
Solow B: Graphical simulation of craniofacial growth. Trans Eur Orthod Soc, London, 1973, pp 516–521.
Solow B, Kreiborg S: Multiprojection cephalometer with laser orientation system. Am J Orthod, 1985 (in preparation).
Tessier P: The definitive plastic surgical treatment of the severe facial deformities of craniofacial dysostosis. Crouzon's and Apert's disease. Plast Reconstr Surg 48:419–442, 1971.
Walker GF: Summary of research report on the analysis of craniofacial growth. N Zealand Dent J 63:31–38, 1967.
Walker GF: A new approach to the analysis of craniofacial morphology. Am J Orthod 61:221–230, 1972.
Walker GF: Kowalski CJ: A two-dimensional coordinate model for the quantification, description, analysis, prediction and simulation of craniofacial growth. Growth 35:191–211, 1971.
Walker GF: Kowalski CJ: Computer-aided diagnosis of craniofacial abnormalities. Medinfo 74. Amsterdam: North-Holland Publishing Company, 1974, pp 553–557.

Dysmorphic Growth and Development and the Study of Craniofacial Syndromes

M. Michael Cohen, Jr.
Dalhousie University, Halifax, Nova Scotia, Canada

> Some general principles of syndromic growth and development useful for cephalometric studies are set forth under the headings of (1) bone age determination, (2) limitations of radiographic assessment in syndromic dysmorphism, (3) dysharmonic maturation and patterned dysmorphism, (4) primary growth deficiency of prenatal onset, (5) asymmetric dysmorphism, (6) problems in diagnostic homogeneity, and (7) problems in ascertainment bias.

Key words: craniofacial syndromes, cephalometric studies, growth deficiency, dysmorphic growth and development, dysharmonic maturation, bone age, patterned dysmorphism, asymmetric dysmorphism, diagnostic homogeneity, ascertainment bias

INTRODUCTION

Sam Pruzansky spent most of his productive professional career studying dysmorphic craniofacial growth and development. As he recognized early on, the study of craniofacial syndromes presented a series of problems that defied classical cephalometric techniques and analyses and required instead modified and sometimes new cephalometric techniques as well as broad-based new types of analyses specifically adapted to the individual problems at hand. Of the approximately 40 syndromes that have been studied cephalometrically to date, Pruzansky (alone or together with his co-workers) has been responsible for 25 of these [Kreiborg, this volume].

In this paper, some general principles of syndromic growth and development useful for cephalometric studies are set forth under the following headings: (1) bone age determination, (2) limitations of radiographic assessment in syndromic dysmorphism, (3) dysharmonic maturation and patterned dysmorphism, (4) primary growth deficiency of prenatal onset, (5) asymmetric dysmorphism, (6) problems in diagnostic homogeneity, and (7) problems in ascertainment bias. These topics have been developed more fully elsewhere [Cohen 1981, 1982].

BONE AGE DETERMINATION

Bone age determination is frequently abused in the assessment of growth, and an understanding of its uses and limitations is essential, especially in assessing dysmorphic syndromes. Radiologic assessment of bone maturation is commonly overrequested, underfilmed, and overread. Otherwise authoritative textbooks promote

---

Address reprint requests to M. Michael Cohen, Jr., D.M.D., Ph.D., Dalhousie University, Halifax, Nova Scotia, Canada B3H 3J5.

© 1985 Alan R. Liss, Inc.

TABLE I. Normal Ranges of Age-At-Appearance of Principal Ossification Centers[1]

Range	Age of child (years)	
	Male	Female
± 3–6 months	0–1	0–1
± 1–1.5 years	3–4	2–3
± 2 years	7–11	6–10
± 2 plus years	13–14	12–13

[1]From Graham [1972].

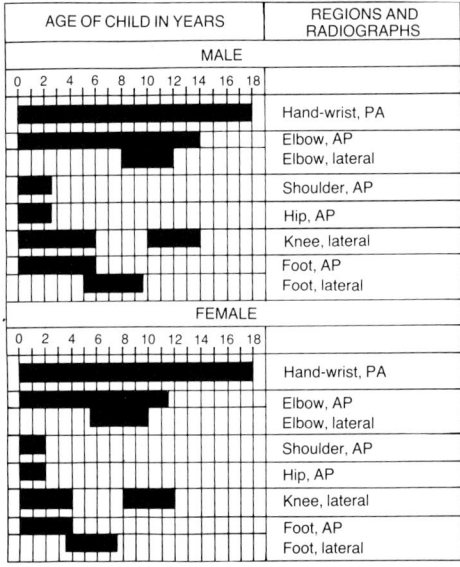

Fig. 1. Bone age sampling method [from C.B. Graham, 1972].

"normal ranges" that are much too narrow, being only one-half or even one-fourth as wide as the actual ranges [Graham, 1972]. Table I shows the normal ranges of the age-at-appearance of the principle ossification centers based on the excellent study of the Fels Research Institute [Garn et al, 1967]. It will be observed that the normal ranges are very broad. For example, a 3-year-old girl with a bone age between 1½ and 4½ years falls within the normal range. Because the estimation of osseous maturation from hand-wrist films alone is often misleading, while the routine study of all the hemiskeletal ossification centers is usually superfluous, a sampling method based on the usual age-at-appearance ranges of the most important ossification centers has been recommended [Graham, 1972] (Fig. 1).

LIMITATIONS OF RADIOLOGIC ASSESSMENT IN SYNDROMIC DYSMORPHISM

Caution is indicated when interpreting the relevance of bone age for syndromes with either growth deficiency or overgrowth of prenatal onset. In syndromes with prenatal onset growth deficiency, a lag in the appearance of various ossification

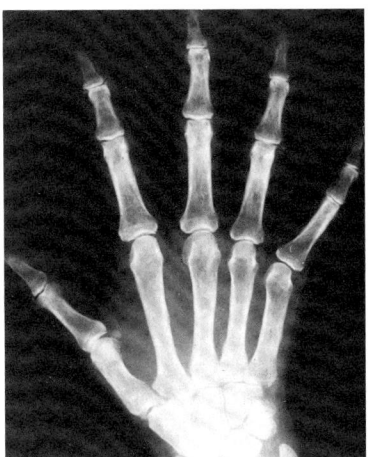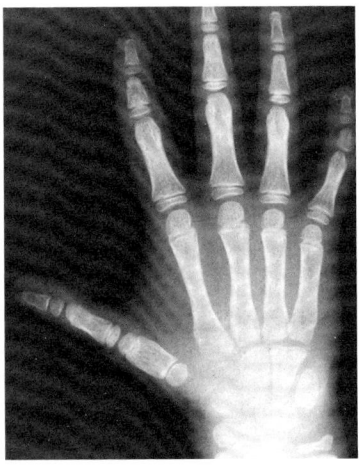

Fig. 2. Radiographs of two patients with the hand-foot-uterus syndrome. Although shortening of various tubular bones is evident on radiographs, metacarpophalangeal profile patterns (illustrated in Fig. 3) are more sensitive indices for detecting similarity of hand radiographs than simple inspection of the radiographs [from Poznanski et al, 1972].

centers does not necessarily mean that such findings are secondary to an abnormality in the maturation rate. Similarly, the precocious bone development in some prenatal onset overgrowth syndromes does not necessarily indicate accelerated maturation; it may indicate a mesenchymal defect that has resulted in early mineralization of ossification centers. With chondrodysplasias, the bones commonly used to assess maturation are part of the disorder, thus rendering bone age determination meaningless. However, complete radiologic assessment of the abnormal configuration of various bones can be extremely helpful in diagnosing the particular chondrodysplasia.

Growth predictions for various syndromes must be based on knowledge of the particular condition in question. For example, stature and final height attainment in achondroplasia can be predicted only from standard curves constructed for that particular disorder [Horton et al, 1978]. The same principle holds for other aspects of dysmorphic growth and development. For example, in normal human development, growth of the maxilla is essentially complete by age 14. In Apert syndrome, as Pruzansky has shown [1977], midfacial growth is arrested because of hypoplasia and faciostenosis, and it would be erroneous to conclude that maxillary growth in this condition continues until age 14.

DYSHARMONIC MATURATION AND PATTERNED DYSMORPHISM

In syndromic dysmorphism, unusual radiographic features may be observed such as bizarre ossification sequences, delay or advance of specific ossification centers, side-to-side asymmetry, abnormal configuration of various bones, and patterned dimensional alterations of various bones [Poznanski et al, 1971, 1972]. For example, a patient with trisomy 18 syndrome who survived to 42 months might have a hand-wrist film with absent carpal ossificiation centers and most of the epiphyses present, representing an unusual ossification sequence not found in the general population. The hand-wrist film of a 6-year-old with Hurler syndrome has such markedly abnormal bone configuration that accurate estimation of skeletal age becomes virtually

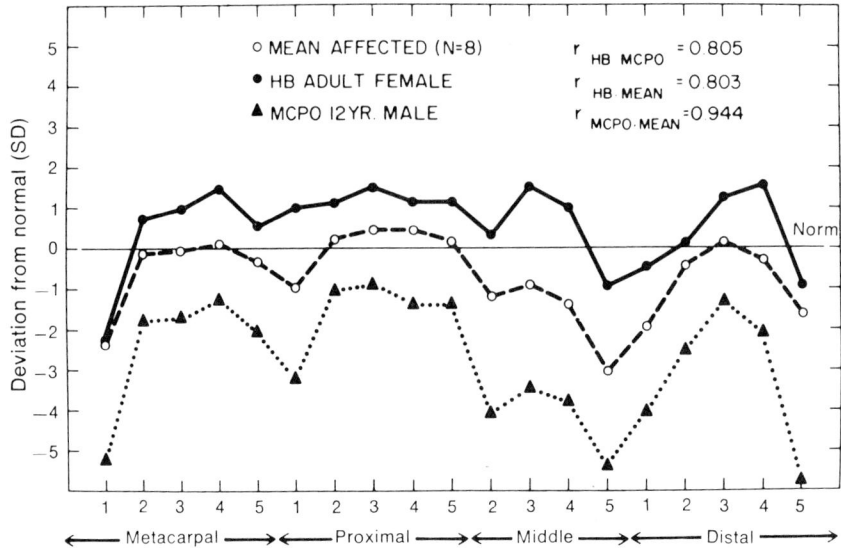

Fig. 3. Hand-foot-uterus syndrome. Metacarpophalangeal profile patterns showing relative shortening of the first metacarpal, first proximal phalanx, second middle phalanx, fifth middle phalanx, and fifth distal phalanx. Since profile patterns are plotted against appropriate standards for age and sex, an affected adult female, an affected 12-year-old male, and a mean profile pattern for eight affected individuals can be compared. All bear strong similarity to one another [from Poznanski et al, 1972].

Table II. Dimensions Used in Craniofacial Profile Pattern Analysis[1]

Dimension	Abbreviation	Landmarks	Landmark numbers
Posterior skull base length	PS	Opisthion-sella	8–7
Total skull base length	TS	Opisthion-glabella	8–6
Anterior skull base length	AS	Sella-glabella	7–6
Sella-nasion	SN	Sella-nasion	7–5
Facial depth	FD	Condylion-nasion	9–5
Palatal length	PL	Anterior-posterior nasal spines	4–11
Superior ramus length	SR	Condylion-coronoid process	9–17
Mandibular corpus length	MC	Gnathion-gonial intersection	1–16
Ramus height	RH	Condylion-gonial intersection	9–16
Mandibular height	MH	Distal M_1 CEJ Point 15[2]	14–15
Symphyseal height	SH	Gnathion-infradentale	1–2
Alveolar height	AH	Supradentale-anterior nasal spine	3–4
Anterior dental height	AD	Infradentale-supradentale	2–3
Posterior dental height	PD	Distal M^1 CEJ-distal M_1 CEJ	12–14
Palate-mandible height	PM	MH line extended to alveolar plane	13–15
Gonion-sella	GS	Gonial intersection-sella	16–7
Posterior facial height	PF	Distal M^1 CEJ-point 10[2]	12–10
Superior facial height	SF	Anterior nasal spine-nasion	4–5

[1]From Garn et al, [1984].
[2]Denotes points defined by intersections. Landmark 10 is a point on the condylion-nasion line from which a perpendicular intersects the distal cemento-enamel junction of the maxillary first molar (Distal M^1 CEJ). Landmark 15 is a point on the inferior mandibular plane from which a perpendicular intersects the distal cemento-enamel junction of the mandibular first molar (Distal M_1 CEJ).

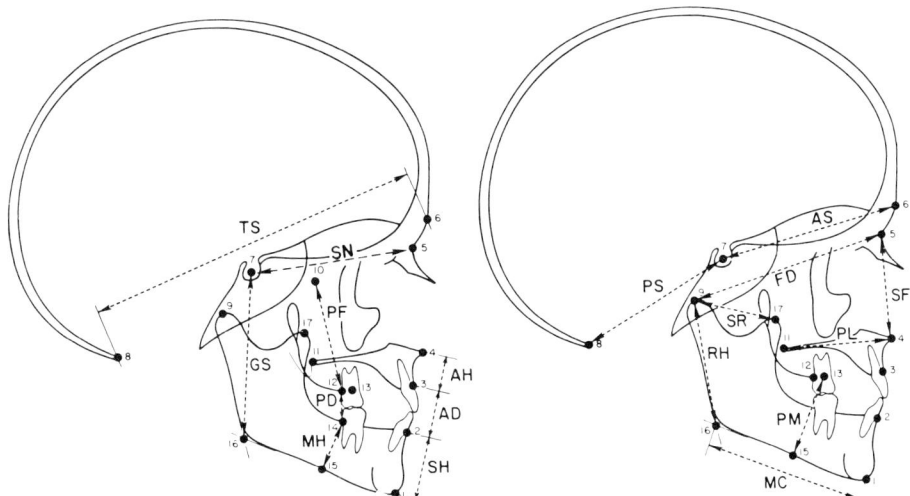

Fig. 4. Selected dimensions used in craniofacial profile pattern analysis. Landmark numbers and dimensions correspond to description in Table II [from Garn et al, 1984].

impossible. The hand-wrist films of two patients with the hand-foot-uterus syndrome are shown in Figure 2. Although relative shortening of various bones can be appreciated to some extent in the radiographs, the patterned dimensional alterations in these x-rays, known as metacarpophalangeal profile patterns (Fig. 3), provide information far beyond the capabilities of the most experienced radiographic observer. In metacarpophalangeal profile pattern analysis, the relationship between the lengths of various tubular bones in the hand can be illustrated graphically. The lengths of the tubular bones in the condition to be studied are plotted in terms of standard deviation units derived from normal tubular bone lengths. Because profiles are plotted against standards for age and sex, they allow comparison between various individuals. For example, in the hand-foot-uterus syndrome graphed in Figure 3, it will be observed that an affected adult female profile pattern, an affected 12-year-old male profile pattern, and a mean profile pattern for eight affected individuals all bear strong similarity to one another.

Profile pattern analysis has recently been applied to the craniofacial region by Garn and his coworkers [1984]. The dimensions used are defined in Table II and illustrated in Figure 4. A craniofacial profile pattern of monozygotic twins with Robin sequence* appears in Figure 5, showing close resemblance, extreme reduction in facial and cranial depths, and above average facial heights. The craniofacial profile pattern of monozygotic twins with oto-palato-digital syndrome (OPD 1) is shown in Figure 6, indicating pronounced syndromic patterning, but large discrepancies in a few of the cranial and facial depths.

The next order of business is to analyze the craniofacial profile patterns of various syndromes with sufficient sample size. I would predict that some conditions

---

*The accepted dysmorphology term for Pierre Robin syndrome.

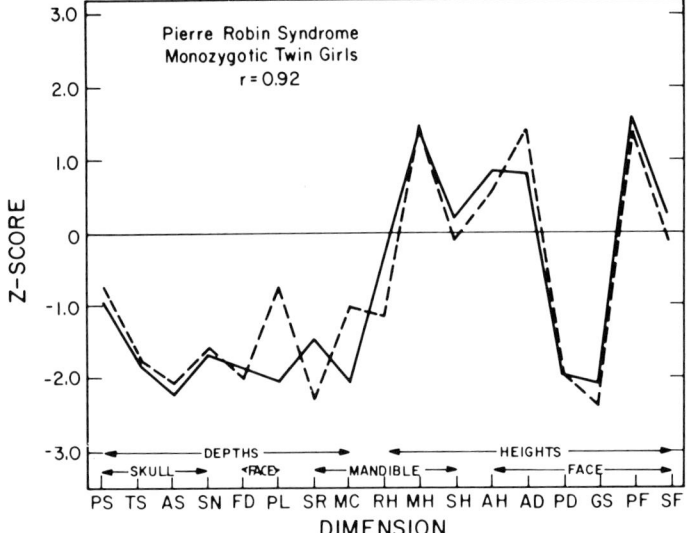

Fig. 5. Close craniofacial pattern profile resemblance ($r_z = 0.92$) in monozygotic twin girls with clinical manifestations of the Pierre Robin syndrome. Extreme reduction of facial and cranial depths and above average facial heights are clearly visible in this representation [from Garn et al, 1984].

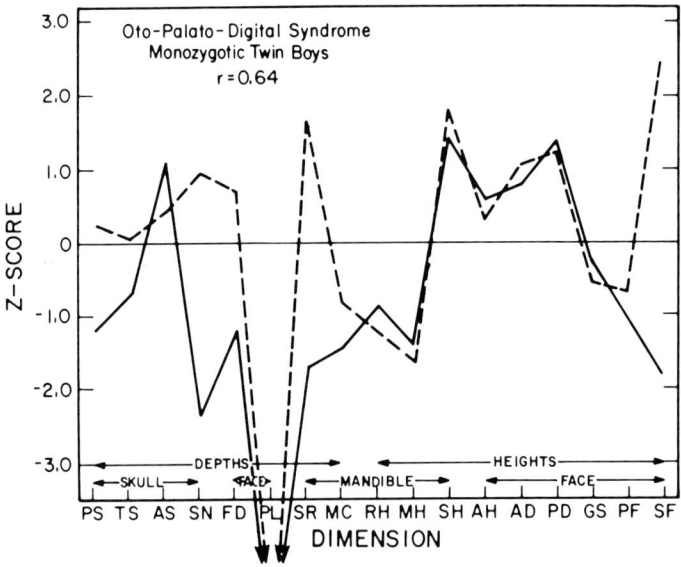

Fig. 6. Strongly patterned craniofacial pattern profiles in a set of twins affected with the oto-palato-digital syndrome. As shown, both twins are highly divergent from norms for age and sex. The twins show a moderate resemblance to each other ($r_z = 0.64$), but the large discrepancies in some cranial and facial depths (SN, SR, SF) indicate independent developmental dysmorphism. Both twins had surgical repair for soft palate clefts, but the values for PL (palatal length) $<5\sigma$ indicate that the hard palate is also extremely underdeveloped [from Garn et al, 1984].

will be syndrome specific, others will be nonspecific, still others will have too much intrasyndrome variability, and finally, some, like the craniosynostosis syndromes, will lend themselves better to other methods of pattern analysis.

Pruzansky [1977] has studied dysmorphic growth and development over time, observing that some syndromes remain essentially static, others improve, and still others grow worse. For example, the underlying osseous abnormalities in mandibulofacial dysostosis remain essentially unchanged throughout the entire postnatal growth period. The curvature of the lower border of the mandible was shown to be syndrome specific and could be defined by a computer-generated polynomial equation [Roberts et al, 1975]. The Pierre Robin mandible was found to have a specific mandibular shape and tongue posture, regardless of age, and was found to exhibit significant catch-up growth postnatally [Pruzansky 1969, 1977]. Finally, extensive studies of the craniosynostosis syndromes have demonstrated an increase in severity over time in both Apert and Crouzon syndromes. Increasing severity was caused by disproportionate growth of the craniofacial structures, which resulted in displacements, compressions, and dysfunctions [Pruzansky, 1973, 1976, 1977].

PRIMARY GROWTH DEFICIENCY SYNDROMES OF PRENATAL ONSET

Growth deficiency of prenatal onset is of special importance in syndromology. In the small-for-gestational-age infant, growth deficiency may be primary, in which the intrinsic capacity of skeletal cells is affected, as in some malformation syndromes and chondrodysplasias, or secondary, in which the cause is exogenous to the skeletal system, as in deformational growth restriction, prenatal infectious disease, and teratogenic growth deficiency.

Let us consider primary growth deficiency associated with both major and minor malformations, especially those of incomplete morphogenesis. If such prenatal onset growth deficiency is regarded as a malformation—that is, as hypoplasia of the whole individual—it is not surprising that other malformations, especially those of incomplete morphogenesis, frequently accompany the growth deficiency [Smith, 1971]. Organ formation and developmental placement are susceptible to malformation if hypoplasia occurs during the period of rapid differentiation and growth. For example, trisomy 18 syndrome, characterized by growth deficiency of prenatal onset, also has many anomalies of organ formation, developmental placement, and insufficient growth such as microcephaly, short palpebral fissures, low-set hypoplastic ears, micrognathia, microstomia, short sternum, and ventricular septal defect.

An expected consequence of a primary growth deficiency syndrome is that cell cultures from affected individuals should manifest the growth deficiency. A preliminary study of the in vitro fibroblast doubling time of three trisomy 18 syndrome patients showed an approximate doubling time of 40 hours compared with the normal doubling time of 27 hours [Pious et al, 1975].

With primary growth deficiency of prenatal onset, the growth deficiency persists into postnatal life as, for example, with de Lange syndrome or with those few trisomy 18 patients who survive into childhood. Unlike humorally mediated growth deficiencies, such as hypopituitarism and hypothyroidism, which respond to replacement therapy, primary growth deficiency has no effective treatment [Smith, 1971].

Another characteristic of primary growth deficiency syndromes is that the features may be correlated. For example, the severity of microcephaly in the de Lange syndrome is correlated with the severity of the growth deficiency [Smith, 1977]. Growth of various parts may also be dysharmonic or dyssynchronous. In the de Lange syndrome, for example, Pruzansky [1976] studied the neurocranial silhouette cephalometrically and confirmed the finding of microbrachycephaly, but also concluded that the posterior cranial fossa was disproportionately reduced in size.

ASYMMETRIC DYSMORPHISM

Mild degrees of asymmetry are a normal state in human development. Paired structures known to be asymmetric include the cerebral hemispheres, humeri, radii, femora, fibulae, clavicles, and ribs, among others [Halperin, 1931; LeMay and Clebras, 1972; Meredith, 1947; Schultz, 1937]. With respect to the face, subtle degrees of normal asymmetry become especially evident when frontal photographs are divided along the median plane and reprocessed, each side being paired with its mirror image yielding two slightly different faces [Peck and Peck, 1970].

Some developmental disturbances not known to produce significantly dysmorphic effects still augment the normal degree of asymmetry. For example, left-right crown size asymmetry of the teeth, evident by measurement but not by visual inspection, is a normal state in the general population [Garn et al, 1966]. In trisomy 21 syndrome, left-right crown size asymmetry of the teeth is definitely increased, although the asymmetry still cannot be appreciated visually [Garn et al, 1970]. Other developmental disturbances seem not to be related to normal asymmetry. For example, preferential laterality is known to occur for various anomalies of paired structures such as limb reduction defects. The predominantly involved side in such limb defects does not correspond to the preferred smaller side in normal development [Schnall and Smith, 1974].

Preferential laterality for some anomalies is striking, as with left-sidedness for cleft lip and postaxial polydactyly or with right-sidedness for inguinal hernia and fibular aplasia [Schnall and Smith, 1974]. To date, no adequate hypotheses to explain such phenomena have been put forth. However, developmental interrelationships may account for similarities or difference in sidedness of at least a few anomalies such as right-sided inguinal hernia and cryptorchidism.

Pruzansky has adapted cephalometric techniques to deal with craniofacial asymmetry. For example, in plagiocephaly the eyes and ears are both asymmetrically placed, and two head films must be taken—one with both ear rods in place, the other with only partial engagement of the ear rods and alignment of the face with respect to the presumed midline. In studies of hemifacial microsomia, cephalometric adaptation must be made for a displaced or absent external auditory meatus on one side [Pruzansky, 1975]. Postero-anterior cephalometric studies have shown that in hemifacial microsomia, the angular deviation from the midline does not increase, but with increasing vertical height of the face, the linear deviation of the chin point from the midline does [Pruzansky, 1973]. With respect to laterality, the right side is observed to be affected almost twice as frequently as the left side [Figueroa and Pruzansky, 1982].

PROBLEMS IN DIAGNOSTIC HOMOGENEITY

It should be obvious that a diagnostically heterogeneous sample will lead to faulty conclusions no matter how sound the cephalometric analysis. It is somewhat like

TABLE III. Conditions Associated With the Robin Sequence[1]

  Monogenic syndromes
    Beckwith-Wiedemann syndrome
    Campomelic syndrome
    Cerebrocostomandibular syndrome
    Diastrophic dysplasia
    Donlan syndrome
    Myotonic dystrophy
    Persistent left superior vena cava syndrome
    Radiohumeral synostosis syndrome
    Spondyloepiphyseal dysplasia congenita
    Stickler syndrome
  Chromosomal syndromes
    Partial trisomy 11q syndrome
  Teratogenically induced syndromes
    Fetal alcohol syndrome
    Fetal hydantoin syndrome
    Fetal trimethadione syndrome
  Unknown-genesis syndromes
    Digitopalatal syndrome
    Femoral dysgenesis-unusual facies syndrome
    Martsolf syndrome
    Robin-amelia syndrome

[1]From Cohen [1982].

studying fruit instead of analyzing apples, oranges, peaches, and pears separately. With craniofacial syndromes, it is not always easy to get a diagnostically homogeneous sample because of the problems inherent in the process of syndrome delineation and the possibility of etiologic heterogeneity [Cohen, 1982]. Let us consider the etiologic and probably pathogenetic heterogeneity of the Robin sequence as an example.

The syndromology perspective on the Robin sequence adds considerably to our understanding of the etiology and pathogenesis. Table III lists some syndromes in which the Robin sequence is one feature. The etiology of each condition is different. Thus, the Robin sequence is probably pathogenetically heterogenous. The autosomal dominantly inherited Stickler syndrome is the most common syndrome associated with the Robin sequence. Since abnormalities of bones and joints occur in the Stickler syndrome, the major pleiotropic effect appears to be on connective tissue. Thus, in this condition, the Robin sequence may result from intrinsic mandibular hypoplasia and failure of connective tissue penetration across the palate. Another condition that may have the Robin sequence is partial trisomy 11q syndrome. With the hypoplastic growth that accompanies most chromosomal syndromes, there may not be significant mandibular catch-up growth in patients with partial trisomy 11q syndrome who survive. Therefore, to include such patients in a mandibular growth study of the Robin sequence would be a study of "fruit" since "oranges" are being confused with "apples."

Some instances of the Robin sequence have been associated with oligohydramnios. It is thought that reduced amniotic fluid results in compression of the chin against the sternum, restricting mandibular growth and impacting the tongue between

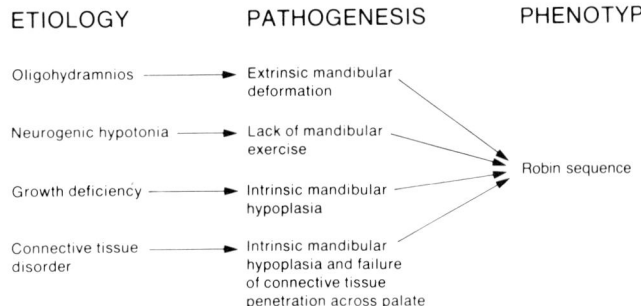

Fig. 7. Etiologic heterogeneity suggests pathogenetic heterogeneity in the Robin sequence. The following pathogenetic possibilities should be considered. (I) Oligohydramnios results in decreased amniotic fluid, compressing the chin against the sternum and thus restricting mandibular growth. (II) If hypotonia restricts mouth opening during early fetal life prior to complete palatal closure, the Robin sequence might result from lack of mandibular exercise. (III) Growth deficiency, as observed in chromosomal syndromes such as the partial trisomy 11q syndrome, may produce the Robin sequence by intrinsic mandibular hypoplasia. (IV) In a connective tissue disorder such as the Stickler syndrome, the Robin sequence may result from intrinsic mandibular hypoplasia and failure of connective tissue penetration across the palate [from Cohen, 1982].

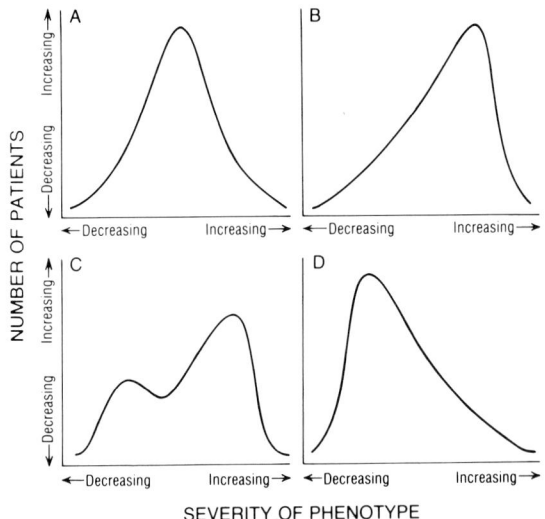

Fig. 8. The phenotypic spectrum of a syndrome. A. The normal phenotypic spectrum that occurs when the syndrome population is ascertained independently of the phenotype, as is possible with a chromosomal syndrome or biochemical disorder. This phenotypic spectrum also occurs when the ascertainment bias has been corrected for in a monogenic disorder by including only affected sibs born after the proband and excluding the proband. B. Syndrome population truncated toward the severe end of the phenotypic spectrum. Such artificial homogeneity occurs when a syndrome population is ascertained by phenotypic features alone. C. Syndrome population with biomodal distribution, emphasizing both severe and mild ends of the phenotypic spectrum. Such a distribution probably occurs in a monogenic syndrome population composed of probands plus previously unrecognized, mildly affected sibs who were born before the proband and actively searched for. D. Syndrome population truncated toward the mild end of the phenotypic spectrum. Such a distribution probably occurs in a monogenic syndrome population composed of previously unrecognized, mildly affected sibs who were born before the proband and actively searched for, the proband himself being excluded in an attempt to correct for ascertainment bias [from Cohen, 1982].

the palatal shelves. Because micrognathia is based on intrauterine molding, mandibular catch-up growth is expected after birth when intrauterine deforming forces are no longer acting. Poswillo [1966] has produced a phenocopy of the Robin sequence in rats by puncturing the amniotic sac prior to palatal closure. Some experimental animals also had deformities of the limbs, ranging from clubfoot to ring constrictions and intrauterine amputations. Such limb abnormalities have also been associated with the Robin sequence in humans.

Finally, the Robin sequence has been associated with congenial hypotonia. If neurogenic hypotonia occurred prior to complete closure of the palate, it is conceivable that the Robin sequence might result from lack of mandibular exercise. [Cohen, 1982].

Different etiologic and pathogenetic possibilities are summarized diagrammatically in Figure 7. Pruzansky was able to delineate a Pierre Robin specific mandibular shape by removing other etiologically specific syndromes from his sample. It should be emphasized that it is not necessary to eliminate any of these categories in a cephalometric study, but *it is essential to separate them in the analysis of data*.

PROBLEMS IN ASCERTAINMENT BIAS

How a cephalometric sample is selected can considerably affect the result. Figure 8A illustrates a given syndrome sample that follows a normal distribution. By this, we mean that, morphometrically, the highest number of cases fall midway between the mildest and most severe cases and that the number of mild and severe cases are approximately equal. The approximation of a normal distribution is desirable in obtaining a cephalometric sample. Also, it is ideal if intrasyndrome population variability of morphometric traits is not either reduced or increased.

Such a sample can be most effectively obtained if the syndrome to be studied can be diagnosed independently of its phenotypic manifestations, ie, from some cytogenetic or biochemical test. For example, if we wish to carry out a cephalometric growth study of trisomy 21 syndrome and all our cases are ascertained through a cytogenetics laboratory that diagnoses the condition by the presence of an extra number 21 chromosome, if our sample size is large enough, the phenotypic spectrum of abnormalities will approach a normal distribution. If, however, we obtain our sample from a mental retardation hospital by selecting patients with trisomy 21 syndrome on the basis of their physical appearance, the distribution will be skewed to the right (Fig. 8B) because we will tend to select the most severe cases. Such a skewed sample will tend to truncate mean values for various cephalometric measurements toward the severe end of the phenotypic spectrum.

If we wish to study a monogenic condition, for example, an autosomal dominant malformation syndrome such as Crouzon syndrome, the diagnosis is made from the physical appearance alone and therefore cannot be ascertained independently of the phenotype. Since there is a greater chance of ascertaining a proband who is severely affected, the total sample will be biased in favor of severely affected patients. Thus, the net affect on the sample will be a distribution that shows some skewness to the left (Fig. 8B). It is possible to correct the ascertainment bias and approximate a normal distribution by subtracting the proband from each family and carrying out the cephalometric study on the remaining cases.

Figure 8C represents a syndrome population with a bimodal distribution, emphasizing both severe and mild ends of the phenotypic spectrum. Such a distribution might occur in an autosomal recessive syndrome population composed of probands plus previously unrecognized, mildly affected sibs who were born before the proband and actively searched for.

Figure 8D represents a syndrome population truncated toward the mild end of the phenotypic spectrum. Such a distribution might occur in an autosomal recessive syndrome population composed of previously unrecognized, mildly affected sibs who were born before the proband and actively searched for, the proband himself being excluded in an attempt to correct for ascertainment bias.

If the etiology of a syndrome is unknown as with de Lange syndrome or Rubinstein-Taybi syndrome, and all or almost all examples occur sporadically, the only way to collect the sample is to diagnose the condition directly from the physical appearance, which will result in the sample's being skewed to the right because severe cases will be diagnosed with certainty and there will be a tendency to exclude mild cases that cannot be diagnosed with assurance. Unlike the situation with monogenic syndromes, there is no way to correct for sampling bias and the sample must be used just the way it is.

It is not our purpose to dismiss or even to modify such studies because of sampling bias. On the contrary, because of the relative rarity of such biologically important syndromes, we wish to encourage the inclusion of all correctly diagnosed cases in a given syndrome sample. It is simply our contention that in all cephalometric studies of dysmorphic syndromes, *a statement of the type of ascertainment bias encountered should be included in the paper together with a discussion of the probable effects on the results* [Cohen, 1981, 1982].

REFERENCES

Cohen MM Jr: A critical review of cephalometric studies of dysmorphic syndromes. Koski Festschrift Proc Finn Dent Soc 77:17–25, 1981.

Cohen MM Jr: "The Child with Multiple Birth Defects." New York: Raven Press, 1982.

Figueroa A and Pruzansky S: The external ear, mandible and other components of hemifacial microsomia. J Max -Fac Surg 10:200–211, 1982.

Garn SM, Cohen MM, Geciauskas MA: Increased crown-size asymmetry in trisomy G. J Dent Res 49:465, 1970.

Garn SM, Lewis AB, Kerewsky RS: The meaning of bilateral asymmetry in the permanent dentition. Angle Orthodont 36:55–62, 1966.

Garn SM, Rohmann CG, Silverman FN: Radiographic standards for postnatal ossification and tooth calcification. Med Radiogr Photogr 43:45–66, 1967.

Garn SM, Smith BH, and LaVelle M: Applications of pattern profile analysis to malformations of the head and face. Radiology 150:683–690, 1984.

Graham CB: Assessment of bone maturation—Methods and Pitfalls. Radiol Clin N Am 10:185–202,1972.

Halperin G: Normal asymmetry and unilateral hypertrophy. Arch Intern Med 49:676–682, 1931.

Horton WA, Rotter JI, Rimoin DL, Scott CI Jr, Hall JG: Standard growth curves for achondroplasia. J Pediatr 93:435–438, 1978.

Kreiborg S: The application of roentgencephalometry to the study of craniofacial anomalies (this volume).

LeMay M, Clebras A: Human brain: morphologic differences in the hemispheres demonstrable by carotid arteriography. N Eng J Med 287:168–171, 1972.

Meredith HV: Length of upper extremities in Homo sapiens from birth through adolescence. Growth 11:1–50, 1947.

Peck H, Peck S: A concept of facial esthetics. Angle Orthodont 40:284–318, 1970.

Pious D, Millis AJT, Sabo K: In vitro growth rates in primary cellular growth deficiency syndromes. Pediatr Res 9:279, 1975.

Poswillo D: Observations of fetal posture and causal mechanisms of congenital deformity of palate, mandible, and limbs. J Dent Res 45:584–596, 1966.

Poznanski AK, Garn SM, Kuhns LR, Sandusky ST: Dysharmonic maturation of the hand in the congenital malformation syndromes. Am J Phys Anthropol 35:417–432, 1971.

Poznanski AK, Garn SM, Nagy JM, Gall JC Jr: Metacarpophalangeal pattern profiles in the evaluation of skeletal malformations. Radiology 104:1–11, 1972.

Pruzansky S: Not all dwarfed mandibles are alike. Birth Defects 5(2): 120–129, 1969.

Pruzansky S: Clinical investigation of the experiments of nature. ASHA Report 8:62–94, 1973.

Pruzansky S: Roentgencephalometry of infants: 1949–1973, Trans 3rd Int Congr Orthodont, 1975, pp 101–117.

Pruzansky S: Radiocephalometric studies of the basicranium in craniofacial malformations. In Bosma JF (ed): "Development of the Basicranium." U.S. Dept. of HEW Pub. No. (NIH) 76-989, Bethesda, MD, 1976, ch 17, pp 278–300.

Pruzansky S: Time: The fourth dimension in syndrome analysis applied to craniofacial malformations. Birth Defects 13(3C):3–28, 1977.

Roberts FG, Pruzansky S, Aduss H: An X-radiocephalometric study of mandibulofacial dysostosis in man. Arch Oral Biol 20:265–281, 1975.

Schnall BS, Smith DW: Nonrandom laterality of malformations in paired structures. J Pediatr 85:509–511, 1974.

Schultz AH: Proportions, variability and asymmetries of the long bones of the limbs and the clavicles in man and apes. Hum Biol 9:281–328, 1937.

Smith DW: Growth deficiency: A new classification into primary cellular growth deficiency and secondary humoral growth deficiency. S Med J 64[Suppl.]:5–15, 1971.

Smith DW: "Growth and Its Disorders." Philadelphia: WB Saunders, Co, 1977.

Regional Specification of Cell-Specific Gene Expression During Craniofacial Development

Harold C. Slavkin
Laboratory For Developmental Biology, Department of Basic Sciences, School of Dentistry, University of Southern California, Los Angeles

> The core problem in craniofacial development is regional specification of cell-specific gene expression. Regional specification is also referred to as pattern formation or spatial organization. During early embryogenesis, regional specification is possibly operant following blastula, and is apparent during gastrulation and thereafter during embryonic and fetal stages of development. Current interdisciplinary approaches toward understanding embryonic development incorporate a number of scientific approaches including those of recombinant DNA technology. Three major advances have significantly enhanced the utility of so-called "genetic engineering," including (i) the discovery of restriction nuclease enzymes that cleave DNA sequences at specific sites; (ii) the discovery of DNA ligase enzymes that facilitate ligation and annealing of DNA sequences to one another, so as to facilitate the joining of foreign DNA sequences with host DNA; and (iii) the discovery of effective techniques for the introduction of foreign DNA sequences into previously refractory organisms. The present discussion analyzes the problem of regional specification of ameloblast-specific gene expression as a paradigm for utilizing recombinant DNA technology in studies of normal and abnormal craniofacial development.

Key words: recombinant DNA technology, ameloblast, enamel gene products, cDNA, gene expression

INTRODUCTION

I first met Professor Samuel Pruzansky through the literature. He was, of course, very prolific, and I found his writing both important and inspiring. Years later, I met him in person while we served together on a government panel to explore critical issues of congenital craniofacial biology. That was in 1973. He was, of course, also inspiring in person; his breadth and depth of knowledge in both the clinical challenges of diagnosis and treatment, as well as his enthusiastic promise for opportunities in research, were both wonderful to experience. Thereafter, we did several projects together. I had the unique and special privilege to write several position papers with Sam in the late 1970s and early 1980s.

Address reprint requests to Harold C. Slavkin, Laboratory For Developmental Biology, Andrus Gerontology Center, Room 314, University Park MC-0101, University of Southern California, Los Angeles, CA 90089-0191.

© 1985 Alan R. Liss, Inc.

For me Sam Pruzansky is a synonym for the genesis of interdisciplinary approaches to problems of congenital craniofacial malformations. His pioneering interdisciplinary efforts were in part captured during his Introduction presentation at the now classic Gatlinburg Conference, held at the Mountain View Hotel in Gatlinburg, Tennessee, on December 6–9th, 1959: "For dental science, congenital malformations of the head offer a challenge and an opportunity. The challenge is in the treatment of such patients and the opportunity is in research. Never before has there been such a gathering of talents and resources as we have here in Gatlinburg. This is an occasion for intellectual ferment, for the cross-pollination of ideas, and for the making of new allies in our common effort against the unknown. ..." [Pruzansky, 1961].

The present communication in this volume is dedicated to Sam's joy and creativity regarding advancement toward the unknown. The opportunities for research in craniofacial biology remain fascinating; in particular, research opportunities in cellular, molecular, and developmental biology problems associated with the craniofacial complex. This review will focus upon the emerging research activities that now utilize recombinant DNA technology to investigate craniofacial developmental biology—in particular, the problem of regional specification of cell specific gene expression.

GENE CONTROLS DURING CRANIOFACIAL DEVELOPMENTAL BIOLOGY

Perhaps the most fascinating current problem in development concerns the processes by which gene activity is regionally specified or controlled. Whereas the structural and functional highlights of genes and gene products have become understandable as a consequence of the last 30 years of research in molecular biology [Crick, 1982; Judson, 1979], in contrast, the mechanisms that control embryonic and fetal development remain elusive. The central problem in development is to understand how cells in different regions of the gastrula, embryo and fetus become directed onto different pathways of development—regional specification of cell-specific gene expression.

The consequences of regional specification are readily apparent. For example, regional specification results in the gene expression of enamel matrix gene products in ameloblasts at specific times and positions during the developmental course of tooth formation [see recent discussions in Kollar, 1983; Slavkin et al, 1984]. What processes invoke the activation of selected structural genes and their expression during craniofacial development? Whereas cell differentiation is of immense importance during development, it remains the result or consequence of regional specification. What regulates cell-specific gene expression during development?

It is evident that following fertilization and the first cleavages, blastula cells are coupled and sustain some type of ionic and metabolic cooperativeness, which changes as these blastula cells lose their potentialities to become individual organisms. Subsequently, regions of the morula, blastocyst, gastrula, and following embryonic stages of development illustrate unique patterns of regional cellular activity. Fate maps, for example, have been constructed that diagram what becomes of each region of the individual organism (ie, using invertebrate as well as vertebrate organisms) in normal development. How the fate of a particular region is irreversibly specified to take a particular fate remains unknown. Therefore, fate maps can be very useful to present a diagrammatic representation of several characteristics of regionalization, but do not provide explanations as to *how* cells become committed for a particular phenotype. For example, when, where, and *how* are enamel structural genes activated and subsequently expressed to a detectable level only in ameloblast cells at specific positions and times during tooth development? Moreover, *how* does regional specification function and result in bilateral symmetry during development (eg, right and left mandibular first molar morphogenesis)?

During the very early stages of development following fertilization, blastula cells are either considered to be nearly equivalent or to possess very small differences between them. With subsequent development these "differences" become increased so that a regional distribution of cells reflects actual differences in the developmental behavior of individually positioned cells. The key question, of course, is *how* gene regulatory molecules become unequally distributed amongst the emerging populations of embryonic cells? Determinants for "differences" allegedly are localized either (i) within the fertilized egg, (ii) progressively partitioned as cytoplasmic determinants, and/or (iii) small putative signals that serve as epigenetic regulators either within or between cells.

What is clear is that cells generally become specialized from a sheet or aggregate within which cells are ionically, electrically, and metabolically coupled. Individual ameloblasts, for example, do not function independently as discrete cells, but appear to be a synchronized sheet of epithelial cells that illustrate remarkably interdependent cooperativeness. In terms of this paradigm, we can ask when, where or *how* do cranial neural crest-derived dental papilla ectomesenchyme cells (or tissue) provide regional specification for the dentition?

STRATEGIES TO INVESTIGATE REGIONAL SPECIFICATION OF CELL-TYPE-SPECIFIC GENE CONTROL

When, where and *how* does regional specification regulate cell-type-specific gene control? For example, how are chick oviduct tubular epithelial cells determined to express ovalbumin genes? How are mammary acinar epithelial cells determined to express casein genes? How are pancreatic acinar epithelial cells determined to express insulin genes? Three strategies seem to be most essential in the pursuit of these questions. However, before one approaches the problem, of course, one must document details of the selected developing system (eg, animal, organ, tissue) to be studied including species, strain, sex, and precise development staging. Confounding variables should be identified and controlled for whenever possible. For example, investigations of morphogenesis using serumless and chemically defined medium for in vitro culture studies provide several obvious advantages.

In terms of the three experimental strategies to investigate regional specification of cell-type-specific gene control, one is the identification of the DNA sequences and non-DNA control molecules (eg, non-histone chromosomal proteins; steroid-like hydrophobic molecules) associated with the particular phenotype under consideration. For example, one can ask, when, where, and how does chromatin become accessible in terms of a promoter sequence for a specified RNA polymerase? Among all of the gene possibilities, a discrete domain of chromatin becomes accessible for the activation of a unique DNA sequence with the subsequent transcription of that sequence into functional mRNA transcripts. In turn, functional mRNA transcripts are translated in the cytoplasm into specific polypeptides (eg, collagens, insulin, enamel proteins,

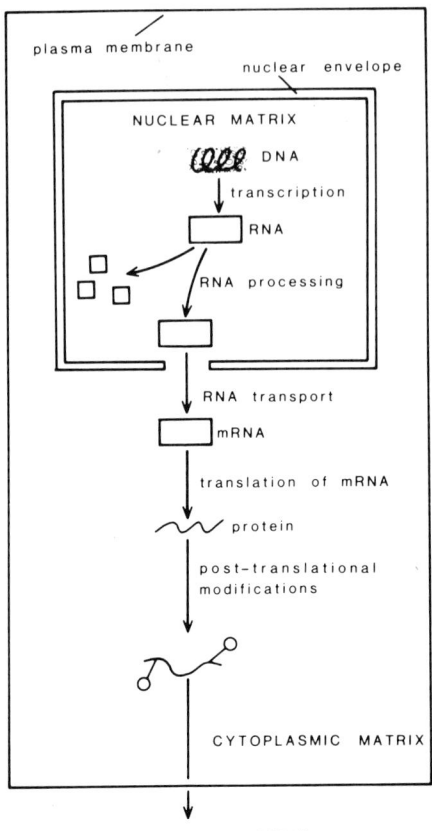

Fig. 1. A generalized scheme for gene expression. Eucaryotic cell types possess three major compartments or matrices, which are closely coupled: (i) nuclear matrix, (ii) cytoplasmic matrix, and (iii) extracellular matrix. Interactions between these matrices appear to mediate regional specification of de novo cell-specific gene expression.

dentine phosphoproteins, amylase). A second strategy is to determine how putative regulatory non-DNA molecules become distributed during development, so as to be accessible in the proper cell type, in the proper position, and at the right time. Finally, a third strategy is to determine if these developmental regulators are partitioned within the cytoplasm during development (and are therefore intrinsic), or do they regulate as extracellular epigenetic signals derived from adjacent yet complementary cell types (Fig. 1).

A CRANIOFACIAL PARADIGM FOR STUDIES OF REGIONAL SPECIFICATION OF CELL-TYPE-SPECIFIC GENE CONTROLS

It is generally accepted that dermal or mesenchyme provide regional specification for adjacent epithelial differentiation [see review by Dhouailly and Sengel, 1983]. Of extreme interest have been the results showing that heterotypic tissue recombinations, such as between non-dental epithelial and dental mesenchyme tissues, result in the formation of teeth with the included expression of ameloblast differentiation and the production of a discrete enamel extracellular matrix [see review by Kollar, 1983]. In order to further investigate mechanisms by which mesenchyme regional specification results in epithelial ameloblast-specific gene expression of enamel gene products, one might carefully consider the fascinating studies described by Kollar and Fisher [1980]. In these studies chick pharyngeal epithelial tissue was combined with mouse dental papilla mesenchyme and cultured as an heterotypic tissue recombinant within a permissive environment. Whereas chick normally do not form teeth nor do they produce enamel gene products (modern birds apparently evolved during the last 110 million years), how can the regional specification of cell-type-specific gene expression be explained? Are there related DNA sequences for enamel gene products within the avian genomic DNA? Did the mouse cap-stage dental papilla mesenchyme provide extracellular epigenetic signals that activated sets of "quiescent" avian genes? What are the mesenchyme-derived putative signals? How do epithelial cells receive these putative signals? How do these regional mesenchyme specification signals mediate de novo structural gene activation and subsequent enamel gene expression?

In order to further investigate this fascinating model, methods and assays are required that, for example, can identify enamel DNA sequences in genomic vertebrate DNA, identify de novo transcription of functional mRNA for enamel gene products (ie, amelogenins and enamelins), and to identify nascent enamel polypeptide production. Of course, suitable selection of animal model systems, and, if possible, localization of these instructive developmental interactions using serumless and chemically-defined medium in tissue or organ culture are additional objectives for this proposed experimental odyssey. It quickly becomes evident that a number of different scientific disciplines working in concert might impinge upon this fascinating and complex developmental problem area.

CONSTRUCTION AND IDENTIFICATION OF MOUSE ENAMEL cDNA CLONES

In 1953 the Watson-Crick model for the structure and suggested function of DNA introduced the molecular investigations of replication, transcription, and translation of nucleic acids [see Alberts et al, 1983; Crick, 1982; Judson, 1979]. The genetic code was deciphered, and it was established that A (adenosine), T (thymidine), C (cytosine), and G (guanosine) were the nucleotide bases that composed the genetic code found in DNA, and that U (uridine) substituted for T in RNA molecules. Each amino acid found in proteins was coded for in DNA and RNA in the form of one or several codons, each codon consisting of three nucleotide bases (eg, GCT, CCT, etc). In addition, specified codons are required for the progressive positioning of amino acids into a primary structure for a protein. Additional codons were identified to be either "start" or "stop" signals. Within genomic DNA, functional coding sequences termed "exons" were found to be interrupted by intervening sequences termed "introns." Segments of DNA including upstream and downstream sequences, as well as included exons and introns, were noted to be transcribed into nuclear RNAs. Restriction nuclease as well as ligase enzymes within the nuclear matrix were discovered to participate in the processing of expressed genetic transcripts to become functional mRNAs for transport from the nucleus to the cytoplasm for subsequent translation into nascent proteins (Fig. 2). These discoveries, as well as the identifica-

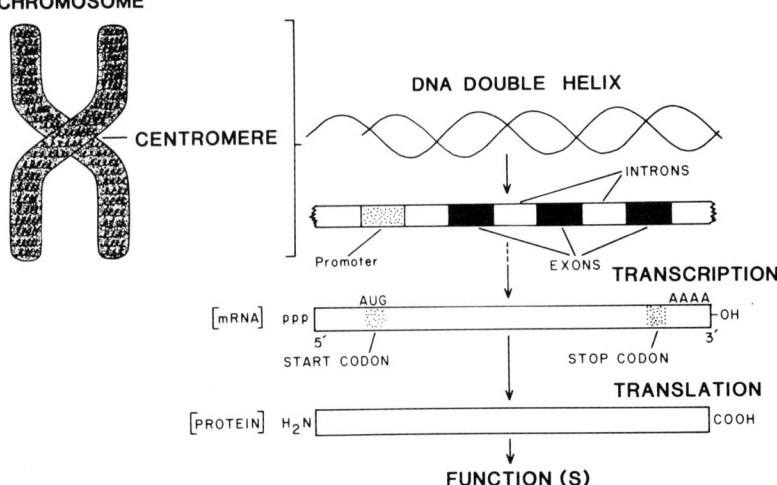

Fig. 2. Schematic drawing of a typical metaphase chromosome and several different orders of functional genetic constituents: (i) the double helix of DNA is approximately 2 nm wide and contains several hundred thousands of gene sequences that are expressed during development; and (ii) a schematic representation of a DNA sequence or "gene" indicating a promoter, start signal, exons, intron, and stop signal sequences. Whereas a great deal of information is known regarding DNA replication (mitosis), transcription, reverse transcription, and translation, very little is known as to how discrete sequences of DNA are activated and then transcribed under regional specification during embryogenesis.

tion of reverse transcriptase enzyme, monospecific antibodies to identify proteins, cell-free translation systems, bacterial genetics, electrophoretic separation methods for DNA and RNA molecules, DNA vectors or plasmids suitable for insertion of "foreign DNA" sequences and subsequent insertion into viable host systems to increase the yield of producing foreign DNA copies, and the advent of eucaryotic cell lines for the expression of "foreign genes" heralded the era of recombinant DNA technology [for detailed discussions see Alberts et al, 1983; Dahl et al, 1981; Johnson, 1983; Steinmetz and Hood, 1983; Williams, 1981]. The intellectual cooperativeness among cellular, molecular, and developmental biologists coupled with mutual interests in both procaryotic (non-nucleated) as well as eucaryotic (nucleated) cells by cell biologists, has forged a unity in biology and remarkable progress in this rapidly evolving field.

During the 1970s, four major advances occurred that made recombinant DNA technology possible. First, restriction endonucleases were identified that cleave the bond between specific nucleotide sequences (Fig. 3). Second, procedures were discovered for introducing specific sequences of DNA into bacterial (procaryotic) cells and for selecting bacteria for the inclusion of exogenous "foreign DNA" sequences (eg, human insulin). Third, enzymes called DNA ligases were discovered that are required for replication, recombination, and repair of DNA. These enzymes enable one to insert and anneal a foreign DNA sequence into a host DNA chromosome. Fourth, methods were discovered for the electrophoretic separation of DNA and RNA fragments and for the visualization of these fragments which both enabled calculation of size as well as nucleotide sequence. This led to rapid advances in determination of the nucleotide base sequence of DNA sequences. It became, therefore, routine to isolate a DNA sequence (eg, produce a double-stranded DNA sequence from a

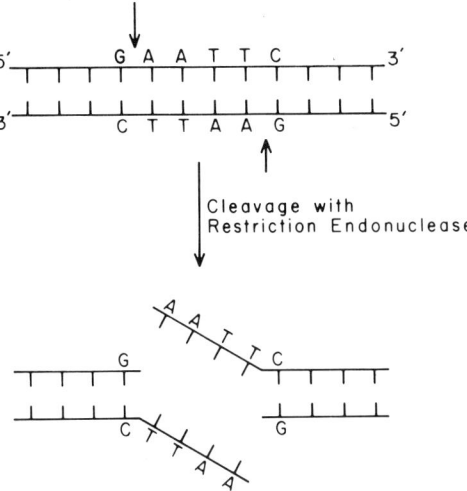

Fig. 3. Diagrammatic representation of restriction endonuclese enzyme cleavage of double-stranded DNA at one specific site or at staggered sites, and a suggested process by which cut ends can join or be annealed together to form unorthodox associations between for example, foreign DNA (eg, human insulin) and host DNA (*Escherichia coli* bacterial DNA).

specific mRNA using reverse transcriptase enzyme) that contains information for a specific gene, introduce the foreign sequence into a vector, produce multiple copies of the gene sequence in host microorganisms, harvest the vector, and then re-isolate the specific gene. This method is termed gene cloning and provides virtually unlimited amounts of a desired gene (Fig. 4).

Between 1980 and 1981 our laboratory began the process of adapting this recombinant DNA technology for proposed studies to investigate regional specification of ameloblast enamel gene expression. Our strategy was to use the embryonic, fetal, neonatal, and early postnatal mouse mandibular first molar tooth organ from genetically defined mouse strains. Our studies were both in vivo as well as in vitro and attempted to develop a suitable organ culture method without serum or other exogenous factors as supplements. This approach resulted in a permissive in vitro environment within which mouse cap stage tooth organs (ie, 17 days of gestation from Theiler stage 24 fetuses) developed into discrete tooth organs and expressed morphogenesis (molariform) and produced both dentine as well as enamel extracellular matrices in serumless and chemically defined medium [Yamada et al, 1980; Slavkin et al, 1982].

During early postnatal development, mandibular first molar tooth organs are actively engaged in secretory amelogenesis and the production of the enamel matrix. For example, approximately 90% of the total ameloblast protein synthesis in 2-day postnatal pups is enamel matrix proteins. This indicated that the mRNAs for enamel proteins were relatively abundant in this differentiated cell type and, therefore, might be readily obtained for the construction and subsequent identification of mouse enamel cDNA (complementary DNA) clones. Mandibular first molar tooth organs from Swiss-Webster strain mice from 2-day-postnatal aged pups were found to be ideal for the isolation of enamel poly (A)RNAs [Slavkin et al, 1982a]. Monospecific polyclonal antibodies directed against mouse amelogenin polypeptides were used to facilitate the identification of the enamel mRNAs using a cell-free translation system [Slavkin et al

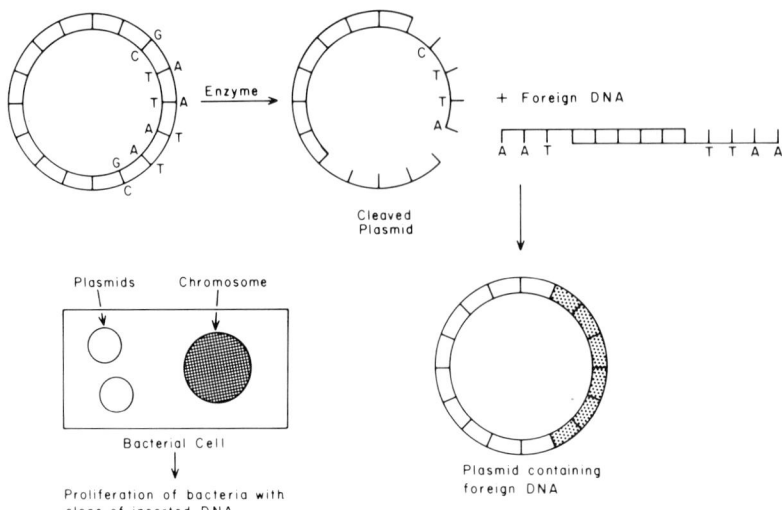

Fig. 4. Diagrammatic representation of the cloning of a gene to illustrate several features of a complex process. The insertion of fragments of eucaryotic DNA (eg, mouse amelogenin cDNA) into bacterial plasmids (ie, a small circle of DNA found in bacterial cells that are capable of autonomous self-replication), followed by cloning (bacterial cell multiplication), facilitates the growing of bacterial cell cultures of any size containing a unique foreign DNA sequence (eg, mouse amelogenin DNA sequence, human insulin, chick collagen type I cDNA sequences, etc).

1982a,b]. Using the isolated mRNA, we then constructed and identified a mouse amelogenin cDNA clone using the methods of recombinant DNA technology [Snead et al, 1983]. This authentic cDNA clone has been used to identify amelogenin DNA sequences in the genomic DNA from rodents (mouse, rat, hamster) as well as human genomic DNA.

DE NOVO ENAMEL GENE EXPRESSION DURING MOUSE MOLAR TOOTH FORMATION

In order to understand gene control during development, several cogent issues must be addressed. First, *when* and *where* are enamel genes expressed during development? Enamel gene expression can be assayed by methods sensitive enough to discriminate between specific mRNAs for enamel production, and other closely related but different mRNA transcripts. The precision of recombinant DNA technology enables such discrimination using a Northern analysis of cytoplasmic RNAs as detected by a specific cDNA probe for enamel gene products. Recently, we were able to define *when* amelogenin gene expression can first be detected during in vivo mouse molar tooth development using these techniques [Snead et al, 1984]. Cytoplasmic amelogenin mRNAs and polypeptides were first detected at birth. Both transcription and translation of enamel gene products appeared to be tightly coupled, in that both were first detected at the same time during molar tooth development. Neither mRNAs or polypeptides for amelogenin gene products were detected during embryonic or fetal stages of mouse development.

Studies are now in progress to determine *where* regional mesenchyme specification for ameloblast cell-specific gene expression takes place in terms of positional information. In situ hybridization using the cloned cDNA probe for mouse amelogenin should be useful to localize the spatial relationships during instructive mesenchyme-directed epithelial differentiation into ameloblasts as assayed by de novo gene expression in histological sections of normal developing tooth organs, as well as in heterotypic tissue recombinations.

Finally, *how* regional specification controls de novo enamel gene expression remains as yet unknown. Cap stage dental papilla mesenchyme is inductive when combined with non-dental epithelial tissues [see review by Kollar, 1983]. It would seem that the next generation of problems in craniofacial developmental biology will benefit from the identification of DNA sequences and non-DNA molecules involved in gene regulation. I further suggest that putative "inductive" signals can be evaluated using defined in vitro environments coupled with stringent conditions for molecular analyses of expressed gene products. In addition, methods to insert interesting structural or regulatory genes into unorthodox eucaryotic cell types may further provide valuable opportunities for research into *how* epigenetic signals invoke the activation and expression of genes during craniofacial development.

PROSPECTUS

It is evident that we are living within a "biological revolution" in which rapid advances are being made toward an understanding of vertebrate development. Useful animal model systems, in vivo and in vitro approaches, production of polyclonal and monoclonal antibodies directed against precise protein structural domains, construction of complementary DNA probes with which to detect genes as well as unique messenger RNAs, exquisite techniques to label and identify specific cell types such as cranial neural crest cells, animal and human genomic libraries, transposable genetic elements, epigenetic signals which mediate cell differentiation, and many other approaches continue to progress at a seemingly exponential rate. A question, for example, is no longer "how" to clone a structural gene, but rather "what" problem in development can best be approached using highly specific cloned sequences of DNA.

The core problem in craniofacial development remains regional specification. How do specific genes become activated and expressed at specific times and in specific positions within the developing individual? Pattern formation remains the intriguing issue. What mechanisms regulate cell-specific and time-specific gene expression during development? This problem must not be confused with cell differentiation—the biosynthesis of a specific collection of gene products and related subcellular and cellular events that clearly enable one cell type to be distinguished from another cell type (eg, keratinocyte versus an erythrocyte). Cell differentiation and the subsequent maintenance of the differentiated cellular state is the result of regional specification and not the cause. To understand the process of craniofacial development during normal as well as abnormal morphogenesis it becomes seemingly prudent to know exactly what, when, and how mediators influence differential gene expression. The challenges and opportunities are immense. Sam would have liked that!

ACKNOWLEDGMENTS

This paper is dedicated to the memory of Professor Samuel Pruzansky. Sam was a remarkable individual who saw beyond the obvious and worked toward the original conceptualization of the hybrid field of craniofacial biology. He was a model for interdisciplinary research, and an inspiration for clinical as well as fundamental scientific research directed toward understanding and helping "experiments of nature."

REFERENCES

Alberts B, Bray D, Lewis J, Raff M, Roberts K, Watson JD: "Molecular Biology of the Cell." New York: Garland Publishing, Inc, 1983.

Crick F: DNA today. Perspect Biol Med 25(4):512–517, 1982.

Dahl HH, Flavell RA, Grosveld FG: The use of genomic libraries for the isolation and study of eucaryotic genes. In: Williamson R (ed): "Genetic Engineering," Vol II. New York: Academic Press, 1981, pp 50–129.

Dhouailly D, Sengel P: Feather forming properties of the foot integument in avian embryos. In: Sawyer RH, Fallon JF (eds): "Epithelial Mesenchymal Interactions in Development." New York: Praeger Publishers, 1983, pp 147–162.

Johnson IS: Human insulin from recombinant DNA technology. Science 219:632–636, 1983.

Judson HF: "The Eighth Day of Creation." New York: Simon and Schuster, 1979.

Kollar EJ: Epithelial-mesenchymal interactions in the mammalian integument: tooth development as a model for instructive induction. In: Sawyer RH, Fallon JF (eds): "Epithelial-Mesenchymal Interactions in Development." New York: Praeger Publishers, 1983, pp 27–50.

Kollar EJ, Fisher C: Tooth induction in chick epithelium: Expression of quiescent genes for enamel synthesis. Science 207:993–995, 1980.

Pruzansky S (ed): "Congenital Anomalies of the Face and Associated Structures." Springfield, IL: Charles C. Thomas, Publisher, 1961.

Slavkin HC, Zeichner-David M, MacDougall M, Bessem C, Bringas P, Honig LS, Lussky J, Vides J: Enamel gene products during murine amelogenesis *in vivo* and *in vitro*. J Dent Res 61:1467–1471, 1982a.

Slavkin HC, Zeichner-David M, MacDougall M, Bringas P, Bessem C, Honig LS: Antibodies to murine amelogenins: Localization of enamel proteins during tooth organ development *in vitro*. Differentiation 23:73–82, 1982b.

Slavkin HC, Honig L, Bringas P: Experimental 'dissection' of avian and murine tissue interactions using organculture in a serumless medium free from exogenous (non-defined factors). In: Dixon A, Sarnat B (eds): "In Factors and Mechanisms Influencing Bone Growth." New York: Alan R. Liss, Inc, 1982, pp 217–228.

Slavkin HC, Snead ML, Zeichner-David M, Bringas P Jr, Greenberg GL: Amelogenin gene expression during epithelial-mesenchymal interactions. In Trelstad RL (ed): "The Role of Extracellular Matrix In Development." New York: Alan R. Liss, Inc, 1984, pp 221–253.

Snead ML, Zeichner-David M, Chandra T, Robson KJH, Woo SLC, Slavkin HC: Construction and identification of mouse amelogenin cDNA clones. Proc Natl Acad Sci, USA 80:7254–7258, 1983.

Snead ML, Bringas P, Bessem C, Slavkin HC: De novo gene expression detected by amelogenin transcript analysis. Dev Biol 104:255–258, 1984.

Steinmetz M, Hood L: Genes of the major histocompatibility complex in mouse and man. Science 222:727–733, 1983.

Williams JG: The preparation and screening of a cDNA clone bank. In: Williamson R (ed): "Genetic Engineering," Vol. I. New York: Academic Press, 1981, pp 2–61.

Yamada M, Bringas P Jr, Grodin M, MacDougall M, Slavkin HC: Developmental comparisons of murine secretory amelogenesis *in vivo*, as xenografts on chick chorio-allantoic membrane, and *in vitro*. Calcif Tissue Int 31:161–171, 1980.

III. OROFACIAL CLEFTING

Timing Cleft Palate Closure—Age Should Not Be the Sole Determinant

Samuel Berkowitz
Cranio-Facial Anomalies Program, University of Miami School of Medicine, Miami, Florida

> Attainment of normal speech, facial and palatal development, and dental occlusion is possible without compromising one objective for another. Although speech development may benefit from early palatal closure, there are instances when cleft closure should be postponed to a later age to permit conservative palatal surgery. Increase in palatal size with the spontaneous narrowing of the cleft space can occur early, late, or not at all, and, in rare instances, the cleft may even widen. Nonphysiological surgery causes facial and palatal maldevelopment by extensive undermining and displacement of mucoperiosteum, fracture of bone, or destruction of blood supply. To avoid these consequences, timing of palatal closure should be related to the anatomical and functional assets in the individual and not determined by age alone. Serial studies of 36 unilateral (UCLP) and 29 bilateral (BCLP) cleft lip and palate cases with good speech demonstrated that conservative palatal surgery is conducive to good speech as well as palate and facial development. Speech appliances may be necessary as an interim device after 2 years of age.

Key words: cleft palate closure, speech, palate and facial development, age, size of cleft space, nonphysiological surgery

INTRODUCTION

Most speech pathologists advocate repair of the cleft palate before 1 year to avoid perverted patterns of speech that require prolonged and difficult reeducation at a later age. For example, Dorf and Curtin [1982] in a study of patients from the Center for Craniofacial Anomalies-University of Illinois Medical Center, convincingly showed that early palatal surgery results in superior speech development. They further stated that surgery to close the palatal cleft might best be performed between 6 and 9 months of age, the child's stage of phenomic development of articulation age. Some past surgical strategies also emphasized early palatal closure and velar lengthening, with the aims of resolving immediate problems with the cleft space and preventing future speech problems associated with hypernasality. In addition, velum lengthening was advocated in the newborn period often without evidence of incompetent function to avoid a possible second surgical procedure.

A review of cleft palate surgical history shows that a single mode of surgery for all cases resulted in severe palatal and midfacial deformities as well as poor speech development. Unfortunately, the same poor results still occur despite the timing of surgery and the skill and experience of the plastic surgeon. This is so because of the

---

Address reprint requests to Samuel Berkowitz, 6601 S.W. 80 Street, South Miami, FL 33143.

failure to define the criteria for timing of palatal surgery and the failure to agree on which surgical procedures interferred with normal growth and development of the structure involved. Poor results were understandable when there were no standardized methods for estimating success or recording the effects of surgery on speech and facial growth and development; these shortcomings no longer exist. Nonetheless, some present-day surgical reports still do not describe adequately the original deformity; thus the efficacy of the surgical effort cannot be evaluated.

After 24 years of data collection, Pruzansky [1973] listed some important findings from his cleft palate research. They are 1) the existence of a wide spectrum of variation within each cleft type; 2) the need to avoid lumping all clefts together when describing treatment results; 3) the age of surgery is not a primary variable in determining the effect on facial growth; and 4) quantitative and qualitative characteristics of the defect, general health of the patient, and genotype are determining factors.

CORRELATION AND CAUSATION

Speech studies of individuals or a small sample of subjects are often sufficient and sometimes essential to solutions of a particular problem being investigated; however, the fact that a correlation exists between two variables (speech proficiency and age) does not indicate or prove causation. While the *age of surgery* may be the sole variable studied, sensory function, genotype, the geometrics of the original deformity, the facial growth pattern and the surgical procedure performed are also factors. It is difficult, and perhaps impossible, to demonstrate the effectiveness of a treatment philosophy in a clinical setting, where many variables cannot be identified, controlled, or manipulated. Therefore conclusions drawn from such investigations should be considered with caution.

CUSTOMIZING TREATMENT PLANS ACCORDING TO THE SEVERITY OF THE CLEFT SPACE

The case for palatal closure within the first year is well presented by Dorf and Curtin [1982]. While speech pathologists are urging earlier palatoplasties, other factors, such as the differential diagnosis and the physical assets and deficits of each case, must also be considered. Long-term serial facial and palatal growth studies by Pruzansky and others show that ideal treatment objectives of good facial and palatal growth need not be compromised to attain excellent speech.

IMPORTANT SURGICAL LESSONS

In 1938 Kilner listed cleft palate treatment aims in order of importance as speech, chewing, and aesthetics. This order of priorities still seems to be preferred by many plastic surgeons. As a result, the surgical history of cleft palate repair is replete with varied attempts to close the cleft space as if it were "a hole," with little or no concern as to the surgical effect on palatal growth and form. Some clinicians criticized the poor results created by the nonphysiological surgical procedure that did too much too soon.

In the 1940s Brophy's forceful palatal compression technique grew out of the mistaken belief that in complete clefts of the lip and palate bringing the laterally dispersed segments into more normal anatomical alignment prior to palatal surgery would encourage normal development after surgery. The opposite occurred due to the destruction of maxillary growth centers by excessive traction forces and extensive mucoperiosteal undermining. The resulting palatal scar tissue led to severe midfacial and palatal deformities with poor occlusion and unintelligible speech. Reacting to these poor results, Slaughter and Brodie [1949] stressed that reduction in blood supply and constriction by scars would jeopardize palatal growth. In addition, they stated that unwarranted trauma to hard and soft tissue, fracturing of bone, and stripping of mucoperiosteum would cause permanent damage to growth sites that were active until 5 years of age. They did not criticize the timing of surgery, only the procedures being performed.

WHEN TO CLOSE THE PALATAL CLEFT

What to do and when to do it were questions that had no universally acceptable answers. While surgeons such as Veau [1931] believed that early closure of the cleft palate improved speech development, there were many who emphasized midfacial-palatal development and recommended that cleft palate closure be postponed until either the deciduous or the permanent dentition. Advocates of delayed palatal closure wanted to avoid secondary malformations to the palate and severe deformities of the maxilla caused by extensive mucoperiosteal undermining associated with exposed lateral areas of denuded bone. Similar malformations were created in animals by Kremenak et al. [1970].

LATE PALATAL CLOSURE AND PROSTHETIC OBTURATION

To avoid the consequences of early surgery, Hotz [1979] and others advocated an obturator in the interim until additional palatal growth occurred. They believed that speech results would not be jeopardized by postponing closure. Bzoch [1980], however, found that use of an obturator for several years prior to closing the cleft space was harmful to speech development due to inadequate seal. He found that early speech therapy corrected speech problems acquired before closure of the palatal cleft between 1 and 3 years of age.

Longacre [1970] closed the palatal cleft between 3 to 4 years of age. Dingman and O'Connor [1973] followed a surgical sequence of lip adhesion at 1 to 2 months, definitive lip closure at 9 to 12 months, soft palate repair between 15 to 18 months, use of an obturator at 2 years, and palatal closure with a vomer flap between 3 and 4 years. They reported good speech and normal palatal growth and development. Blockman [1975] found that after early mucoperiosteal flap closure palates looked excellent at 5 years of age, but showed serious growth arrest in the teens. He advocated a surgical sequence similar to Dingman, but did not use a prosthetic obturator as an interim device.

Schweckendick's primary goal [1979a,b] was to achieve full palatal growth without interference from surgery. He stressed the importance of a functional soft palate between 6 to 8 months of age. The palate was closed between 12 to 24 months

TABLE I. Complete Unilateral Cleft Lip and Palate, Cleft Lip on Right Side

Name	Case	Class I Neutrooclusion		Class II Distooclusion		Tooth in Cross-bite					
						Right palatal			Left palatal		
		Right	Left	Right	Left	C	D	E	C	D	E
A.A.	AE-70		X	X		X	X	X			
M.B.	SS-47	X	X			X					
M.B.	AC-64	X	X			X	X	X			
D.C.	PP-20	X	X								
M.D.	AM-17	X	X			X	X				
R.F.	AJ-07	X	X			X	X				
B.G.	ZZ-12	X			X						
S.G.	AL-58	X	X			X	X				
J.L.	AF-80	X	X			X	X				
S.R.	AC-12	X	X								
A.R.	AF-87		X	X		X	X	X			
T.S.	EE-15		X	X		X	X	X			
R.S.	SS-71	X	X			X					
J.Z.	AE-32	X	X			X					

All had conservative palatal cleft closure ranging between 8 months to 5 years of age. At 5 years of age 70% had good overall speech while 30% had some degree of articulation and hypernasality problems. Competency of velopharingeal closure does not appear to be related to the timing of hard palate closure or to the degree of distortion of the original deformity. Significantly, only 5 of 36 cases had a complete bucal cross-bite which was correctable by simple orthodontics. Cuspid cross-bite is the most frequent occurrence and is due to palatal rotation as well as to ectopic eruption. Distribution here and in Table II is according to cross-bite and anteroposterior dental relationship (Angle classification). C, cuspid; D, first deciduous molar; E, second deciduous molar.

of age, when the "growth of the palate was virtually completed." An obturator was utilized until the secondary palate was closed. He recognized that the speech results were fair with this method and were usually better following early palatal closure. Since the primary concern was with palatal and midfacial development, he was willing to accept a lesser speech result.

RESULTS OF CUSTOMIZING THE SURGICAL CLOSURE OF THE PALATAL CLEFT ACCORDING TO THE SEVERITY OF THE CLEFT DEFECT (TABLES I–III)

Our longitudinal facial growth studies of complete unilateral (UCLP) and bilateral (BCLP) cleft lip and palate children show excellent midfacial and palatal development following a regime of two-stage palatal closure. Millard [1980] generally unites the lip between 1 to 3 months and then simultaneously closes the soft and hard palates between 12 to 24 months of age. If the cleft space is wide, he prefers to wait until additional growth narrows the cleft dimension to avoid extensive mucoperiosteal undermining and wide denuded lateral areas.

In our series of 36 complete UCLP and 29 complete BCLP, neonatal orthopedics or obturators were never utilized, yet good speech developed. The surgical procedures chosen to close the cleft space varied according to its size and shape. Some clefts were so narrow at 12 months that the edges were brought together by simple mucosal approximation. In another instance a conservative von Langenbeck closure was performed following Kremenak's suggestion that the lateral incisions be made at least

TABLE II. Complete Unilateral Cleft Lip and Palate, Cleft Lip on Left Side[1]

Name	Case[2]	Class I neutroocclusion		Class II Distoocclusion		Tooth in Cross-bite					
						Right Palatal			Left Palatal		
		Right	Left	Right	Left	C	D	E	C	D	E
D.M.	JJ-75	X			X				X		
L.L.	AG-60	X	X						X		
C.M.	AC-33	X			X				X		
G.O.	AL-96			X	X				X	X	
A.S.	UU-96	X			X				X		
C.S.	MM-30	X			X				X		
D.V.	LL-27	X			X						
J.Z.	SS-50	X			X				X	X	
L.C.	AH-60	X			X				X		
D.W.	VV-70		X	X					X		
M.A.	CO-25	X			X				X		
C.C.	AF-38	X			X				X		
K.C.	ZZ-01	X			X				X	X	
E.D.	AF-04	X	X						X	X	
P.D.	AI-97	X	X						X	X	X
E.G.	TT-63	X	X						X		
M.G.	SS-11	X	X						X		
R.G.	KK-55			X	X				X		
B.G.	AH-66	X			X				X	X	
B.K.	RR-55	X			X				X	X	
V.E.	II-91	X			X				X		
J.K.	AF-64	X	X						X	X	

[1]For details, see footnote 1 to Table I.
[2]Total number of cases, 22; male, 17; female, 5.

5 mm palatal to the buccal teeth, leaving very little exposed bone. If a very wide cleft space was present, a vomer flap was utilized and joined to a conservatively undermined mucoperiosteal flap. Fortunately, we did not encounter the failure in transverse palatal development that was reported by Prydsø et al [1974]. In some cases only a simple vomer flap was utilized to avoid mucoperiosteal undermining. The dental occlusion in both cleft types was generally excellent, with most cases having only a cuspid crossbite. Cases are presented in Figures 1–4 to demonstrate various geometric changes that occur if palatal growth is allowed to proceed without interference. In those cases when Millard used an *Island Flap*, either as a primary or secondary velar lengthening procedure, there was extensive palatal and midfacial maldevelopment due to extensive mucoperiosteal undermining (Fig. 5). The Island Flap has been abandoned in cleft cases until the age of seven because of these adverse long-term effects.

DISCUSSION
Spontaneous Closure of Cleft Palate Clefts

Pruzansky [1953] analyzed cleft types and found great variation between different types and within a single type. Although clefts may be similarly classified, the palatal segments vary in size, shape, and relationship to each other and to the other contiguous skeletal parts. After the molding action of the laterally displaced palatal segments

TABLE III. Complete Bilateral Cleft Lip and Palate[1]

Name	Case	Class I neutroocclusion Right	Class I neutroocclusion Left	Class II Distoocclusion Right	Class II Distoocclusion Left	Right Palatal C	Right Palatal D	Right Palatal E	Left Palatal C	Left Palatal D	Left Palatal E
D.A.	MM-89			X	X	X			X	X	
P.A.	DD-96	X	X			X	X	X	X	X	X
R.B.	AB-45			X	X	X				X	X
D.B.	KK-92	X			X	X			X		
P.B.	EE-12			X	X						
S.B.	AJ-42			X	X	X					
L.B.	CC-44			X	X	X			X		
K.B.	AI-59	X	X			X	X	X			
A.F.	AB-93	X	X						X		
B.G.	AH-62	X		X					X	X	
R.G.	AJ-22			X	X					X	
C.H.	II-64			X	X	X					
D.K.	AI-31			X	X	X			X		
L.L.	OO-68			X	X						
M.L.	KK-56			X	X					X	
V.L.	AI-53		X	X		X			X	X	X
C.M.	AC-66	X	X			X			X		
D. Mc.	AD-80	X	X						X	X	X
W. Mc.	AD-81		X	X		X	X				
P.M.	KK-22			X	X	X					
B.P.	KK-78	X			X				X	X	
O.S.	VV-60		X	X		X			X		
R.S.	AN-62	X	X								
C.S.	AF-48	X	X			X	X	X	X		
E.S.	EE-34	X	X								
T.S.	AK-31	X	X			X			X		
J.W.	AF-27	X	X			X			X		
T.W.	II-92	X	X								
J.Z.	AR-47	X	X								

[1]In all cases the lip was closed in one procedure before 3 months of age. The hard palatal clefts were operated on between 1 to 5 years either using a von Langenbeck procedure with or without a vomer flap or a vomer flap alone. In most cases the anterior cleft space was completely reduced by 1 year of age due to premaxillary ventroflexion and appositional bone growth. The hard palatal cleft after 1 year varied greatly in size and shape. Analysis of the occlusion showed that five cases had one side in complete buccal cross-bite. A bilateral cross-bite existed in only one instance; six cases had no cross-bite. The remaining had only cuspid cross-bites. Distribution is according to cross-bite and anteroposterior dental relationship (Angle classification). Total number of cases, 29. C, cuspid; D, first deciduous molar; E, second deciduous molar.

in complete clefts of the lip and palate is completed, the remaining closure of the cleft space is due to the appositional bone growth at the medial border of the palatal segments (Fig. 6).

Burston [1958] and others stated that lateral activity in the midpalatal suture was greatly diminished by 18 months, and had essentially ceased by 2 years of age. Therefore, they recommend early palatal closure. They seemed to have discounted the importance of palatal size and cleft width in determining the proper time to close

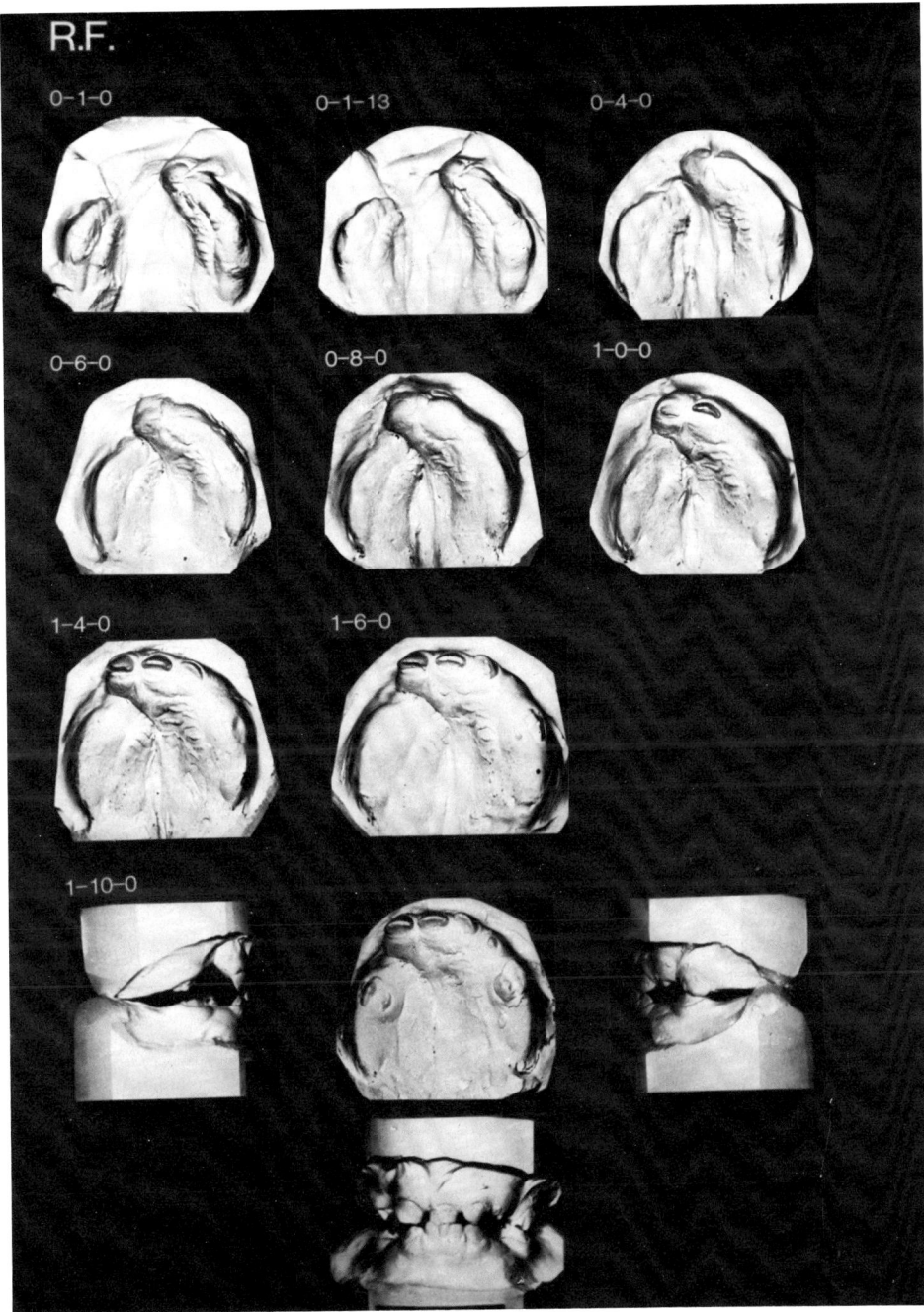

Fig. 1. Case R.F. AJ-7 late palatal closure, complete unilateral cleft lip and palate. The lip was repaired at 3 months and the soft palate by 9 months of age. The molding action brought the laterally displaced segments medially. The cleft space continued to narrow by appositional bone growth at the medial border of palatal segments. By 1 year of age, the cleft space was triangular in shape, 4 mm at its greatest width. This cleft continued to narrow and at 1 year 10 months it was less than 1 mm, at which time it was closed by simple mucosal approximation. The slight anterior cross-bite is due to palate tooth displacement rather than the existance of maxillary hypoplasia.

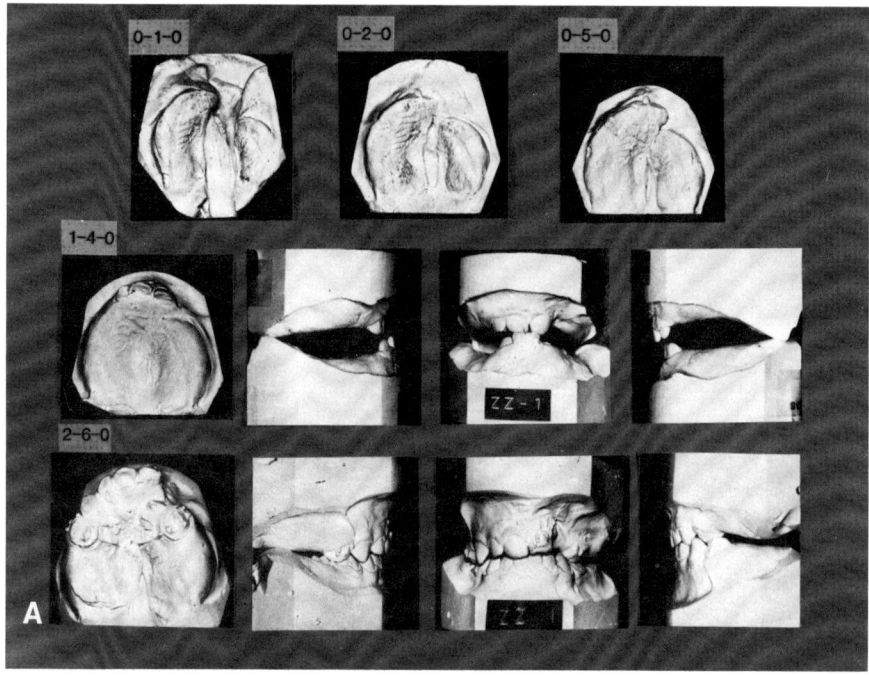
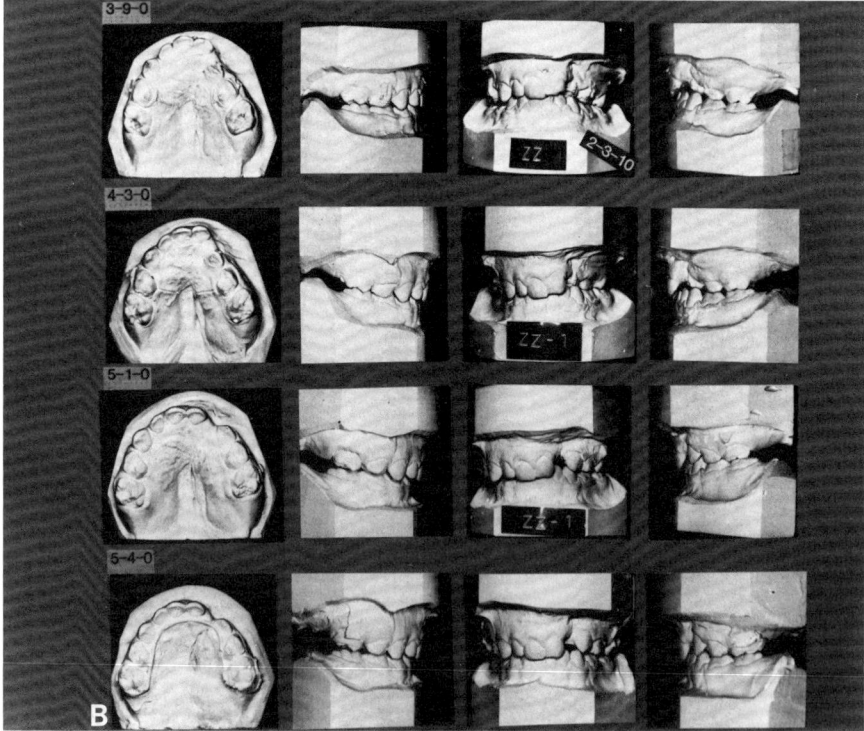

Fig. 2. A,B) Case K.C. ZZ-1. Early palatal cleft closure, complete unilateral cleft lip and palate. Two stage closure. The lip was closed by 18 days and the soft palate at 45 days. By 5 months a 2-mm cleft space remained which was surgically closed at 6 months by simple mucosal approximation. The cleft left segment rotated medially with the cuspid cross-bite occurring. Both the anterior and cuspid cross-bites were corrected by 5 years of age and a palatal holding arch was used to maintain the new arch form. The remaining small anterior palatal fistula did not cause a speech problem.

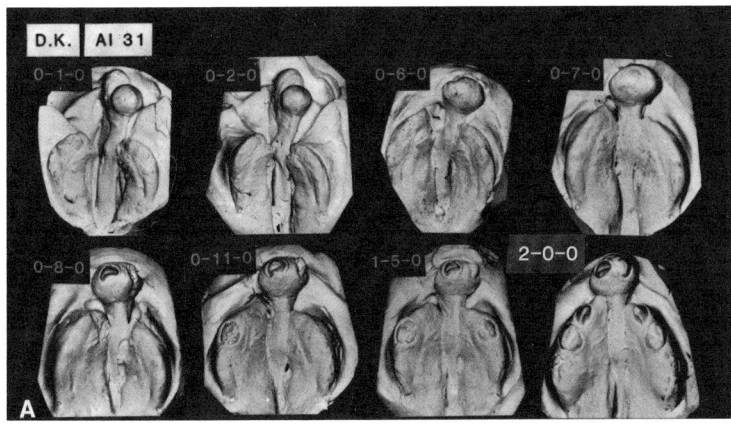

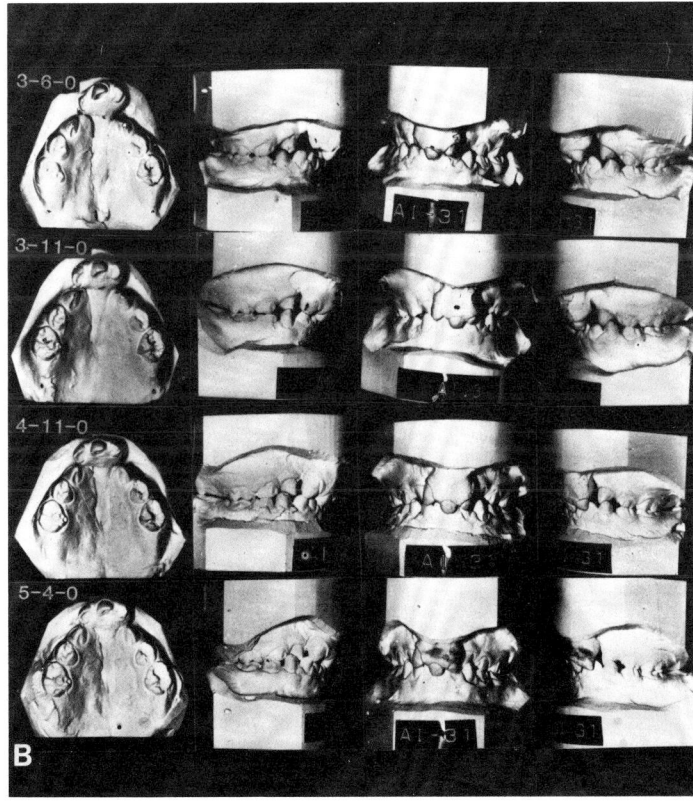

Fig. 3. A,B) Case D.K. AI-31. Complete bilateral cleft lip and palate, late palatal cleft closure. This case demonstrates that good arch development can occur without the need to use neonatal manipulation. The anterior and posterior palatal clefts narrowed first as a result of medial movement of the palatal segments and later by appositional bone growth to the 3 palatal segments. The posterior one half of the hard palatal cleft was closed with a von Langenbeck procedure. Only the cuspids are in cross-bite. Even though the anterior palate was still cleft, good speech developed. The inferior surface of the vomer appears to obturate the anterior cleft space thus limiting the amount of air escape.

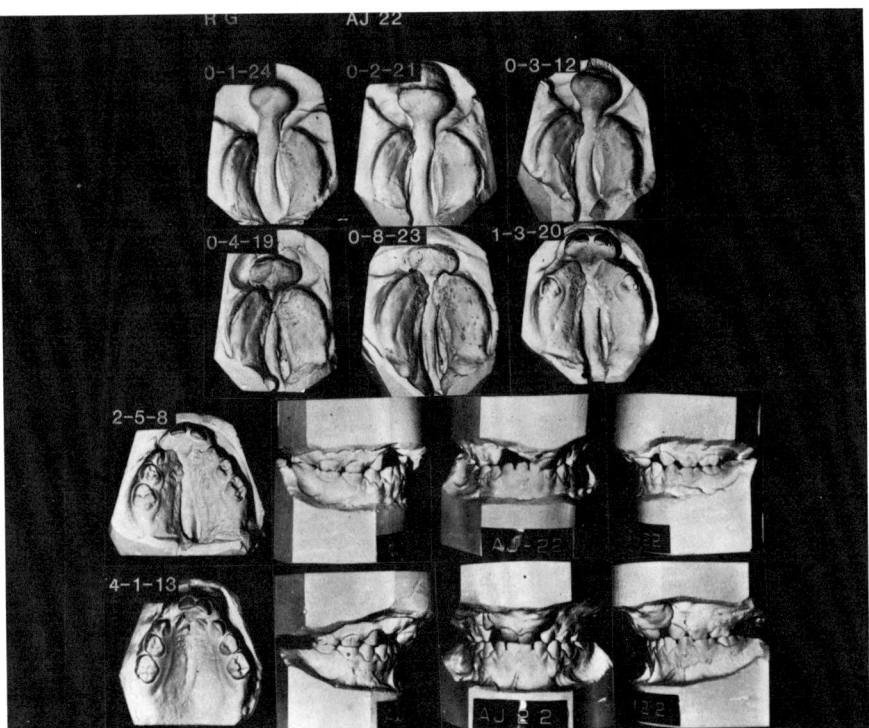

Fig. 4. Case R.G. AJ-22. Late palatal closure, complete bilateral cleft lip palate. The lip was united at 4 months. The cleft space was still wide open at 2 years 5 months. The cleft space was closed by a conservative von Langenbeck and vomer flap procedure at 2 years 7 months. Comments: Extensive lateral releasing incisions would have been necessary prior to 1 year 3 months due to the presence of a very wide cleft space. The buccal segments were in normal occlusal relationship at 5 years of age and there was no reason to believe that his occlusal relationship would change with further growth and development.

the cleft space. Maisels [1966], following the reasoning of Burston and others, concluded that there were no adverse effects on palatal growth by the tethering action to transverse palatal scar. Our growth records have shown their conclusion to be in error; the cleft space can continue to narrow up to 5 years of age, and scar tissue can cause palatal malformation.

Can the Cleft Space Be Stimulated to Close More Rapidly?

Berkowitz [1977] has contradicted the thesis of Burston [1958] and others that neonatal maxillary orthopedic appliance could stimulate midfacial growth and thereby hasten and increase the amount of growth at the border of the cleft space. Pruzansky [1953], Bishara [1973], Berkowitz [1977], and others have stated that spontaneous cleft space closure is part of the "catch up growth" phenomenon which characterizes most of the cleft palate population. They support the thesis that the developing palate cannot be stimulated to increase in size beyond its inherent growth potential but it can be retarded by nonphysiological surgery.

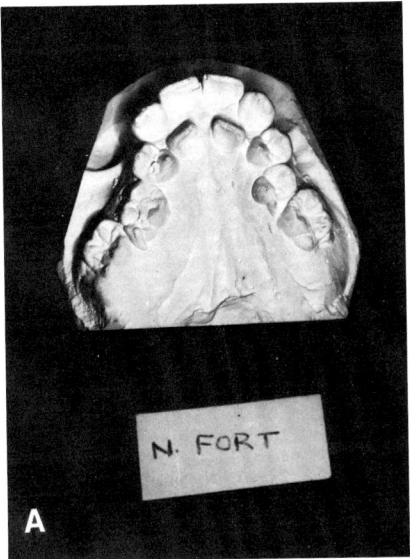 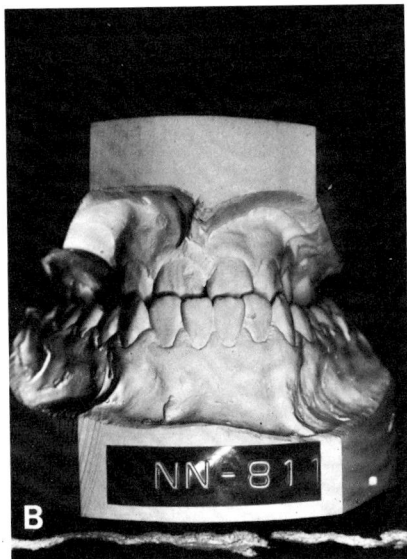

Fig. 5. A) Isolated cleft palate repaired with an early Island Flap procedure (severe mucoperiosteal undermining with wide releasing incisions). Palatal view of palate at 11 years of age showing the distoring effect of transpalatal scarring on arch form. The narrowed collapsed arch caused the lateral incisors to erupt palatally. B) The same case in occlusion showing anterior and bilateral cross-bite. This patient ultimately needed a LeFort I advancement procedure.

Isolated Cleft Palate—Normal or Deficient In Mass (Fig. 7)

There are rare instances where the cleft width does not diminish with time and remains wide open into adulthood. This may indicate localized osteogenic tissue deficiency rather than a hypoplastic maxilla. Kaplan [1981] was in error by stating that *isolated cleft palate* children exhibit midfacial hypoplasia related to an inherent limitation of growth, and that surgery has minimal effects on facial growth. Our serial growth records show the opposite to be true. Even when the cleft space width remains large, the midface can still grow and develop normally with conservative surgery. The relative retrussive position of point A, the anterior limit of the maxilla, signifies that the maxilla may be posteriorly positioned within the skull rather than be hypoplastic, as interpreted by Kaplan. Nonphysiological surgery in these cases, as well as in other cleft types, can adversely effect the anteroposterior development of the midface and cause severe malocclusion and speech impediment.

Speech and Neonatal Orthopedics

Over two decades ago McNeil introduced the concept of neonatal palatal manipulation. His chief supporters, Burston [1958], Graf [1979], Latham [Millard, 1980], and Rosenstein et al [1982], have claimed many benefits from this technique. Some have added that palatal obturation also improves speech production and reduces middle ear disease. No convincing data exist to support these claims [Berkowitz, 1977].

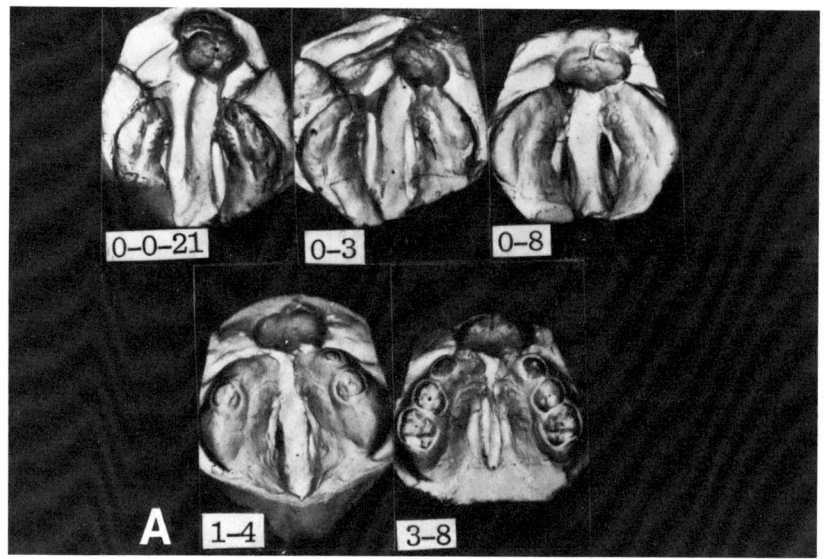

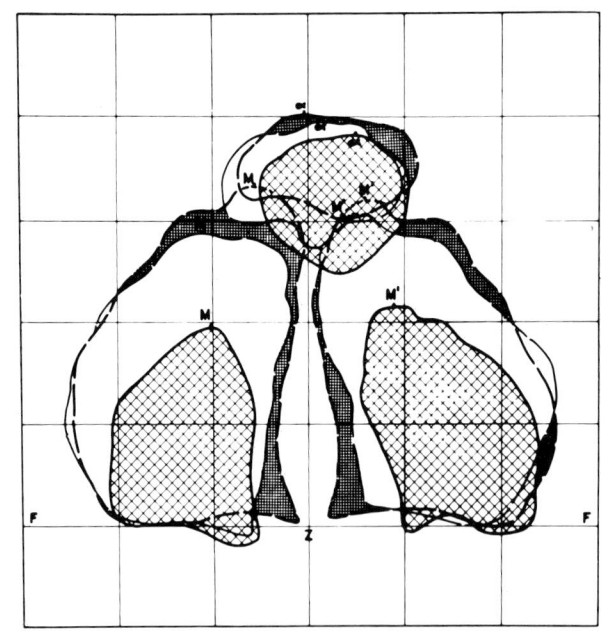

Antero-posterior growth changes of the midface showing the premaxilla and maxillay outlines of each age superimposed on base line F–F, and registered on point Z.

M = Most anterior part Maxilla by inspection
◂ = Most anterior part Premaxilla by inspection

0-0-21
1-5-0
3-8-4

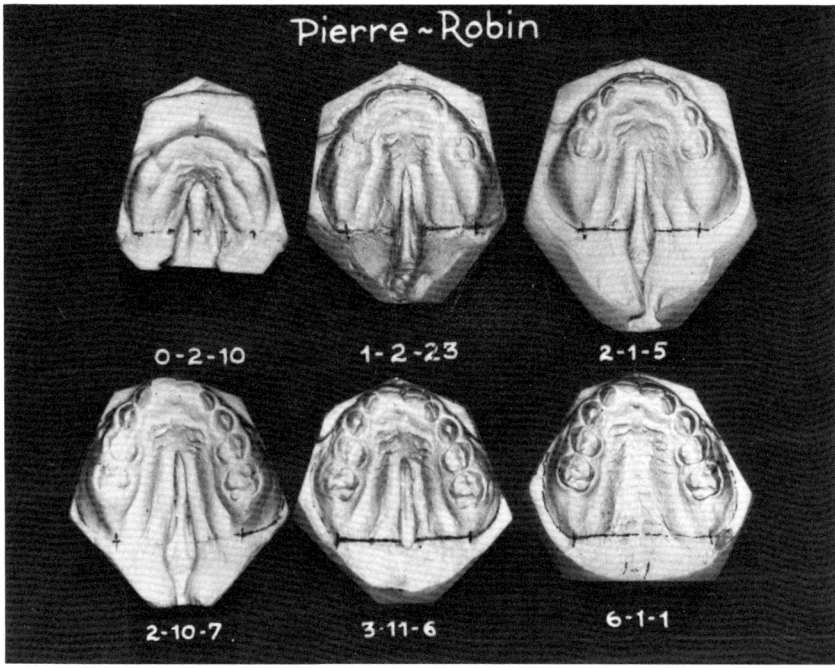

Fig. 7. Pierre Robin sequence. The cleft space length increases equally with the anteroposterior palatal growth. However, the growth at the border of the cleft appears to be more rapid than that seen elsewhere. This very *rapid* spontaneous cleft growth is generally not seen in other isolated cleft palate cases; however, similar reduction in cleft space width can be predicted in most cases.

Feeding

In addition to speech, there are other benefits to early closure of the palatal cleft space. Swallowing patterns can be altered by the absence of an anatomic and functional separation of the oral from the nasal cavity. Deglutition occurs without the assistance of the positive pressures available in an intact oral cavity and is dependent on positioning and gravity, especially during infant feeding. Although feeding is complicated by the inability to suck efficiently, we have found that children with open cleft palates do well when the parents are properly instructed. However, there is no justification for early palatal closure on the basis of feeding alone.

Fig. 6. A) Complete bilateral cleft lip and palate, two stage lip repair. The hard palate cleft was closed at 3 years 8 months of age. The anterior cleft space closure is brought on by ventroflexion of the premaxilla coupled with appositional bone growth of the lateral palatal segments. B) Superimposition of the outlines of three casts, ages 0-0-21, 1-5-0, and 3-8-4. All of the casts are superimposed on the base line which represents the posterior limits of the hard palate. Appositional bone growth is responsible for the closure of the cleft space after the premaxilla has been ventroflexed by the force of a reconstructed lip musculature. Note that the premaxilla has been restrained in its forward growth as the palatal process grew up to it. These growth phenomena are characteristic of most complete bilateral cleft lip and palate individuals.

Palatopharyngeal Action

Function is dependent on form. The muscle movements of the soft palate and pharynx must be integrated for normal speech. The soft palate must make contact with the posterior pharyngeal wall and must be coordianted with the lateral pharyngeal wall and posterior superior pharyngeal constrictor muscle movements. Therefore, the requirements for effective palatopharyngeal function are as follows: 1) intact palate with adequate length, 2) mobile soft palate, 3) appropriate movements of lateral and posterior pharyngeal muscles, and 4) integrated muscle actions. Nonphysiological surgery interferes with some or all of the above.

Indication, Timing, and Procedures in Palatal Surgery

Pruzansky's statement [Lis, et al, 1956] of thirty years ago is still true today: Surgical procedures on the palate must be related not only to the quantity and quality of tissue available at any given time but also to the possibility that more favorable circumstances in terms of structure and function may develop at a later stage in the child's development. Timing of all therapeutic procedures becomes an individual matter. Each child must be observed longitudinally so that prescription of treatment is based on a careful assessment of the assets and deficits and their pattern of changes with growth.

All surgeons need be concerned with the objectives of good anatomic closure, normal speech, and palatal and midfacial development. To achieve these goals they must avoid injury to growing structures. The mere closure of the cleft space is not sufficient to assure functional success in all cases. Pruzansky's explanation for variable results of identical procedures in the hands of the same surgeon was the considerable variation in the severity of the deformity within the same cleft type and in the facial growth pattern between individuals. Because of this, *timing of surgery for an individual is related to the anatomical and functional assets present in the patient and should not be determined by age alone.* Early palatal surgery does not jeopardize palatal and facial development provided conservative surgical methods are employed. Early repair of the cleft space facilitates development of normal speech. This is generally accepted even by those who choose speech appliances instead of early surgical closure. Advocates of an interim device claim that speech intelligibility is often good, sometimes without benefit of formal speech training. In the South Florida Cleft Palate Clinic speech appliances have not been used before palatal surgery. Speech results have been determined to be equal to those who have used similar treatment sequences. From our experience and that of others, we have concluded that speech appliances may be necessary as an interim device. When the deformity is so severe as to preclude surgery, the appliance needs to be modified with the growth of the palate.

CONCLUSION

Poor speech is the single most handicapping aspect of a cleft palate. It cannot be hidden and should be avoided. The thesis of this report favors consideration of the total emotional and physical health of the child with a cleft based on attainment of a cosmetically attractive face, dental function, and respiration, as well as speech. Many surgical, medical, and dental therapies may be necessary. As long as the surgeon *individualizes the treatment plan*, with care to do no harm to growing structures, *all goals are obtainable*.

REFERENCES

Berkowitz S: State of the art in cleft palate-Section III. Orofacial growth and dentistry. Cleft Palate J 14:288–301, 1977.
Berkowitz S, Pruzansky S: Stereophotogrammetry of serial casts of cleft palate. Angle Orthod 38:136–149, 1969.
Bishara SE: The influence of palatoplasty and cleft length on facial development. Cleft Palate J 10:390–398, 1973.
Blocksma R, Lenz CA, Mellerstig KE: A conservative program for managing cleft palates without the use of mucoperiosteal flaps. Plast Reconstr Surg 55:160, 1975.
Bzoch KR: In: Millard DR (ed): "Cleft Craft—The Evaluation of Its Surgery, III, Alveolar and Palatal Deformities." Boston: Little Brown Co., 1980.
Burston WR: Early orthodontic treatment of cleft palate conditions. Dental Pract 9:41, 1958.
Dingman RO, O'Conner JE: A conservative program of surgical management of the Cleft lip and cleft palate patient. Presented at The Second International Congress on Cleft Palate, Copenhagen, 1973, Abstract, p 262.
Dorf SD, Curtin JW: Early cleft palate repair and speech outcome. Plast Reconstr Surg 70:74–79, 1982.
Graf B: Early orthopaedic treatment. In: Kherer B, Slongo T, Graf B, et al (eds): "Long-Term Treatment in Cleft Lip and Palate With Coordinated Approach." Bern: Hans Huber, 1979, pp 208–211.
Hotz MM: 22 years of experience in cleft palate management and its consequences for treatment planning. In: Kherer B, Slongo T, Graf B, et al (eds): "Long-Term Treatment in Cleft Lip and Palate With Coordinated Approach." Bern: Hans Huber, 1979, pp 208–211.
Kaplan EN: Cleft palate repair at three months. Ann Plast Surg 7:179–190, 1981.
Kremenak CR, Huffman WC, and Olin WM: Maxillary growth inhibition by mucoperiosteal denudation of palatal shelf bone in non-cleft beagles. Cleft Palate J 7:817–825, 1970.
Lis EF, Pruzansky S, Koepp-Baker H, Kobes HR: Cleft lip and cleft palate—Perspectives in management. Pediatr Clin North Am 3:995–1028, 1956.
Longacre JJ: In: Millard DR (ed): "Cleft Craft—The Evaluation of Its Surgery, III, Aveolar and Palatal Deformities". Boston: Little Brown Co., 1970.
Maisels DO: The timing of various operations required for complete alveolar clefts and their influence on facial growth. B J Plast Surg 20:230–243, 1966.
Millard DR (ed): "Cleft-Craft—The Evaluation of Its Surgery, III, Aveolar and Palatal Deformities." Boston: Little Brown Co., 1980.
Pruzansky S: Description, classification, and analysis of unoperated clefts of the lip and palate. Am J Orthod 39:590, 1953.
Pruzansky S, Aduss H, Berkowitz S, Friede H, Ohyama K: Monitoring growth of the infant with cleft lip and palate. Trans Eur Orthod Soc 538–546, 1973.
Prydsø U, Holm P, Dahl E, Fogh-Andersen P: Bone formation in palatal clefts subsequent to palatovomer plasty. Scand J Plast Reconstr Surg 8:73—78, 1974.
Rosenstein SW, Monroe CW, Kernahan DA: The case for early bone grafting in cleft lip and palate. Plast Reconstr Surg 70:297–309, 1982.
Schweckendick W: Two stage closure of cleft palate. Rationale for its use. In: Kherer B, Slongo T, Graf B, et al (eds): "Long-Term Treatment in Cleft Lip and Palate with Coordinated Approach." Bern: Hans Huber,, 1979a, p 254.
Schweckendick W: Speech development after two stage closure of cleft palate. In: Kherer B, Slongo T, Graf B, et al (eds): "Long-Term Treatment in Cleft Lip and Palate With Coordinated Approach." Bern: Hans Huber, 1979b, p 307.
Slaughter WB, Brodie AG: Facial clefts and their surgical management in view of recent research. Plast Reconstr Surg 4:311–332, 1949.

Excess of Parental Non-Righthandedness in Children With Right-Sided Cleft Lip: A Preliminary Report

F.C. Fraser and A. Rex

Division of Community Medicine, Memorial University, St. John's, Newfoundland (F.C.F.), and Department of Medical Genetics, The Montreal Children's Hospital, Montreal, Quebec (A.R.), Canada

> Parents of children with right-sided cleft lip are more likely to be non-right-handed than parents of children with left-handed or bilateral cleft lip. The implications are discussed.

Key words: cleft lip, handedness, biological laterality, left-handedness, right-handedness

INTRODUCTION

There has been a recent surge of interest in the phenomenon of biological laterality in general and handedness in particular [Geschwind and Behan, 1982; Myslobodsky, 1983]. An increase in non-right-handedness has been reported in a wide range of individuals including those in either tail of the intelligence distribution [Gottfried and Bathurst, 1983], those with schizophrenia [Boklage, 1977], and those with autoimmune diseases [Geschwind and Behan, 1982]. Our interest in the subject was rekindled by a paper of Charles Boklage's [1981] demonstrating an increase in non-right-handedness in the parents of twins, either mono- or dizygotic. He suggested that the determination of sidedness requires a developmental program that, when it is destabilized, may result in a variety of deviations from normality ranging from situs inversus viscerum, through twinning, to non-right-handedness. The reader is referred to Boklage's papers for an elaboration of this hypothesis.

Since twinning is thought to be associated with neural tube defects [Layde and Edmonds, 1982]—at least by some authors [Elwood, 1980]—we wondered if there might also be an increase in non-right-handedness in the parents of children with neural tube defects. For many years, one author (F.C.F.) had been recording handedness routinely in family histories taken in the Department of Medical Genetics at The Montreal Children's Hospital. So had (with varying degrees of consistency) colleagues, residents, and graduate students at the hospital. Review of these records showed that parents of children with neural tube defects were, indeed, more often

---

Address reprint requests to Professor F.C. Fraser, Division of Community Medicine, Memorial University, Health Sciences Center, St. John's, Newfoundland, A1B 3V6 Canada.

© 1985 Alan R. Liss, Inc.

non-right-handed than parents of children with various Mendelian disorders [Fraser, 1983].

This raised the question of whether other malformations resulting from early developmental instability might show the same phenomenon. Cleft lip, with or without cleft palate (CL/[P]), seemed an obvious candidate [Fraser, 1984].

MATERIALS AND METHODS

Family histories of probands with CL(P) in the files of the Department of Medical Genetics at The Montreal Children's Hospital were reviewed. Cases in which the cleft was part of a known syndrome were omitted. The handedness of the parents was recorded as noted in the chart. Parents recorded as left-handed, ambidextrous, or left-handed originally but having been "switched" to right-handed, were classified as non-right-handed.

RESULTS

The results are presented in Table I. The proportion of non-right-handedness is much higher in the parents of children with right-sided clefts (16.4%) than in parents of left-sided (7.1%) or bilateral (9.0%) clefts. The difference is highly significant ($p<0.01$). The latter two groups do not differ significantly from each other, or from parents of children with pancreatic cystic fibrosis (7.8%) or Down syndrome (7.2%) [Fraser, 1984].

The frequency of non-right-handedness in probands shows no association with side of cleft (Table II). (Values for probands in our data are consistently high, perhaps because the trait is age-related).

TABLE I. Non-Right-Handedness (NRH) in Parents of Children With CL(P) According to Side of Cleft

Side of cleft	No. of parents	No. of NRH	NRH (%)
R	128	21	16.4
L	226	16	7.1
RL	100	9	9.0

TABLE II. Non-Right-Handedness (NRH) in Probands With CL(P) According to Side of Cleft

Side of cleft	No. of probands	No. of NRH	Percent non-right-handed		
			Present	Tisserand	Rintala
R	40	8	20.0	26.9	4.7
L	77	18	23.3	10.5	14.5
RL	31	7	22.5		12.6
Total	146	45	146	156	459

DISCUSSION

How are we to explain the curious fact that the frequency of non-right-handedness is higher in the parents of children with right-sided cleft lips (the right being the least often affected side) than in parents of children with left-sided or bilateral clefts?

The difference is so large that it is very unlikely to be a statistical fluke, but further data are being collected to test this possibility. A bias of sampling is also unlikely, since the data were collected without respect to any hypothesis related to parental handedness, and the comparison does not involve external controls.

Several hypotheses could account for this phenomenon. First, the reversal of laterality expressed as left-handedness may also affect the developing lip, so that left-handed children predisposed to cleft lip are more likely to have it on the right, rather than the left, side; left-handed children are also more likely to have left-handed parents.

Second, a genetic factor impairing developmental homeostasis may be expressed as a malformation (including cleft lip), or twinning, or non-right-handedness. The type of cleft lip would have to be free of whatever constraint it is that makes the usual type of cleft preferentially left-sided. This hypothesis would explain not only the excess of non-right-handedness in parents of children with cleft lip, but in parents of twins and of children with neural tube defects [Fraser, 1983] and other malformations arising early in development [Fraser, unpublished observations]. It would also (unlike the first hypothesis) be relevant to the increase in neural tube defects in the sibs of children with CL(P) or with various other malformations [Fraser et al, 1982].

Both hypotheses would imply an excess of non-right-handedness in the cleft-lip probands and this does not seem to be so in the present data; the frequency of non-right-handedness is the same for all types of cleft proband (Table II). It should be noted, however, that the frequency of non-right-handedness is highest in the parents of non-right-handed probands with right-sided clefts (5/16 = 31%), but the numbers involved are too small to be considered reliable.

Only two relevant observations have been found in the literature, and they conflict. More left-handedness was reported in a series of French patients with right-sided (26.9%) or bilateral (29.6%) than left-sided (10.6%) cleft lip [Tisserand, 1944]. (This was the study that originally inspired F.C.F. to begin recording handedness in family histories.) On the other hand, a recent Finnish study [Rintala, 1985] reports that patients with left-sided (14.6%) or bilateral clefts (12.6%) are more likely to be left-handed than are patients with right-sided clefts (4.7%). It is clear that the question requires further study.

REFERENCES

Boklage CE: Schizophrenia, brain symmetry development and twinning. Biol Psychol 12:19–35, 1977.

Boklage CE: On the distribution of non-right-handedness among twins and their families. Acta Genet Med Gemellol 30:167–187, 1981.

Boklage CE: Differences in protocols of craniofacial development to twinship and zygosity. J Craniofac Genet Dev Biol 4:151–169.

Elwood JM, Elwood JH: "Epidemiology of Anencephalus and Spina Bifida." New York: Oxford University Press, 1980.

Fraser FC: Association of neural tube defects and parental non-right-handedness. Am J Hum Genet 35:89A, 1983.

Fraser FC: Is non-right-handedness a sign of developmental instability. Proc Greenwood Genet Center 3:138, 1984.

Fraser FC: Czeizel A, Hanson C: Increased frequency of neural tube defects in sibs of children with other malformations. Lancet ii:144–145, 1982.

Geschwind N, Behan P: Left-handedness: Association with immune disease, migraine, and developmental learning disorder. Proc Natl Acad Sci USA 79:5097–5100, 1982.

Gottfried AW, Bathurst K: Hand preference across time is related to intelligence in young girls, not boys. Science 221:1074–1076, 1983.

Layde PM, Edmonds LD: Epidemiology of birth defects in twins. In Persaud TVN (ed): "Advances in the Study of Birth Defects." New York: Alan R Liss, Inc., Vol 5, 1982, pp 197–203.

Myslobodsky MS: "Hemisyndromes: Psychobiology, Neurobiology, Psychiatry." New York: Academic Press, 1983.

Rintala AE: The correlation between the side of the cleft and the left-right-handedness of the patient. Cleft Palate J (in press).

Tisserand Mlle: Dominance Latérale et bec de Lièvre. Arch Fr Pédiatr 2:166–167, 1944–45.

An Investigation to Relate the Overall Size of the Maxillary Arch and the Area of Palatal Mucosa in Cleft Lip and Palate Cases at Birth to the Overall Size of the Upper Dental Arch at Five Years of Age

Arnold G. Huddart and Angela M. Huddart
West Midlands Regional Plastic Unit, Wordsley Hospital, Wordsley, Near Stourbridge, West Midlands, England

> The area of palatal mucosa and the size of the maxillary arches were measured in a group of 30 newborn infants with unilateral clefts of the lip and palate. The overall size of the maxillary arch together with the arch width and arch height were also measured when the children had reached 5 years of age. For comparison purposes, a group of 30 newborn normal children and 30 normal 5-year-old children were similarly measured. The cleft children were found to have a mean deficiency of palatal mucosa of 16.41% at birth, although the overall size of their maxillary arches was 17.08% greater than normal. In the cleft cases there was no significant correlation between the area of palatal mucosa at birth and the overall size of the arch at 5 years of age. A significant correlation did exist between the overall size of the arch at birth and the overall size when the child was 5 years old. The significance of this and other findings is discussed.

Key words: palatal mucosa, maxillary arch size, unilateral cleft lip and palate, birth, 5 years

INTRODUCTION

As a preliminary to assessing the effect of a particular method of treatment on the development of the occlusion in cleft lip and palate cases, it is necessary to identify any other factors that might influence the eventual size and shape of the maxillary dental arch. It has been shown that in cleft subjects, there is an outward displacement of the maxillary segments and a deficiency of palatal mucosa at birth [Huddart et al, 1969; Huddart, 1970, 1979]. Either or both of these factors could be of importance in relation to the development of a maxillary arch of adequate shape and size and the creation of a functionally efficient occlusion. The present investigation, therefore, was designed to measure the area of palatal mucosa and the overall size of the maxillary arch in a group of newborn cleft palate infants in order to relate these factors to the size and dimensions of the maxillary arch when the children had reached 5 years of age.

Address reprint requests to Arnold G. Huddart, Dental Department, The Corbett Hospital, Stourbridge, West Midlands, DY8 4JB England.

© 1985 Alan R. Liss, Inc.

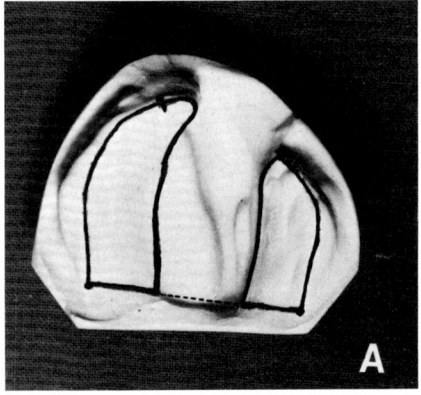 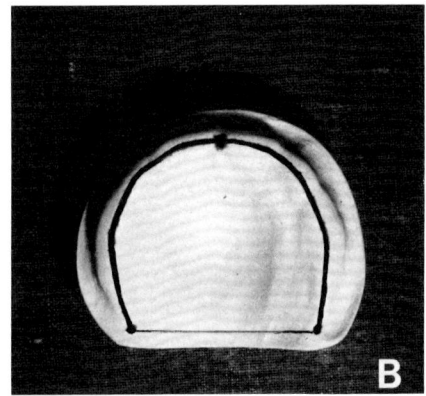

Fig. 1. A. Model of the maxillary arch of a newborn cleft palate infant showing the outline of the palatal mucosa to be measured. On each segment, the line starts at postgingivale and runs along the crest of the alveolar ridge to the alveolar cleft; it then runs along the margins of the alveolar and palatal clefts to a line joining postgingivale on the lesser segment and postgingivale on the greater segment; the outline then proceeds back along this line to postgingivale on the same segment. B. Model of the maxillary arch of a newborn normal infant showing the outline of the palatal mucosa to be measured. The line extends from postgingivale on the left side along the crest of the alveolar ridge to postgingivale on the right and then straight across the back of the palate to postgingivale on the left again.

MATERIALS

Materials consisted of plaster models of the maxillary arches of—

1) Thirty newborn infants (aged 0–14 days) with complete unilateral clefts of the lip, alveolus, and palate seen at the West Midlands Regional Plastic Unit.

2) The same 30 children at 5 years of age (4 years 9 months–5 years 3 months). All these children had complete deciduous dentitions with the occasional exception of the lateral incisor on the margin of the cleft.

The lips and palates had all been repaired by one or other of two plastic surgeons and following surgical closure of the clefts, no treatment of any kind had been carried out prior to the taking of the models at 5 years of age.

3) Thirty newborn normal infants (aged 0–14 days) with intact palates.

4) Thirty normal children at 5 years of age with intact palates and complete deciduous dentitions.

METHODS

This involved measuring the maxillary models at (1) birth and (2) 5 years of age.

Birth

Area of palatal mucosa. The outline of the area of palatal mucosa to be measured was marked in pencil on the models as shown in Figure 1A for the cleft subjects and Figure 1B for the normal infants. The posterior limit of the area was bounded by a line joining postgingivale on each side. All the models were marked by the same person (A.G.H.), and the area of palatal mucosa was measured by the

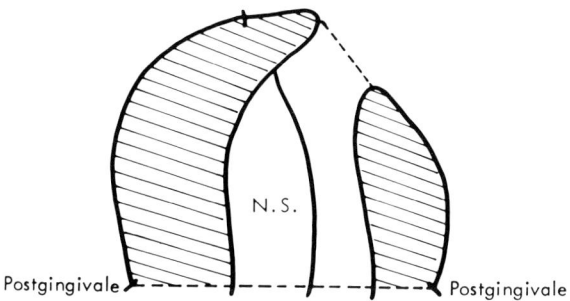

Fig. 2. Measurements at birth: Diagrammatic representation of a photocopy of the maxillary arch of a cleft lip and palate subject. The location of the outline is described in the legend to Figure 1A. The posterior border is formed by a line joining postgingivale on each side. The overall arch size (two dimensions) is the area enclosed by the peripheral outline. The area of palatal mucosa (shaded) involves three dimensions because of the slope of the palatal shelves. N.S. = nasal septum.

vacuum adaptation technique [Huddart et al, 1978]. For comparison purposes, 30 newborn normal children whose palatal surface areas had been measured in an earlier study [Huddart et al, 1978; Huddart, 1979] were included in the investigation. This data had also been obtained by the vacuum adaptation method.

Overall arch size. Unlike measurement of palatal mucosa, which has a three-dimensional connotation owing to the sloping sides of the palate, measurement of the overall size of the arch is a purely two-dimensional concept. Models of the newborn infants with their palatal outlines marked as in Figure 1A for the cleft cases and Figure 1B for the normals were photocopied under standardised conditions to give an exact one-to-one reproduction [Huddart, 1967, 1979]. On each photocopy, the posterior limit of the area to be measured was formed by a line joining postgingivale on each side, whilst in the cleft subjects, the alveolar defect was bridged at its narrowest point by a line joining the mesial and distal margins (Fig. 2). The overall area (the area enclosed by the outline) was then measured using a planimeter. In the normal subjects, this data had already been obtained as part of an earlier study [Huddart, 1979].

Five Years of Age

In both the cleft and normal children, the palatal gingival margins of the teeth were outlined in pencil on the models and the following points marked (Fig. 3):

i) The tip of the cusp of the deciduous canine on each side

ii) The centre of the distal marginal ridge of the second deciduous molar on each side

iii) The crest of the alveolar ridge midway between the deciduous central incisors. The models were then photocopied as described previously and the following measurements carried out:

Overall arch size (Fig. 4A). The posterior limit of the area to be measured was formed by a line joining the distal margins of the upper second deciduous molars. The enclosed area was then measured using a planimeter.

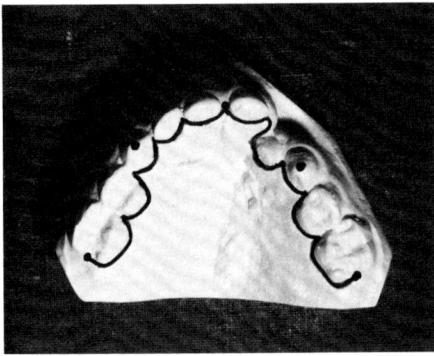

Fig. 3. Model of the maxillary arch of a unilateral cleft palate subject aged 5 years. The palatal gingival margin has been marked, together with the tip of the cusp of the deciduous canines, the midpoint of the distal marginal ridge of the second deciduous molars, and the crest of the alveolar ridge between the central incisors to facilitate their location after the model has been photocopied (see Fig. 4A, B).

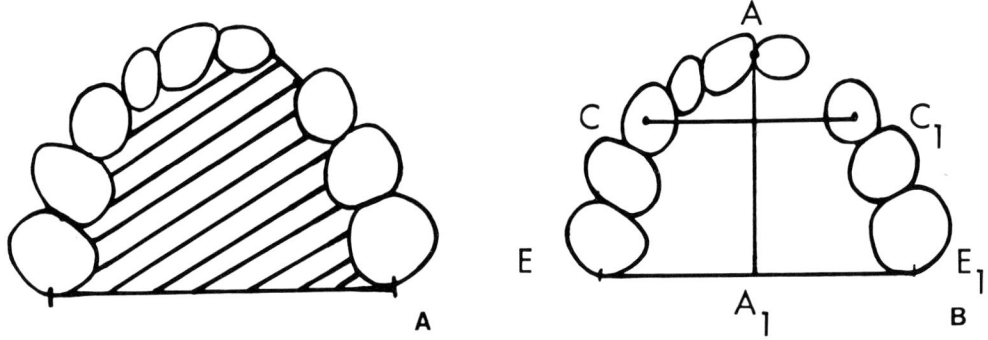

Fig. 4. Five-year measurements: Diagrammatic representation of a photocopy of the maxillary arch of a unilateral cleft lip and palate case at 5 years of age. A. Overall arch size (two dimensions): The area to be measured is shaded and bounded posteriorly by a line joining the distal surface of the second deciduous molars. B. Linear arch measurements: $C-C_1$ = intercanine width; $E-E_1$ = intermolar width; $A-A_1$ = arch height. (See legend to Figure 3 and the text for definitions of the landmark points.)

Linear arch dimensions (Fig. 4B).

i) Intercanine width—the distance between the tips of the cusps of the deciduous canines ($C-C_1$)

ii) Intermolar width—the distance between the centres of the distal marginal ridges of the second deciduous molar ($E-E_1$).

iii) Arch height—the length of the line from midway between the central incisors to where it meets a line joining the posterior margins of the second deciduous molars at 90° ($A-A_1$)

All the measurement data was statistically analysed by the Department of Statistics, West Midlands Regional Health Authority.

TABLE I. Birth Measurements (mm^2)

	Clefts (SD) (mm^2)	Normals (SD) (mm^2)	Difference (mm^2)	Significance	Cleft as % of normal
Overall arch size	747.00 ± 79.83	638.05 ± 45.80	108.95	P < 0.001 t = 6.86	117.08
Area of palatal mucosa	624.50 ± 71.80	747.10 ± 55.57	−122.60	P < 0.001 t = 7.96	83.59

TABLE II. 5 Year Measurements

	Clefts (SD) (mm^2)	Normals (SD) (mm^2)	Difference (mm^2)	Significance	Cleft as % of normal
Overall arch size	546.33 ± 63.81	631.00 ± 55.61	−84.67	P < 0.001 t = 5.90	86.58
Intercanine width (C-C$_1$)	25.36 ± 2.83	29.22 ± 1.97	−3.86	P < 0.001 t = 6.43	86.79
Intermolar width (E-E$_1$)	40.24 ± 3.35	41.22 ± 2.34	−0.98	Not significant t = 1.38	97.62
Arch height (A-A$_1$)	24.60 ± 2.30	26.98 ± 1.29	−2.38	P < 0.001 t = 5.17	91.12

RESULTS

Birth Measurements

The mean values and standard deviations for the cleft and normal infants at birth with respect to overall arch size and the area of palatal mucosa are given in Table I. This also gives the differences between the two groups and their significance. The cleft values are also expressed as a percentage of the normal values.

Five Year Measurements

Table II gives the mean values and standard deviations for the cleft and normal children at 5 years of age with respect to overall arch size, intercanine width, intermolar width, and arch height. It also gives the differences between the two groups and their significance. The cleft values are also expressed as a percentage of the normal values.

DISCUSSION

The results confirmed earlier investigations [Huddart et al, 1969; Huddart, 1979] that a significant deficiency of palatal mucosa exists in unilateral cleft cases at birth (P < 0.001, Table I). The mean deficiency of tissue was equivalent to 16.41% of the surface area of a normal palate. Nevertheless, the cleft infants had an overall arch size on average 108.95 mm^2 (SD ± 79.83 mm^2) or 17.08% greater than the normal newborn babies (P < 0.001, Table I).

Some correlation (r = 0.52, P < 0.01) was found to exist between the overall size of the arch and the area of palatal mucosa. The larger the arch at birth, the greater the area of palatal mucosa even though the mucosal area in the clefts was always less than in the normals. By 5 years of age, the situation had become reversed. The maxillary arches of the cleft children had now become significantly smaller than in the normal chldren, the mean overall arch size in the clefts being 84.67 mm^2 less ($P < 0.001$, Table II).

From being approximately 17% larger at birth, the clefts were now just over 13% smaller (Table II). This was important because overall arch size, as measured by the amount of space within the dental arch, has a bearing on how much room is available for the tongue to function. It is also one of the factors that influences the functional efficiency of the occlusion as well as the total length of the dental arch and hence the degree of crowding which may exist.

Somewhat surprisingly, no correlation was found to exist between the area of palatal mucosa at birth in the cleft children and the overall size of the maxillary arch at 5 years of age. There was however, a correlation between the overall size of the maxillary arch at birth and its overall size at the age of 5 ($r = 0.41$, $P < 0.05$). The bigger the arch at birth, the bigger it was likely to be at 5 years of age.

Measuring the arch width and the arch height showed that in the cleft subjects, although the arches were wider than normal at birth, particularly across the back of the mouth [Huddart et al, 1969; Huddart, 1979], by 5 years of age when the lip and palate had been repaired, these measurements had become much reduced.

Whilst in the 5-year-old children the posterior arch width (E-E$_1$, Table II) was almost normal, the intercanine width (C-C$_1$, Table II) was significantly ($P < 0.001$) less, being in fact only 86.79% of the width in a normal child. The investigation also revealed a significant correlation between the intercanine width and the overall arch size at 5 years of age ($r = 0.70$, $P < 0.001$). There was, however, no significant correlation between molar width and the overall arch size. This suggests it is the factors affecting the intercanine width at the 5-year level that are important in relation to the overall size of the arch at that age and that these factors in turn could effect tongue function and occlusal efficiency. The findings support the view that lip and palate repair creates a new balance of muscle forces that imposes a constricting influence on the maxillary arch.

This is particularly noticeable anteriorly and suggests that repair of the lip is perhaps a more important operation than palate repair so far as the production of a good arch form and dental occlusion is concerned. If the changes noted between birth and 5 years of age were due to an impairment of growth either because of the presence of the cleft or because the defect had been closed surgically, it would be expected that the maxillary arch deformity and the relationship between the upper and lower arches would become *progressively* worse. Clinical observation, however, suggests that at least up to 5 years of age this is not the case. The changes in the size and shape of the arch appear to occur quickly following lip and palate repair and then after a few weeks and months become stable again. From then on, the situation appears to remain reasonably constant in the majority of cases until the child is 5 years of age.

The investigation also showed that the amount of palatal mucosa present at birth is not as important as was previously thought so far as the development of a good maxillary arch at the 5-year level is concerned. In this connection, it is perhaps significant that all but one of the cleft cases had had presurgical maxillary orthopaedic treatment prior to lip repair, and because of this, some caution must be exercised in interpreting the findings of the investigation. It must also be mentioned that although presurgical treatment was originally thought to narrow the palatal cleft by stimulating growth of palatal mucosa, an earlier study [Huddart, 1979] has cast doubt on this assumption. Instead, presurgical treatment appears to work by reducing the lateral segmental displacement present at birth. In this way, the palatal cleft can be reduced by up to 50%, and the alveolar cleft sometimes completely eliminated prior to lip and palate repair. By reducing the displacement, however, presurgical treatment may in fact be predisposing to a *narrower* arch at 5 years of age than would otherwise be the case. This is the exact opposite to what was the original intention of such treatment.

It must be emphasised that no evidence exists at present to confirm or deny this speculation. If presurgical treatment does have this effect, however, it is likely to be only minimal, as otherwise the consequences would already have been observed and brought to the attention of workers in this field. Furthermore, any such effect must be set against the benefits of presurgical treatment such as the more normalised tongue tip function and improved speech found in these cases [Stuffins, 1979].

A great deal more needs to be known about the effects of treatment on the development of the maxillary arch and face generally in cleft cases, and it is important that surgeons should critically examine the results of any procedures carried out. To do this, more long-term studies of the type pioneered by Dr. Pruzansky at the Center for Craniofacial Anomalies in Chicago will have to be undertaken, and for logistical reasons, more inter-centre co-operation will be required if these are to be effective. Because of the length of time necessary to obtain an acceptable series of treated cases, such studies should ideally be commenced early in the career of an investigator whilst he is still relatively young; and they would also have to be of an ongoing nature. It is only by doing this that the management of cleft conditions can be put on a more rational basis and our dependence on an empirical approach reduced. Dr. Pruzansky, by his enterprise and foresight, showed how this should be done. It is up to those of us who follow to take up his work where it was left off and follow the path he charted.

ACKNOWLEDGMENTS

This investigation was carried out under the auspices of the Research Committee, West Midlands Regional Health Authority.

The authors wish to thank their colleagues at the West Midlands Regional Plastic Unit for their help and advice during this investigation.

We would also like to thank the Department of Statistics, West Midlands Regional Health Authority, for the statistical analysis of the results; Mr. S. Forster and his staff, Department of Photography, The Royal Hospital Wolverhampton, for the illustrations; and Mrs. K.M. Randle for the preparation of the manuscript.

REFERENCES

Huddart AG: An analysis of the maxillary changes following presurgical dental orthopaedic treatment in unilateral cleft lip and palate cases. Trans Eur Orthodont Soc 229–314, 1967.
Huddart AG, MacCauley FJ, Davis MEH: Maxillary arch dimensions in normal and unilateral cleft palate subjects. Cleft Palate J 6:471–487, 1969.
Huddart AG: Maxillary arch dimensions in bilateral cleft palate subjects. Cleft Palate J 7:137–155, 1970.
Huddart AG, Crabb J, Newton I: A rapid method of measuring the palatal surface area of cleft palate infants. Cleft Palate J 15:44–48, 1978.
Huddart AG: Presurgical changes in unilateral cleft palate subjects. Cleft Palate J 16:147–157, 1979.
Stuffins G: Speech and mental attitudes in the older presurgical child. In: Kehrer B et al, (eds): "Long Term Treatment in Cleft Lip and Palate With Co-ordinated Team Approach." Bern: Hans Huber, 1979, pp 199–205.

Velopharyngeal Inadequacy in the Absence of Overt Cleft Palate

Sally J. Peterson-Falzone
Center for Craniofacial Anomalies, University of Illinois College of Medicine, Chicago

Velopharyngeal inadequacy in the absence of overt cleft palate may be due to any one, or any combination, of the following: (a) intraorally visible stigmata associated with submucous defects (any combination of bifid uvula, muscular diastasis of the soft palate, bony defect of the hard palate); (b) "occult" anatomical defects of the levator palatini or musculus uvulae, detectable only by nasopharyngoscopy or by operative dissection; (c) anatomic disproportion between the size of the nasopharynx and the length of the hard and/or soft palate; (d) mechanical inteference with motion of the velopharyngeal system occurring as a result of scarring or contracture, and possibly as a result of interposition of the upper poles of the faucial tonsils between the velum and the posterior pharyngeal wall; (e) a wide variety of neuromotor deficits, either congenital or acquired, causing reduced and/or incoordinated movement of the velopharyngeal musculature; (f) a learning error of unknown origin which results in velopharyngeal inadequacy only on specific phonemes with all other pressure consonants emitted orally. Submucous defects of the secondary palate do not necessarily produce velopharyngeal inadequacy. Thus, our estimates of both the incidence of submucous defects and of the frequency of genes for clefting in any given population are undoubtedly low. Finally, "stress velopharyngeal inadequacy" in wind instrument players has been linked to a variety of anatomic findings and is not necessarily accompanied by velopharyngeal inadequacy in speech. This paper will review the historic aspects of velopharyngeal inadequacy and will discuss and analyze the causes outlined above.

Key words: velopharyngeal inadequacy, submucous cleft, structural, anatomic, neuromotor, stress VPI, phoneme-specific VPI

PREFACE

Velopharyngeal inadequacy in the absence of overt cleft palate was a topic which intrigued Samuel Pruzansky throughout the last half of his professional career. His approach to the analysis of such cases was not the one utilized in this paper, but the clinical data he amassed did provide the bulk of this author's experience with the problem. The following is an attempt to organize the rather unwieldy collection of disparate information available in the literature.

Address reprint requests to Dr. S. Peterson-Falzone, Center for Craniofacial Anomalies, University of Illinois College of Medicine, Box 6998, Chicago, IL 60680.

© 1985 Alan R. Liss, Inc.

INTRODUCTION

Velopharyngeal inadequacy[1] in the absence of overt cleft palate has been described in the medical literature for over 150 years. While much of this literature has focused on various forms of submucous palatal defects, there has also been a steady stream of reports of both (a) hypernasal or "cleft palate" speech in the absence of observable anatomical deformity, and (b) conversely, anatomical anomalies in individuals free of any speech defect. Historically, the former led to frequent applications of the label "functional" and even "hysterical" hypernasality. With the development of more sophisticated examination techniques, however, the mystery of hypernasal speech in the absence of immediately observable anatomical deformity has gradually been replaced by a growing body of knowledge regarding the many factors that, alone or in combination, can produce these clinical entities.

The attempt to categorize disorders of velopharyngeal function in the absence of overt cleft palate has absorbed a considerable amount of time and effort, with conflicting and unsatisfactory results [ie, Calnan, 1957b, 1959, 1961a, 1976; Minami et al, 1975; Pitt and Ingram, 1975a; Pruzansky et al, 1977; Randall et al, 1960]. The basic problem is that authors have attempted to derive mutually exclusive categories, failing to deal with the possibility of two or more factors operating in the same speaker. This problem shows in the classification systems offered by Calnan [1957b, 1959, 1961a, 1976] and by Pitt and Ingram [1975a]. The system offered by Randall et al [1960] was addressed solely to neurologic disorders of velopharyngeal function and was labeled "causes of levator paralysis," ignoring the possibility of any contribution to velopharyngeal closure by any other muscle. Minami et al [1975] did recognize that a wide range of conditions could lead to velopharyngeal inadequacy, but the documentation for some of their categories (ie, "mimicry") in the literature is poor if existent at all. In addition, this system, like that of Calnan [1957b, 1959, 1961a, 1976] shows some confusion regarding "congenital" versus "acquired" conditions. Pruzansky et al [1977] divided cases into two broad categories based only on the presence or absence of the intraorally detectable stigmata of bifid uvula, muscular dehiscence of the soft palate, and bony defect of the hard palate, with no attempt to deal either with anatomical abnormalities detectable only by specialized means of observation (ie, radiography, nasopharyngoscopy) or with combinations of anatomic and neurologic disorders. Cotton and Nuwayhid [1983] offered a somewhat simplified classification system for "velopharyngeal insufficiency," which did recognize the possibility of combinations of causal factors.

It is not surprising that older concepts and classification systems are gradually invalidated, at least in part, as newer examination techniques reveal previously unsuspected anatomical differences and/or neurologic deficits. In a similar vein, increasing sophistication in the analysis of speech output differentiates more contemporary reports from the older literature, the latter sometimes confusing "hyponasal" with "hypernasal" speech and rarely offering more than the broadest of descriptions or judgmental labels. Only in more recent literature has phoneme-specific velopharyn-

---

[1]In most of the literature, the terms "velopharyngeal inadequacy," "insufficiency," and "incompetency" are used synonymously. The author has chosen to follow the suggestion of Trost [1981b] that the term "insufficiency" be reserved for insufficiency of tissue, "incompetency" for deficiencies of movement, and "inadequacy" for cases of mixed or undiagnosed origin. The term "inadequacy" is also applied here as a generic or umbrella term, reserving the other two terms for more specific types.

geal inadequacy been delineated ([Trost, 1981a,b]; less complete descriptions were provided by Lawson et al, [1972] and by Peterson [1975]). In the latter, no true physiologic inadequacy is present and one again suspects that speakers exhibiting this phenomenon were historically among those who were assigned to the "functional" category, a label that is incomplete if not blatantly inaccurate.

This paper will focus first upon a variety of anatomic findings that have been described in speakers with velopharyngeal inadequacy and also in some speakers with no speech problem. This will lead to a discussion of the effect of tonsils and adenoids—and of their removal—on velopharyngeal function. We will then undertake a limited discussion of neurologic disorders affecting the velopharyngeal system. Finally, we will discuss phoneme-specific velopharyngeal inadequacy and velopharyngeal dysfunction reported in musicians playing wind instruments. Throughout, the reader is asked to be mindful of the fact that this is not an attempt to develop yet another system of categorizing these cases. Rather, the intent is to draw attention to the probable futility of such systems because nearly any combination of factors is possible, and information will be lost both to the patient and to the investigator when that fact is ignored.

ANATOMIC PATHOLOGY
Submucous Defects of the Secondary Palate

Introduction. In 1966, Winters set out to trace "the written history of congenital velo-pharyngeal incompetence." The confusion regarding this topic is perhaps nowhere better typified than by the fact that he entitled the article "Some Historical Remarks on Congenital Short Palate" and then devoted most of the text to submucous cleft palate. Winters searched the literature to find who was responsible for the first report of "nasal speech without evident cleft of the palate."[2] Most other writers had credited Roux, with considerable confusion between the two reports this French physician published in 1825 and 1835. Roux's case in 1825 was a submucous extension of an overt cleft, while that of 1835 was a palatal fistula. Calnan [1954] and others who followed cited that 1835 date as the first description of a submucous cleft, confusing either the date or the case description. Winters dismissed both of Roux's cases because of the palatal anomalies they did show, but then settled on a rather odd choice of his own if he was truly searching for a case without "evident cleft of the palate." He selected a case described in two successive reports [1862, 1865] by Passavant. The report of 1862 described a woman with ". . .a cleft lip and a spontaneously healed small cleft in the soft palate." The 1865 description of the same patient described the velum as closed and the hard palate as showing "a broad and deep submucous cleft", with the patient exhibiting "an open nasal speech." Winters [1966] mentioned ". . . the conviction of the surgeons of that era [mid-1800s] that late spontaneous closure of palatal clefts was a frequent occurrence, without or after incomplete or unsuccessful surgical intervention. . .[3]" but did not comment upon the accuracy of Passavant's case description of 1862. In 1865, Passavant also described a patient with a submucous cleft of the hard palate, a supposedly intact velum, a small

---

[2]Note how our concept of "evident cleft of the palate" has changed over the past 150 years.

[3]A conviction illustrated further in a case description by Trelat [1867, 1868].

bifid uvula and "a heavy open nasal speech." Because Winters was looking only for cases in which velopharyngeal inadequacy was in fact documented by nasality of speech, he discounted the autopsy findings of Demarquay [1846] in which the palatal muscles were reportedly absent in the midline and there was a defect in the midline of the posterior part of the hard palate. Demarquay was, it appears, the first to describe submucous defects of the hard *and* soft palate.

Lermoyez [1892] shared with his predecessors and contemporaries the convicton that a congenitally short palate occurred only in association with a submucous cleft of the hard palate and a bifid uvula, Gutzmann [1899] being a rare dissenter. Kelly's article of 1910 described both (a) congenital velopharyngeal inadequacy without demonstrable submucous cleft and (b) submucous cleft without velopharyngeal inadequacy, flying in the face of virtually all the case reports and opinions appearing in previous literature. Kelly was the first English author to attempt to clarify this diagnostic problem, earlier reports in the English literature having been sporadic case descriptions [ie, Berans, 1983; Coues, 1906; Foster, 1895; MacKenzie, 1890; Means, 1894; Metcalf, 1908; Ohmann-Dumesmil, 1897; Shufeldt, 1885; Somers, 1896; Stimson, 1909] similar to those in the French and German literature of the 1800s. Most of these reports are of abnormalities of the uvula alone.

The "classic" submucous cleft. Based only on the findings of direct intraoral visual inspection and digital palpation, with occasional data from lateral radiographic studies or intraoperative examination, a lengthy series of descriptions of submucous cleft palates appeared from the 1860s into the 1970s [Calnan, 1954, 1957b, 1976; Crikelair et al, 1970; Fara and Weatherly-White, 1977; Fara et al, 1971; Gylling and Soivio, 1965; Kaplan, 1975; Kelly, 1910; Lowry et al, 1973; Means, 1894; Passavant, 1862, 1865; Porterfield et al, 1976; Pruzansky et al, 1977; Rees-Wood-Smith et al, 1967; Stewart et al, 1971; Thaler and Smith, 1968; Trelat, 1867, 1868, 1870a,b; Weatherley-White et al, 1972; Weatherley-White, 1976].[4] Investigators typically have described varying combinations of the three intraorally visible stigmata of bifid uvula, muscular diastasis of the soft palate, and bony defects of the hard palate. Understandably, clinical descriptions have varied in completeness depending upon the examination techniques. A more thorough examination of some of those patients described in the 1800s as exhibiting bifid uvulae, for example, might have revealed muscular deficiency extending into the velum itself. The more current literature reflects yet another problem, namely, a lack of agreement on just what features must be present in order for the label "submucous cleft" to be applied. For example, Weatherley-White et al [1972] insisted on the presence of all three of the classical stigmata and ignored or discarded cases showing only one or two of the defects in an investigation of the incidence of submucous clefts among school children. Most investigators, by contrast, consider each of the three intraorally visible stigmata to constitute an anatomical abnormality of the secondary palate,[5] and devote attention to the variable

---

[4]Combinations of overt and submucous defects are seen, the submucous defect continuing forward from the anterior margins of the overt defect [Crikelair and Cosman, 1977; Crikelair et al, 1970; Demarquay, 1846; Roux, 1825; Veau, 1931]. In addition, a submucous cleft of the secondary palate may appear in combination with an overt cleft of the primary palate [Calnan, 1954; Kono et al, 1981; Massengill and Fetterolf, 1968].

[5]Shapiro et al [1971], however, considered bifid uvula to "fall in the borderland between malformation and normal development."

concordance among them. Submucous defects of the hard palate or hard and soft palate with a clinically intact uvula have been reported [Calnan, 1954; Fara et al, 1971; Shprintzen et al, 1983]. Calnan's schematic diagrams of 12 cases [1954] illustrated the variability of findings in the uvula, soft palate, and hard palate, as did the report of Pruzansky et al [1977].

The point cannot be made too often that some speakers with one or more of the visible stigmata of bifid uvula, muscular diastasis of the soft palate, and bony defect of the hard palate do *not* demonstrate velopharyngeal inadequacy [Beeden, 1972; Blakeley, 1965; Calnan, 1954, 1976; Kaplan, 1975; Kelly, 1910; Lowry et al, 1973; Massengill et al, 1973; Porterfield et al, 1976; Saad, 1975; Shprintzen et al, 1983; Starr et al, 1971; Stewart et al, 1972; Tolarova et al, 1967a,b; Weatherley-White, 1976; Weatherley-White et al, 1972]. In fact, estimates of the incidence with which submucous defects occur *without* a speech defect [ie, Kaplan, 1975:1–10%] are undoubtedly far too low, since we have literally no way of knowing how many people present with one or more of the visible stigmata in the absence of velopharyngeal inadequacy. For that matter, we also have no way of knowing how many people may in fact have congenitally deep pharynges or even neuromotor deficits of the velopharyngeal mechanism that remain undetected because of a substantial adenoid pad or other structural augmentation of the nasopharynx.

The fact that (1) any one or all three of the intraorally visible stigmata can be present without causing a speech defect, placing many of these "patients" outside our clinical reach, and (2) most investigators consider submucous defects as microforms of cleft palate [ie, Meskin et al, 1964, 1965, 1966] means that two vital sets of figures are probably severely underestimated in the literature: those for incidence of submucous defects and those for frequency of genes for clefting in any given population.

"Occult" muscular deficiencies. Investigators—particularly surgeons—writing about submucous clefts have typically described abnormal orientation and insertion of the velar musculature, primarily the levator palatini [Calnan, 1954; Dorrance, 1930; Fara and Weatherley-White, 1977; Kaplan, 1975; Trier, 1983]. In his 1975 article, however, Kaplan described such muscular abnormalities in 26 patients who showed none of the three classic intraorally visible stigmata. This condition was definitively diagnosed only on the operating table, and was labeled "occult submucous cleft palate."[6] Trier [1983] also described abnormal insertion of the levator both in patients with visible stigmata and in patients whose palates apparently seemed normal on intraoral inspection.

The advent of nasopharyngoscopy [Pigott, 1969] allowed examination of the nasal surface of the velum and the opportunity to view the velopharyngeal port from above. Using this technique, Pigott et al, [1969] described deficiency in the bulk of the musculus uvulae in four patients with repaired clefts. While a midline deficiency in muscular bulk may not have been a surprising finding in repaired clefts, for these patients the hypernasality heard in their speech was directly attributable to a type of postoperative velopharyngeal insufficiency that would not have been detected on intraoral examination or by lateral radiography. Subsequently, extensive nasopharyngoscopic studies [Croft et al, 1978; Lewin et al, 1980] showed a similar central

---

[6]Kaplan also described some characteristic facies in both occult and classic submucous cleft which were mindful of descriptions published earlier by Calnan [1971a], Fara et al [1971], Sedlackova [1955], Sedlackova et al [1973], and Szabo et al [1974]. This topic will be discussed later in this paper.

muscular deficiency in hypernasal speakers whose palatal morphology appeared normal on intraoral inspection. Earlier, Chaco and Yules [1969] used electromyography to diagnose midline muscular deficiencies (which they than labeled "submucous clefts") in six of nine patients who developed hypernasal speech following adenotonsillectomy.

Pigott et al [1969], Croft et al [1978] and Lewin et al [1980] all viewed this muscular deficiency as a lack of bulk of the musculus uvulae, which they felt contributed substantially both to the muscular bulk of the velum and to the area of the "velar" eminence on palatal elevation. This view was substantiated by anatomical studies [Azzam and Kuehn, 1977] showing the musculus uvulae to be a paired muscle, with each bundle taking origin from the tendinous palatal aponeurosis posterior to the hard palate (*anterior* to the insertion of the levator palatini), converging with its counterpart in an area overlying the levator sling, and coursing over the dorsum of the soft palate to divide again into two separate bundles terminating at the uvula proper. Trier [1983], however, took issue with this viewpoint. Noting that none of the authors using nasopharyngoscopy had validated their "hypothetical absence of a uvular muscle" via surgical exploration of the velar muscles, Trier placed greater faith in the anatomical descriptions of Fara and Dvorak [1970] and of Kriens [1969, 1975], in the state-of-the-art reviews of Dickson et al [1974] and of Maue-Dickson [1977, 1979], and in his own intraoperative findings and those of Kaplan [1975] in stating that the crucial muscular deficiency in both classic and occult submucous clefts was in the levator and not the musculus uvulae.

Congenital Palatal Fistulae[7]

There have been several reported cases of overt clefts or congenital fistulae in the hard palate or anterior soft palate, with reported "integrity" of the remainder of the soft palate and presumably the uvula. As pointed out previously, the case described by Roux in 1835 actually exhibited a palatal fistula and not just a submucous cleft. Metcalf [1908] reported autopsy findings on an infant with a cleft of the anterior hard palate extending one centimeter posterior to the incisive foramen, with the remainder of the hard palate, soft palate, and uvula described as "otherwise normal." In cases reported by Trelat [1870a,b], Veau [1931], Calnan [1954], and Thaler and Smith [1968], the thin mucosa over a submucous bony defect was perforated, although whether the perforation was present at birth or acquired thereafter was either unknown or undocumented. In five cases described by Fara [1971], congenital fistulae in the palatal vault were contiguous with submucous clefts extending from the incisive foramen to the uvula (no further description of the uvulae in these patients is given in the text, but the illustrations suggest that they were bifid). In the case reported by Mitts et al, in 1981, the "non-cleft" (authors' term) soft palate posterior to the fistula actually showed abnormal muscle insertion and a bifid uvula. Smiley [1972] presented a similar case, supplied to him by Pruzansky, in support of a theory of abnormal epithelial adherence as the cause of clefts of the secondary palate.

To accept the concept of congenital palatal fistulae with true anatomic integrity of the structures posterior to the defect requires a considerable leap of faith, given our knowledge of embryology of the palatal structures. It is easier to conceptualize a perforation of poorly developed palatal mucosa thinly stretched over a submucous cleft, although both the timing and the cause[s] of such perforations remain unknown.

---

[7]Many readers would consider these cases to fall into the realm of "overt cleft."

Abnormalities of the Faucial Pillars

Before leaving the topic of rather unusual anatomic findings, it is worthwhile to briefly discuss congenital abnormalities of the faucial pillars. Such anomalies have been described in the literature since the 1800s [see Newcomb, 1897]. In 1908, Fridenburg described a patient with a "supernumerary anterior faucial pillar" that ran from the lateral margin of the soft palate to the dorsum of the tongue on each side, "entirely free of the oral or pharyngeal wall." The anterior pillars themselves were also separated from the lateral pharyngeal walls. Speech was described as having "a decided nasal twang. . . certain consonants have the metallic timbre usual with cleft palate." Oldfield and MacNaughtan [1946] described one case of congenital absence of an anterior pillar, and one case in which the posterior pillars formed a thin diaphragm extending from the posterior pharyngeal wall to the posterior border of the soft palate, with an elliptical hiatus in the middle. Speech was affected in both cases. Longacre [1951] described an infant similar to the second case: the soft palate was continuous with the base of the tongue at the level of the foramen cecum, the

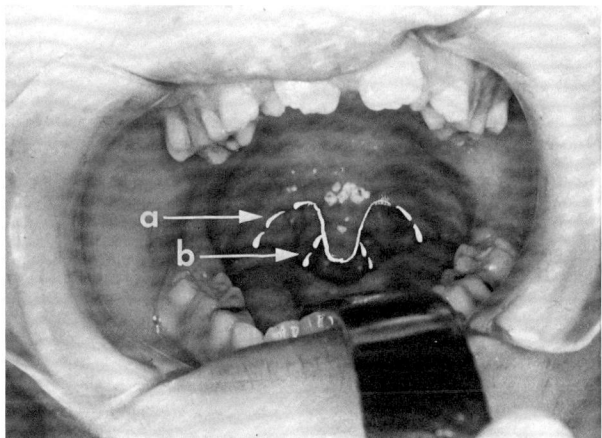

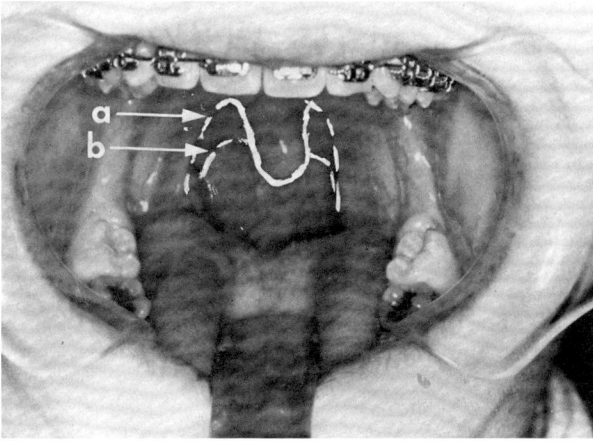

Fig. 1. Uvula placed anterior to the posterior faucial pillars in two normal speakers (a, anterior pillar; b, posterior pillar).

opening into the oropharynx described as being a partial cleft of the velum. Infants with similar findings were also described by Kouyoumdjian and McDonald [1951]; Hub and Jirasec [1961]; Seghers [1966]; and Chandra et al [1974]. Several of these authors labeled the condition "persistent buccopharyngeal membrane." Hoffman [1979] used the same label in describing a patient with a severe speech problem in whom a membrane reached from anterior pillar to anterior pillar and from the soft palate to the base of the tongue, with a small opening centrally. Crikelair et al [1964] described two patients with "cleft palate speech" in whom the velum was anchored inferiorly by abnormalities of the pillars, secondary to massive lymphangioma of the floor of the mouth in the first case and to post-tonsillectomy scarring in the second. Warren et al [1978] described two cases of posterior pillar webbing behind the uvula and a third case of webbing with palatopharyngeal displacement, all with limitation in velar motion and hypernasal speech.[8]

Palatopharyngeal Disproportion

A number of authors have described disproportion between the size of the palate and the size of the nasopharynx as a cause of velopharyngeal insufficiency [Birrell, 1966; Calnan, 1954, 1956, 1961b, 1971a; Cotton and Nuwayhid, 1983; Cotton and Quattromani, 1977; Crikelair et al, 1964; Dorrance, 1930; Dorrance and Shirazy, 1933; Fara et al, 1971; Kaplan, 1975; Jackson et al, 1980; Kelly, 1910; Porterfield et al, 1966; Sedlackova et al, 1973; Stueber and Wilhelmsen, 1984; Winters, 1966, 1975]. It should be noted that in many cases reported by these authors, a foreshortened palate and/or overly large pharynx coexisted with other anatomical abnormalities, such as a classic submucous cleft. In fact, Lermoyez [1892] felt that the short velum in what he termed "L'insuffisance velo-palatine" was healthy and of normal shape but invariably associated with a submucous defect of the hard palate and bifid uvula. Winters [1966] observed that belief in an absolute correlation between "congenital velopharyngeal insufficiency" and a submucous cleft of the hard palate was characteristic of all earlier writers except Gutzmann [1899] until Kelly proved otherwise. Kaplan [1975] reported that 75% of his 240 cases of velopharyngeal inadequacy had a short soft palate but that all of these were subsequently shown to have either classic or occult submucous clefts.

Crikelair et al [1964] pointed to foreshortening of the hard palate, with consequent anterior displacement of the points of insertion of the velar musculature, as a cause of velopharyngeal insufficiency. However, foreshortening of the hard palate has most often been described in conjunction with either classic submucous clefts [Kelly, 1910; Ricketts, 1954] or occult submucous clefts [Kaplan, 1975; Kelly, 1910].

Palatopharyngeal disproportion, with or without the presence of either a classic or occult submucous cleft, may remain undetected so long as an adenoid pad is present in the nasopharynx. The subject of post-adenoidectomy velopharyngeal inadequacy will be discussed in the following section of this paper. However, the point should be made that unless the surgery was careless or overly aggressive, causing a structural change in an otherwise normal nasopharynx, post adenoidectomy palatopharyngel disproportion should in fact be viewed as a *congenital* condition, the presence of which is simply unmasked by—not caused by—the adenoidectomy. This point is well illustrated by three case reports of such disproportion apparently unveiled

---

[8]I have examined several speakers with apparent forward displacement of the uvula, the posterior pillars appearing to converge behind it (Fig. 1). In none of these cases was speech affected.

as the result of normal adenoid involution. Goode and Ross [1972] described a 14-year-old with "a five-year history of hypernasal speech of gradual onset" in whom the palate was reportedly normal. There was no history of adenoidectomy, but no adenoid tissue was present on examination. Radiographic studies showed the nasopharynx to be "relatively large." Massengill and Quinn [1974] described an 18-year-old with hypernasality and a problem of nasal air leakage while playing wind instruments. Comparison of lateral x-rays taken at the ages of 10 years and 18 years revealed "a substantial decrease" in what had been a large adenoid mass. And in 1980, Shapiro reported a 11½-year-old boy who had a history of hypernasality for the previous 1½ years. Lateral x-rays showed "a very deep nasopharynx with a virtual absence of adenoidal tissue and a slight shortness of the palate" (no measurements given). Shapiro concluded, "This case report demonstrates that it is possible for velopharyngeal insufficiency to develop spontaneously at puberty in the presence of a short palate and a deep nasopharynx."

TONSILS, ADENOIDS, AND VELOPHARYNGEAL FUNCTION

Although both the tonsils and the adenoids are lymphoid tissue and both are parts of Waldeyer's ring, they have disparate embryologic origins and cytology [Pruzansky, 1975]. The size of one is not predictive of the size of the other [Mason and Warren, 1980; Pruzansky, 1975]. Both have been implicated in problems of velopharyngeal function, and in rather confusing fashion.

Subtelny and Koepp-Baker [1956] determined that the adenoid pad is generally visible in radiographic views of the nasopharynx by 6 weeks of age and progresses in size thereafter. The literature is inconclusive regarding the age at which the pad reaches its maximum size, seeming to indicate two possible peak ages. Subtelny and Koepp-Baker [1956] reported ". . . as early as 9 to 10 years of age and . . . as late as 14 to 15. . ." Handelman and Osborne [1976] cited the data of Subtelny and Koepp-Baker as "[following] Scammon's lymphatic cycle" [Scammon et al, 1930]. Following suit, Mason and Warren [1980] said, "Adenoid growth generally peaks arond 12 years. This is consistent with peak growth periods for other lymphoid tissue of the body" and cited "Scammon, 1930." However, five years earlier, Pruzansky [1975] had already pointed out the fallacy of applying the lymphoid growth curve reported by Scammon et al to tonsils and adenoids, since this curve was derived from postmortem data on a population subject to infectious diseases no longer prevalent, and these data did *not* include measurement of tonsils and adenoids. Pruzansky stated at that time, "The facts are that we know little about the variations in size and growth pattern of tonsils and adenoids." His own radiographic data on 291 normal children aged 4 to 16 years showed considerable variation in adenoid size in all age groups. What *is* known about the adenoid pad is that it decreases in size after the peak has been reached, undergoing natural and gradual involution until, by the adult years, it has usually disappeared.

While the adenoid pad is first increasing and then decreasing in size, growth of the craniofacial complex is producing other changes affecting the capacity of the nasopharynx.[9] The primary change is the descent of the hard palate away from the base of the skull, carrying the soft palate with it. This descent means an increase in

---

[9]As pointed out by Ricketts [1968] and by Gavron [1981], the actual size of the adenoid pad is not as crucial as the available space it fills.

the vertical size of the nasopharynx [Subtelny and Koepp-Baker, 1956] and an increasing distance between the velum and the gradually disappearing adenoid in later stages of development. In the earlier stages of development, this descent normally allows adequate space for nasal respiration despite the rapidly growing adenoid, although most clinicians have encountered children in whom these two factors have not remained in balance and a hypertrophied adenoid has resulted in mouthbreathing,[10] reduced exercise tolerance, noisy breathing at night, and possibly even sleep apnea.

Many clinicians have focused on the natural role of the adenoids in "velopharyngeal" (actually "velum-adenoid") closure in childhood [Calnan, 1957a; Fletcher, 1960; Mason, 1973; Neiman and Simpson, 1975; Pruzansky, 1975; Subtelny and Koepp-Baker, 1956; Vrticka, 1977] and on the inadvisability of adenoidectomy in children with overt clefts, submucous clefts, or the less obvious conditions of foreshortened velum, deep pharynx or neuromotor problems [Ashley et al, 1961; Beeden, 1972; Bergstrom and Hemenway, 1971; Berner, 1962; Blackfield et al, 1962; Calnan, 1953, 1954, 1956, 1957a,b, 1959, 1961a,b; 1971b; 1976; Chaco and Yules, 1969; Cotton and Nuwayhid, 1983; Cotton and Quattromani, 1977; Dey, 1969; Drettner, 1960; Croft et al, 1981; Freud, 1959; Gibb, 1958; Glover, 1961; Goode and Ross, 1972; Holborow, 1962; Jackson et al, 1980; Lubit, 1967; Linthicum et al, 1959; Mattucci, 1979; McWilliams and Musgrave, 1965; Miller, 1959; Morris, 1975; Minami et al, 1975; Nelson, 1978; Paradise, 1983; Paradise and Bluestone, 1976; Parkins and Barbero, 1975; Pickrell et al, 1976; Pruzansky, 1954, 1960, 1968, 1975; Ricketts, 1954; Roberts, 1959; Saad, 1975; Seeman, 1924; Severeid, 1978; Skolnik, 1958; Subtelny and Koepp-Baker, 1956; Thaler and Smith, 1968; Van Gelder, 1974; Vinicoff, 1960; Vrticka, 1977; Wallner et al, 1968; Whaley, 1957]. Over the years, this concern has given rise to two clinical dilemmas:

a) *Must speech be compromised if chronically enlarged or infected adenoids are affecting auditory tube function—and thus the health of the middle ear—in a child with a known abnormality of the velopharyngeal system?*

The medical literature of the 1950s and 1960s frequently advocated adenoidectomy to protect otologic health in children with clefts, even when the authors acknowledged the potential threat to speech [Baker, 1962; Beatty, 1951; Chalat, 1965; Fahey, 1965; Graham, 1963; Graham and Lierle, 1962; Halfond and Ballenger, 1956; Loeb, 1964; Miller, 1959; Sataloff and Fraser, 1952; Whaley, 1957]. This recommendation still appears sporadically [Goldstone and Horton, 1971; Panis, 1980] and is based on the assumption that it is indeed adenoid tissue that is the primary cause of tubal dysfunction in such children. This assumption has been undermined by information gleaned from both cleft and non-cleft patient populations. As early as 1940, Gaines reported a higher incidence of diseased and enlarged tonsils and adenoids in a normal control group than in a group of patients with clefts, despite the fact that the latter cases had a higher incidence of acute middle ear inflammations and both suppurative and non-suppurative otitis media [Gaines, 1940]. Holmes and Reed [1955] found *no* relationship between hearing and the presence or absence of adenoid tissue in their cleft palate patients. We now know that the principal cause of auditory tube

---

[10]Possible effects of reduced nasal respiratory function on facial growth have been the focus of considerable controversy. See Linder-Aronson [1963, 1970, 1979], Linder-Aronson and Backstrom [1960], McNamara [1979, 1981], O'Ryan et al [1982], Quick and Gundlach [1978], Warren et al [1969].

dysfunction in children with clefts resides in the anatomic and physiologic differences in the tube and contiguous structures, including the intimate relationship between tubal musculature and that of the velum [Bluestone, 1971; Bluestone et al, 1972; Dickson and Dickson, 1972; Doyle et al, 1980; Holborow, 1962; Maue-Dickson and Dickson, 1980; Maue-Dickson et al, 1976; Rood and Doyle, 1982; Seif and Dellon, 1978; Shprintzen and Croft, 1981]. While this evidence was evolving, otolaryngologists were expressing growing dissatisfaction with adenoidectomy as a treatment for ear disease [Dey, 1969; Graham, 1978; Stool and Beery, 1979]. From a retrospective study of adenoidectomy and otitis media in 160 patients with clefts, Severeid [1972] concluded that improved tubal function was more clearly related to increase in age than to adenoidectomy.[11] In 1983, Paradise cited ". . . the lack of convincing evidence that tonsillectomy and adenoidectomy, in the conditions for which they are usually undertaken, are superior in efficiency to conservative management."

In summary, then, the question of speech versus otologic health in patients with known abnormalities of the velopharyngeal system no longer appears to be meaningful. Otologic literature in the last decade has largely discarded adenoidectomy as a primary treatment for ear disease in either cleft or non-cleft patients, the preferred approach to tubal dysfunction being tympanic (myringotomy and ventilating tubes) [Graham, 1978; Paradise and Bluestone, 1976; Severeid, 1978; Stool and Beery, 1979]. If an adenoidectomy or adenotonsillectomy is deemed necessary (ie, for problems of chronic airway obstruction), extreme caution in both patient selection and operative technique is advocated [Mattucci, 1979; Paradise, 1983; Severeid, 1978; Stool and Beery, 1979].

b) *In the individual with no known abnormality of the velopharyngeal system, how can the risks of post-adenoidectomy velopharyngeal inadequacy be minimized?*

Temporary post-adenoidectomy velopharyngeal inadequacy has been frequently mentioned in the literature [Ashley et al, 1961; Calnan, 1954, 1976; Morris, 1975; Porterfield et al, 1966; Roberts, 1959; Subtelny and Koepp-Baker, 1956; Wallner et al, 1968] but has unfortunately been poorly documented with regard to both cause and duration. Some clinicians have attributed this phenomenon to unconscious inhibition of motion in reaction to pain or swelling [Gibb, 1969; Roberts, 1959] while others have described it as a period of adjustment during which the velum is somehow "learning" to move over a greater distance [Morris, 1975]. Estimates of how long this temporary condition may last range from "days or hours" [Morris, 1975] to "a day or two" [Morris et al, 1982] to "within one month" [Goldstone and Horton, 1971] to "two to three weeks" [Calnan, 1954] to "four to six weeks" [Greene, 1957]. When the condition persists, panic sets in for patient, family and physician.[12]

---

[11]The weaknesses of both retrospective and prospective studies of the indications for, and benefit of, adenotonsillectomy have been reviewed by Paradise [1972, 1976, 1983] and by Paradise and Bluestone [1976].

[12]Although he was writing about the possibly deleterious effects of tonsillectomy and adenoidectomy in children with repaired clefts, Glover's narrative [1961] is worth repeating: "The parents become frantic at the thought of impending deafness, and the adenoids and tonsils are whisked out. All is quiet for a few weeks until edema subsides, then everyone is unhappy. The child who was ready for school with an excellent pattern of speech has lost it all, and his utterances are nasal and difficult to understand. The child becomes depressed, the parents hysterical, the pediatrician despondent, and the otolaryngologist looks up his liability insurer."

Roberts [1959] listed the possible causes of post-adenoidectomy velopharyngeal inadequacy as (1) "poor development of the soft palate from disuse" (owing to the hypertrophied adenoid); (2) congenitally short soft palate, congenitally deficient muscle and nerve development; (3) "[possible] creation of a larger than normal pharynx"; (4) "trauma to palatal and pharyngeal musculature";(5) emotional or psychological factors; and (6) neurologic disorders. Assuming (a) that the surgeon recognizes and routinely examines for the three intraorally visible stigmata associated with a submucous defect, and (b) that he or she automatically exercises the utmost care in operative technique, the effort to avoid postoperative velopharyngeal inadequacy evolves down to a decision as to what minimal diagnostic steps should be included in the preoperative examination to detect other predisposing structural or neurologic conditions. A foreshortened velum and/or hard palate or a congenitally deep pharynx [Ashley et al, 1961; Berner, 1962; Calnan, 1971a, 1976; Gibb, 1958; Jackson et al, 1980] will not always be recognized on intraoral examination alone, and requires, at least, lateral still radiographs for diagnosis.[13] Detection of muscular deficits on the nasal side of the velum requires nasopharyngoscopy [Croft et al, 1981]. Deficits in palatal and pharyngeal motion are best visualized on fluoroscopy [Ashley et al, 1961; Croft et al, 1981] or nasopharyngoscopy [Pigott et al, 1969], but not even these studies can ascertain whether a lack of velar motion in the presence of an enlarged adenoid pad is due to lack of room for movement or to a neuromotor deficit. Ashley et al [1961] went to something of an extreme in recommending that "cinefluorographic lateral x-ray examination should be a prerequisite in all potentially incompetent patients, such as . . . preoperative tonsillitis and adenoiditis . . ." Croft and co-authors [1981] were more realistic: "We feel that the minimum preoperative evaluation would include digital palpation of the hard and soft palate, observation of the uvula and palate, and a lateral radiographic view of the nasopharynx with the soft palate in phonation."[14]

A review of the literature reveals a substantial number of children subjected to adenoidectomy (usually not by the authors) in the presence of (1) intraorally visible stigmata associated with submucous defects [Calnan, 1954; Croft et al, 1981; Dey, 1969; Gibb, 1958; Van Gelder, 1974] and/or (2) other "well-documented abnormalities" [the terminology of Blackfield et al, 1962] such as a foreshortened velum [Blackfield et al, 1962; Gibb, 1958; Greene, 1957; Jackson et al, 1980; Lawson et al, 1972]. More jarring is the number of times an adenoidectomy was performed when speech was already known to be hypernasal [Dey, 1969; Gibb, 1958; Greene, 1957; Mazaheri et al, 1964; Morris et al, 1982; Owsley et al, 1967]. If some of these procedures were performed by physicians confused between hypernasality and hyponasality, our post hoc criticism should be tempered by the fact that such confusion is not limited to physicians.

---

[13]The cephalometrician attempts to estimate the postoperative depth of the pharynx by "subtracting" the adenoid mass in the tracings of the films.

[14]The soft palate does not phonate. One assumes that the authors meant a lateral film exposed during production of a sustained vowel or consonant. In this context, it is worthwhile to point out that there is a substantial body of literature indicating that velar elevation is greater during production of consonants requiring high intraoral air pressure than during vowels, and greater during production of voiceless as opposed to voiced consonants. The only high-pressure consonants that can be sustained (as for exposure of a still radiograph) are the voiceless /f, θ, s, $\int$/ and the voiced /v, ð, z, ʒ/.

In summary, the recommendations of Croft et al [1981] appear to offer the practicing otolaryngologist reasonable guidelines for a preoperative workup of the potential adenoidectomy patient. One might add an evaluation by a certified speech pathologist in view of the fact that physicians are not trained to evaluate speech. Regardless of the steps taken, however, no one should offer patients or parents a guarantee of no postoperative velopharyngeal inadequacy. Particularly when velar movement is reduced or absent in the presence of an obstructing adenoid mass, the clinician must be aware of the limitations of each type of preoperative examination and convey those limitations to patients and parents.

The literature of the 1950s and 1960s was somewhat preoccupied with estimating the frequency of occurrence of post-adenoidectomy velopharyngeal inadequacy, perhaps in tacit acknowledgment of a lack of sufficient diagnostic tools allowing the clinician to detect many predisposing conditions preoperatively. Greene [1957] reported an incidence of 7.2% (25 of 347 cases) after adenotonsillectomy and 10% (3 of 30 cases) after adenoidectomy alone. However, one case in the first group had had nasal escape before surgery, and another developed nasal speech as a result of bulbar polio one month after surgery.[15] Eliminating these two cases, Greene's figures become 6.6% for the post-adenotonsillectomy group and 6.9% for both groups combined. The condition persisted in only four cases, reducing incidence to .01% if the above two cases are eliminated. A similar problem appears in the article of Gibb [1958], who reported post-adenotonsillectomy hypernasality in 19 of 27,734 cases (.006%). However, four of these were hypernasal preoperatively, and another four had bifid uvulae but normal speech preoperatively. The condition persisted in six cases (.002%, or .001% if the four who were hypernasal preoperatively are excluded). In a later article, Gibb [1969] estimated that hypernasality probably occurs at least once in every 2,000 adenotonsillectomies (.005%). Van Gelder [1974] estimated an occurrence of once in 3,000 cases (.003%). In his own experience with a reported 10,000 patients, he found postoperative velopharyngeal inadequacy in four cases after adenoidectomy (.004%) and in the same number of cases after tonsillectomy.[16]

In summary, estimates of the frequency of velopharyngeal inadequacy following adenoidectomy or adenotonsillectomy range from a low of .001% to a high of 10%, but the derivation of these numbers appears to have been contaminated by (1) inclusion of patients with known anatomic problems and/or hypernasal speech preoperatively and (2) questionable computation.

Enlarged tonsils can obstruct the oropharynx just as enlarged adenoids obstruct the nasopharynx, in extreme cases causing forward carriage of the tongue and an

---

[15]An extremely important point in reviewing these studies is whether the author[s] examined the patient before surgery, or whether the assumption of normal speech preoperatively is based on reports of parents or the patients themselves. For example, Croft et al [1981] relied on case histories to report "no evidence of hypernasality prior to adenotonsillectomy" in 48 cases, and Morris et al [1982] relied on mailed questionnaires to make the same assumption about 28 cases of congenital palatal incompetence, 14 of whom were unmasked by adenoidectomy.

[16]The incidence figures given throughout Van Gelder's article are not consistent. For example, despite the report of 4/10,000 cases of adenoidectomy, he states that the incidence following this procedure is approximately 1/10,000. Also, he does not clarify if the population figure of 10,000 means 10,000 cases *each* of adenoidectomy and tonsillectomy.

altered head-to-neck posture to protect the airway. Although, as Morris [1975] pointed out, not much is known about the effects of enlarged tonsils on speech, there are scattered reports and clinical conjectures in the literature. Clinicians have noted that hypertrophied tonsils may either "aid" in velopharyngeal closure by pushing the velum upwards and backwards [Freud, 1959; Gibb, 1958, 1969; Leung, 1981] or mechanically interfere with motion of the velum [Goldstone and Horton, 1971]. Calnan [1958] questioned whether tonsillectomy could ever give rise to hypernasality, and Mason [1973] stated that removal of tonsils was "not linked to deterioration in velopharyngeal competency." However, others have commented on postoperative scarring of the velum and/or faucial pillars leading to restriction in velopharyngeal motion [Crikelair et al, 1964; Croft et al, 1981; Freud, 1959; Goldstone and Horton, 1971; Gibb, 1958, 1969; Mattucci, 1979; Stool and Beery, 1979; Vinicoff, 1960]. In fact, Beatty [1951] warned against tonsillectomy in cleft palate patients but not against adenoidectomy! Gibb and Stewart [1975] attributed their case of post-tonsillectomy hypernasal speech to "hysterical aetiology" because of the patient's complex emotional symptomatology. Richstein and Jonas [1981] drew a questionable conclusion of "an increase of durable open nasal speech after tonsillectomy but not after adenoidectomy" in a study of patients with class III malocclusions. This statement was based on a margin of one patient (1/7 after adenoidectomy, 2/7 after tonsillectomy). Of 13 who underwent a combined procedure, 3 showed "detectable" and 2 "audible" rhinolalia aperta. Of greater curiosity than the conclusion that the authors drew, however, is that out of 33 *unoperated* cases 5 showed "detectable" and 3 showed "audible" rhinolalia aperta, exceeding the percentages among the operated cases.

In summary, the threat of adenoidectomy as a causal factor in velopharyngeal inadequacy appears to be on a decline as otolaryngologists opt for more conservative and apparently more effective approaches to the treatment of chronic ear disease. Concerns about tonsillectomy have generally been minimal by comparison and center upon risks of scarring and contracture. Nevertheless, the majority of current articles on velopharyngeal inadequacy continue to report a certain percentage of cases as having been "unmasked by T&A."

NEUROMOTOR DEFICITS

Neurologic deficits affecting motor speech production [17] are generally categorized into (a) the dysarthrias (there are several forms), which are characterized by abnormalities of muscular strength, range of motion, speed, accuracy and tonicity; and (b) dyspraxia (more commonly called "apraxia"), which is characterized by an impairment of programming of articulatory movements [Noll, 1982]. The dysarthrias may encompass coexisting disorders of respiration, phonation, resonation, articulation and prosody [Darley et al, 1975; Rosenbek and LaPointe, 1978]. A patient with extensive neurologic damage may exhibit a combination of dysarthria and dyspraxia.

There is very limited information regarding any effect of apraxia on velopharyngeal function. To date, only one study of apraxia has focused on velar motion [Itoh et al, 1977, 1978]. The single patient in this study showed marked variation in velar movement and abnormal movement patterns, including lack of coordination (inappro-

---

[17]Neurologic problems of motor speech production are distinguished from problems in verbal symbolic manipulation (aphasia).

priate timing) of velar movements with those of other articulators, but neither report mentions hypernasality or nasal emission. Noll [1982] speculated that the apparent paradox may have been due to the subtlety of the abnormalities of velar motion, being so minor as to have no perceived effect on speech. Logically, apraxia could indeed affect velopharyngeal function since this system is in fact an "articulator" (responsible for the nasal/non-nasal contrast), the programming for which could be affected just as the programming for the rest of the articulatory system is affected.

Extensive information is available on velopharyngeal incompetency in various types of dysarthrias, a large portion of it found in textbooks on neurologic disorders of speech. In reviewing clinical reports in the literature, one finds authors describing two phenomena:

1) Neuromuscular problems *apparently* affecting primarily the velopharyngeal system[18] or this system together with "other muscle complexes of the oral-facial-pharyngeal-laryngeal complex" [Johns and Salyer, 1978]. For example, Worster-Drought [1956] stated, "The most frequent example of congenital suprabulbar paresis affecting a single peripheral organ, I believe to be that of paralysis or weakness of the soft palate; this may be accompanied by an increased jaw jerk, but by no other manifestation of the disorder. Paresis of the soft palate may also co-exist with only a minor degree of weakness of the tongue or of the orbicularis oris. . . I have come to regard an isolated congenital palsy of the soft palate as a manifestation of a mild form of congenital suprabulbar paresis." Paresis or paralysis of the velum alone or together with the pharyngeal musculature has also been described by Ardran and Kemp [1975]; Ashley et al [1961]; Blackfield et al [1962]; Calnan [1975b, 1959, 1961a, 1976]; Cohn et al [1982]; Crikelair et al [1964]; Hoopes et al [1970a,b]; Jackson et al [1980]; Jafek et al [1979]; Kelly [1910]; Keogh [1956]; Lawshe et al [1971]; Mazaheri et al [1964]; Minami et al [1975]; Owsley et al [1967]; Pitt and Ingram [1975a,b]; Pollack et al [1979]; Shprintzen et al [1977]; Stueber and Wilhelmsen [1984]; and Sturim and Jacob [1972]. The impairment in velopharyngeal motion may be bilateral or may be unilateral, as often seen in cases of hemifacial microsomia [Luce et al, 1977; Shprintzen et al, 1980].

Also of interest are a number of reports of "palatal myoclonus" or "nystagmus" [Alajouanine et al, 1944; Alfaro, 1950; Baruk et al, 1945; Belman, 1947; Bender et al, 1952; Bjork, 1954; Bollinger et al, 1974; Davison et al, 1936; Dobson and Riley, 1941; Faure-Beaulieu and Garcin, 1940; Foix et al, 1926; Freeman, 1933; Gallet, 1927; Garcin et al, 1945; Guillain, 1938; Guillain and Mollaret, 1931; Guillain et al, 1933a,b; Herrmann et al, 1956; Hillemand et al, 1935; Jacobson and Gorman, 1949; Jonesco-Sisesti and Hornet, 1949; Langworthy and Grimmer, 1939; Leshin and Stone, 1931; Lhermitte and Sigwald, 1941; Nathanson, 1956; Riley and Brock, 1933; Shy and Carmichael, 1949; Spencer, 1886; Swanson et al, 1962; van Bogaert and Bertrand, 1928]. In the majority of these papers, speech is only vaguely described.

Finally, reduced motion of the velopharyngeal system associated with reduced facial expression and minor morphologic differences in the face has been described by a number of authors [Calnan, 1971a; Fara et al, 1971; Kaplan, 1975; Kruk and Tronczynska, 1978; Pitt and Ingram, 1975a; Saad, 1980; Sedlackova, 1955; Sedlackova et al, 1973; Shprintzen et al, 1978; Szabo et al, 1974] in a syndrome—or

---

[18]Some investigators [i.e., Netsell, 1983] have seriously questioned the existence of neuromotor deficits affecting the velopharyngeal system exclusively.

TABLE I. Categorizing Neuromotor Deficits Affecting the Velopharyngeal System

By type of dysarthria[1]
    Ataxic [Darley et al, 1969a,b, 1975]
    Flaccid [Darley et al, 1969a,b, 1975]
    Hyperkinetic [Darley et al, 1969a,b, 1975; Rosenbek and LaPointe, 1978]
    Hypokinetic [Darley et al, 1969a,b, 1975]
    Mixed (flaccid + spastic) [Darley et al, 1969a,b, 1975; Rosenbek and LaPointe, 1978; Wertz, 1978]
    Spastic [Canter, 1967; Darley et al, 1969a,b, 1975; Schweiger et al, 1970]

By level of site of damage
    Cerebellar [Darley et al, 1969a,b, 1975]
    Extrapyramidal [Canter, 1967; Darley et al, 1969a,b, 1975; Randall et al, 1960; Rosenbek and LaPointe, 1978; Wertz, 1978]
    Lower motor neuron [Canter, 1967; Darley et al, 1969a,b, 1975; Randall et al, 1960; Rosenbek and LaPointe, 1978; Wertz, 1978]
    Mixed (upper + lower) [Darley et al, 1969a,b, 1975]
    Pyramidal [Canter, 1967]
    Upper motor neuron [Darley et al, 1969a,b, 1975; Randall et al, 1960; Wertz, 1978; Worster-Drought, 1956, 1968]

By disease process[2]
    Amyotrophic lateral sclerosis [Darley et al, 1969a,b, 1975; Hirose et al, 1982; Minami et al, 1975; Randall et al, 1960; Rosenbek and LaPointe, 1978]
    Bulbar palsy [Darley et al, 1969a,b, 1975; Honjow et al, 1969; Rosenbek and LaPointe, 1978; Pitt and Ingram, 1975a]
    Bulbar poliomyelitis [Blackfield et al, 1962; McWilliams and Musgrave, 1965; Minami et al, 1975; Pitt and Ingram, 1975a; Worster-Drought, 1968]
    Cerebral palsy [Blackfield et al, 1962; Hardy et al, 1961, 1969; Hegarty, 1960; Heller et al, 1974; Jackson et al, 1980; Kent and Netsell, 1978; McWilliams and Musgrave, 1965; Netsell, 1969; Owsley et al, 1967; Pitt and Ingram, 1975a; Randall et al, 1960; Worster Drought, 1968]
    Chorea [Hoopes et al, 1970a, 1970b]
    Congenital suprabulbar paresis [Worster-Drought, 1956, 1968]
    Dystonia [Hoopes et al, 1970a, 1970b]
    Gilles de la Tourette [Rosenbek and LaPointe, 1978]
    Moebius syndrome [Henderson, 1939; Languth, 1972; Meyerson and Foushee, 1978; Pitt and Ingram, 1975a, 1975b; Rubin, 1976]
    Multifocal eosinophilic granuloma (Hand-Schuller-Christian disease) [Chon et al, 1982]
    Multiple sclerosis [Rosenbek and LaPointe, 1978]
    Muscular dystrophy [McCoy and Zahorski, 1972; Minami et al, 1975; Mullendore and Stoudt, 1961; Randall et al, 1960; Rosenbek and LaPointe, 1978]
    Myasthenia gravis [Canter, 1967; Honjow et al, 1969; Minami et al, 1975; Wolski, 1967]
    Myoclonus [Rosenbek and LaPointe, 1978]
    Myotonic dystrophy [Pitt and Ingram, 1975a; Leach, 1962; Pollack et al, 1979; Weinberg et al, 1968]
    Neurofibromatosis [Hoopes et al, 1970a,b; Minami et al, 1975; Pollack and Shprintzen, 1981]
    Parkinson's [Darley et al, 1969a,b, 1975]
    Post-diphtheria [Minami et al, 1975; Randall et al, 1960; Worster-Drought, 1968]
    Pseudobulbar palsy [Darley et al, 1969a,b, 1975; Hirose et al, 1982; Hoopes et al, 1970a,b; Minami et al, 1975; Pitt and Ingram, 1975a,b; Pollack et al, 1979; Randall et al, 1960]
    Syringomyelia [Randall et al, 1960]
    Wilson's disease [Rosenbek and LaPointe, 1978]

[1]Authors do not agree on a standardized system for categorizing types of dysarthria. For a different system, see Canter [1967].
[2]Care has been taken to use exactly the same medical label used by the authors.

possibly a related family of syndromes—involving a range of palatal defects (including overt and submucous clefts), minor ear malformations, cardiac findings and problems of intellectual development. Prior to 1978, the term "Sedlackova syndrome" was frequently applied to this grouping of anomalies. After the article by Shprintzen et al [1978], the term "velo-cardiofacial syndrome" became more popular. The association of palatal anomalies and facial findings is the one common thread running through the reports cited above; description of other findings has varied, suggesting that this may not be a single entity.

2) Abnormalities of velopharyngeal muscular motion occurring as part of a generalized neurologic deficit [Blackfield et al, 1962; Calnan, 1959; Crikelair et al, 1964; Darley et al, 1969a,b, 1975; Hardy et al, 1961, 1969; Hegarty, 1960; Hellar et al, 1974; Hirose et al, 1982; Honjow et al, 1969; Hoopes et al, 1970a,b; Jackson et al, 1980; Johns and Salyer, 1978; Kent and Netsell, 1978; Leach, 1962; McCoy and Zahorski, 1972; McWilliams and Musgrave, 1965; Minami et al, 1975; Mullendore and Stoudt, 1961; Netsell, 1969; Owsley et al, 1967; Pitt and Ingram, 1975a; Pollack and Shprintzen, 1981; Randall et al, 1960; Rosenbek and LaPointe, 1978; Schweiger et al, 1970; Weinberg et al, 1968; Wolski, 1967; Worster-Drought, 1968].

Two problems are encountered in attempting to review and organize information on neuromotor deficits affecting the velopharyngeal system. First, there is a lack of consistency in how some neurologic disorders are labeled by different authors. Second, the information is sometimes presented in relation to type of dysarthria, sometimes in relation to the level or site of neurologic damage, and sometimes in relation to the disease process itself. Table I illustrates these three approaches to categorization, listing some key references.

A number of investigators have described the occurrence of hypernasality in mentally retarded or developmentally delayed speakers [ie, Daly and Johnson, 1974; Heller et al, 1974; Hoopes et al, 1970a,b; McWilliams and Musgrave, 1965]. The adequacy of neuromotor function is of course suspect in such speakers. In addition, any sizable sample of mentally retarded speakers may well include patients with genetic or chromosomal abnormalities showing either subtle or overt craniofacial dysmorphology, possibly affecting the velopharyngeal system. Thus, there are several possible links between mental retardation and either structural or neuromotor velopharyngeal inadequacy.

More obscure is the occasionally suggested link between psychological factors and impaired velopharyngeal function. Current literature still contains references to "psychogenic" or "psychoneurotic" disorders [Minami et al, 1975] and "emotional disturbance" [Heller et al, 1974] as bases for hypernasality. However, the nature of the cause-effect relationship, if any, between emotional disturbances and such a change in speech behavior has never been well delineated.

STRESS VELOPHARYNGEAL INADEQUACY

In 1970, Weber and Chase described an oboe player who developed "continuous nasal snorting" after the first 10 minutes of playing. This phenomenon occurred only during playing and not during speech. No structural abnormality of the velopharyngeal mechanism could be detected on oral exam, oral endoscopy, or cineradiographic examination, although the ratio of palatal length to pharyngeal depth (30/31 mm) on cephalometric films was not discussed by the authors and *may* have indicated a marginal mechanism, based on Subtelny's norms [1957]. Weber and Chase labeled this phenomenon "stress velopharyngeal incompetence."[19] A similar problem was described in a bassoon/saxophone player by Massengill and Quinn in 1974. In the latter case, the liability was attributed to progressive adenoid involution, but such involution is normal and if this normal process results in velopharyngeal inadequacy some underlying mechanism is present. Of the two cases reported by Dibbell et al [1979], one had a submucous cleft, while the other showed "herniation" of the soft palate into the nasopharynx under the stress imposed by the high intraoral pressures required for playing a wind instrument: with continuous playing the soft palate was literally blown into the nasopharynx. Argamaso and Shprintzen [1983] described velopharyngeal inadequacy in a trumpet player who had undergone a tonsillectomy which resulted in scarred musculature. In the single case seen by the present author, a clarinet player with normal speech developed nasal leakage after approximately 30 minutes of playing. Interestingly, this first occurred only after she enrolled as a music major in college and began playing 6 to 8 hours a day. Nasopharyngoscopy revealed a slight V-shaped defect on the nasal surface of the velum, resulting in a small inconsistent central velopharyngeal gap.

Reviewing the few cases of stress velopharyngeal inadequacy in musicians reported to date, it is apparent that some actually did have at least some minor structural defect. Others may have had either a structural defect which was undetected or some predisposing minor muscular weakness that became symptomatic only under sustained use of extremely high intraoral pressures (see Dibbell et al [1979] for a table of required pressures in wind instrument playing).

PHONEME-SPECIFIC VELOPHARYNGEAL INADEQUACY

In 1972, an article by Lawson and co-authors contained the following statement: "For some patients, the nasal emission appeared only on specific phonemes or combinations." In 1975, I described "nasal emission as a component of the misarticulation of sibilants and affricates" both in children who had been treated for cleft palate or other forms of structural velopharyngeal inadequacy and in children for whom no history of such inadequacy could be documented. In all cases, all pressure consonants except /s/ and /z/, all four sibilants, or the sibilants and affricates together were free of nasal distortion.[20] Aberrant lingual position for these phonemes could be identified on lateral radiographic films. Trost [1981a], in describing "posterior nasal frication," commented upon "a notable occurrence in non-cleft velopharyngeal disorders, including the neurogenic problems of the dysarthrias and phoneme-specific velopharyngeal inadequacy." She used the latter term ". . . to define the occurrence of nasal air emission and audible posterior frication on cetain pressure consonants only."

In the clinical experience of this author, this pattern has been observed in speakers as young as 3 years and as old as 23 years. In some speakers, the nasal emission or

---

[19]I have chosen to use the term "inadequacy," in accordance with the categorization described earlier, because some of these cases have in fact been shown to have at least minor structural findings while others have not.

[20]The perceptual consequence of the phoneme-specific inadequacy was limited to the label "nasal emission" in the 1975 article but may also be heard as "posterior nasal frication" [Trost, 1981a].

frication is heard as a "co-articulation" with correct or distorted (ie, interdentalized) oral placement, while in others it *replaces* the oral gesture. In the latter cases, the lips may be entirely closed during the /s/, /z/, etc., virtually assuring that nothing but nasal production can occur. One speaker in my experience was so "specific" in his substitution of nasal emission for /s/ that he used it only in prevocalic /st-/ blends. When nasopharyngoscopy is performed, one sees velopharyngeal gaps only on those phonemes produced with either nasal emission or posterior nasal frication [Peterson-Falzone, 1981].

To date, we have no information to tell us why phoneme-specific inadequacy develops. Why is the speaker unaware or unconcerned that he is emititng these consonants nasally while all others are appropriately produced orally? What type of breakdown in learning has occurred, and when? These questions await examination in further studies of this phenomenon. The key point to be made for the present, however, is that, unlike other forms of this problem, correction of phoneme-specific velopharyngeal inadequacy is the task of the speech pathologist, not the surgeon or prosthodontist.

ACKNOWLEDGMENTS

This work was sponsored in part by a grant from the National Institutes of Health, NINCDS 1 RO1 19879.

REFERENCES

Alajouanine T, Thurel R, Wolfrom R: Myoclonies rythmees du voile, de la glotte et du diaphragme, survhant par acces periodiques et se traduisant par du hoquet. Revue Neurologique 76:96–97, 1944.
Alfaro F: Palatal myoclonous. Arch Otolaryngol 51:65–72, 1950.
Ardran G, Kemp F: Radiology in the study of neurological diseases affecting the pharynx and larynx. Proc Soc Med 68:641–44, 1975.
Argamaso R, Shprintzen R: Fanfare for a pharyngeal flap. Videotape presentation before the American Cleft Palate Association, Denver, May, 1983.
Ashley F, Sloan R, Hahn E, Hanafee W, Miethke J: Cinefluorographic study of palatal incompetency cases during deglutition and phonation. Plast Reconstr Surg 28, 4:347–364, 1961.
Azzam N, Kuehn D: The morphology of musculus uvulae. Cleft Palate J 14:78–87, 1977.
Baker D: The tonsillectomy and adenoidectomy problem. Pediatr Clin N Am November, 1962, pp 1138–1146.
Baruk H: Owsianik, Borenstein (no initials given): Myoclonies velo-palato-laryngees consecutives a l'ectro-choc: Remarques critiques sur cette method therapeutique. Revue Neurologique 77:319–320, 1945.
Beatty H: Relation between tonsil and adenoid operations and cleft palate. J Am Med Assoc 145, 6:379–381, 1951.
Beeden A: The bifid uvula. J Laryngol Otol 86:815–819, 1972.
Belman E: Traumatic velopalatine myoclonus. Nevropatologiya i psikhiatriya 16:43–44, 1947.
Bender M, Nathanson M, Gordon G: Myoclonus of muscles of the eye, face and throat. AMA Arch Neurol Psychiatr 67:44–58, 1952.
Berans C: Anomalies of the uvula. Philadelphia Med Bull 15:177–179, 1893.
Bergstrom L, Hemenway W: Otologic problems in submucous cleft palate. Southern Med J 64, 10:1172–1177, 1971.
Berner R: Hazards of adenotonsillectomy in the child with cleft palate. J Am Med Assoc 181, 6:558–559, 1962.
Birrell J: Palatal disproportion in children. J Laryngol 80:706–717, 1966.
Bjork H: Objective tinnitus due to clonus of the soft palate. Acta Oto-laryngologica [Suppl] 116:39–45, 1954.
Blackfield H, Miller E, Owsley J, Lawson L: Cinefluorographic evaluation of patients with velopharyngeal dysfunction in the absence of overt cleft palate. Plast Reconstr Surg 30:441–451, 1962.

Blakeley R: Variations in the soft palate of school children. Presented before the American Speech and Hearing Association, Chicago, 1965.

Bollinger M, Menkes H, Benjamin J, Ball W: The syndrome of rhythmic palatal myoclonus: A cause of significant extrathoracic airway obstruction. Am Rev Respir Dis 110:803–806, 1974.

Bluestone C: Eustachian tube obstruction in the infant with cleft palate. Ann Otol Rhinol Laryngol [Suppl] 2, 80:1–30, 1971.

Bluestone C, Wittel R, Paradise J: Roentgenographic evaluation of eustachian tube function in infants with cleft and normal palates. Cleft Palate J 9:93–100, 1972.

Calnan J: Congenital large pharynx: A new syndrome with a report of 41 personal cases. Brit J Plast Surg 24:263–271, 1971a.

Calnan J: Diagnosis, prognosis, and treatment of "palato-pharyngeal incompetence," with special reference to radiographic investigations. Br J Plast Surg 8:265–282, 1956.

Calnan J: Investigation of children with speech defect, with particular reference to nasality. Br Med J March 29, 1958, pp 737–740.

Calnan J: Modern views on Passavant's ridge. Br J Plast Surg 10, 2:89–113, 1957a.

Calnan J: Movements of the soft palate. Br J Plast Surg 5:286–296, 1953.

Calnan J: Palatopharyngeal incompetence in speech. In: Pruzansky S (ed): "Congenital Anomalies of the Face and Associated Structures." Springfield, IL: C.C. Thomas, 1961a.

Calnan J: Permanent nasal escape in speech after adenoidectomy. Br J Plast Surg 24:197–204, 1971b.

Calnan J: Submucous cleft palate. Br J Plast Surg 6:264–282, 1954.

Calnan J: Surgery for speech. In: Calnan J (ed): "Recent Advances in Plastic Surgery, I." Edinburgh: Churchill Livingstone, 1976.

Calnan J: The investigation of nasality (nasal escape) in speech. Speech 21:59–74, 1957b.

Calnan J: The mobility of the soft palate: A radiological and statistical study. Br J Plast Surg 14:33–38, 1961b.

Calnan J: The surgical treatment of nasal speech disorders. Ann R Coll Surg Engl 25:119–141, 1959.

Canter C: Neuromotor pathologies of speech. Am J Phys Med 46:659–666, 1967.

Chaco J, Yules R: Velopharyngeal incompetence post tonsillo-adenoidectomy. Acta Oto-Laryngologica 68:276–278, 1969.

Chalat N: Tonsillectomy, adenoidectomy and the cleft palate clinic. Laryngoscope 75:408–427, 1965.

Chandra R, Yadava V, Sharma R: Persistent buccopharyngeal membrane. Plast Reconstr Surg 54:678–679, 1974.

Cohn E, Garver K, Metz H, McWilliams B, Skolnick M, Garrett W: Velopharyngeal incompetence in a patient with multifocal eosinophilic granuloma (Hand-Schuller-Christian disease). J Speech Hearing Dis 47:320–323, 1982.

Cotton R, Nuwayhid N: Velopharyngeal insufficiency. In: Bluestone C, Stool S (eds): "Pediatric Otolaryngology, Vol. 2." Philadelphia: W.B. Saunders, 1983.

Cotton R, Quattromani F, Lateral defects in velopharyngeal insufficiency. Arch Otolaryngol 103:90–93, 1977.

Coues W: A case of double uvula in a child. Boston Med Surg J 154:706–707, 1906.

Crikelair G, Cosman R: On submucous cleft palate (letter to the editor). Plast Reconstr Surg 59:424–425, 1977.

Crikelair G, Kastein S, Fowler E, Cosman B: Velar dysfunction in the absence of cleft palate. N Y State J Med January 15, 1964, pp 263–269.

Crikelair G, Striker P, Cosman B: The surgical treatment of submucous cleft palate. Plast Reconstr Surg 45:58–65, 1970.

Croft C, Shprintzen R, Daniller A, Lewin M: The occult submucous cleft palate and the musculus uvulae. Cleft Palate J 15:150–154, 1978.

Croft C, Shprintzen R, Ruben R: Hypernasal speech following adenotonsillectomy. Otolaryngol Head Neck Surg 89:179–188, 1981.

Daly D, Johnson H: Instrumental modification of hypernasal voice quality in retarded children: Case reports. J Speech Hearing Dis 39:500–507, 1974.

Darley F, Aronson A, Brown J: Clusters of deviant speech dimensions in the dysarthrias. J Speech Hear Res 12:462–496, 1969a.

Darley F, Aronson A, Brown J: Differential diagnostic patterns of dysarthria. J Speech Hear Res 12:246–269, 1969b.

Darley F, Aronson A, Brown J: "Motor Speech Disorders." Philadelphia: W.B. Saunders Co., 1975.

Davison C, Riley H, Brock S: Rhythmic myoclonus of the muscles of the palate, larynx and other regions. Bull Neurolog Inst NY 5:94–126, 1936.

Demarquay J: Tissue fibrineux remplacant au voile du palais et a la voute palatine les muscles palatine. Bull Soc Anatomique de Paris 21:11–13, 1846.

Dey D: Nasal speech, adenoidectomy and the Hynes' pharyngoplasty. Med J Australia September 13, 1969, pp 553–555.

Dibbell D, Ewanowski S, Carter W: Successful correction of velopharyngeal stress incompetence in musicians playing wind instruments. Plast Reconstr Surg 64, 5:662–664, 1979.

Dickson D, Dickson W: Velopharyngeal anatomy. J Speech Hear Res 15:372–381, 1972.

Dickson D, Grant J, Sicher H, DuBrul E, Poltau J: Status of research in cleft palate and anatomy and physiology. Part I. Cleft Palate J 11, 3:471–492, 1974.

Dobson J, Riley H: Rhythmic myoclonus: A clinical report of 6 cases. Arch Neurol Psychiatr 45:145–150, 1941.

Dorrance G, Shirazy E: "The Operative Story of Cleft Palate." Philadelphia: W.B. Saunders, 1933.

Dorrance G: Congenital insufficiency of the palate. Arch Surg 21:185–248, 1930.

Doyle W, Cantekin E, Bluestone C: Eustachian tube function in cleft palate children. Ann Otol Rhinol Laryngol [Suppl 68] 89:34–40, 1980.

Drettner B: The nasal airway and hearing in patients with cleft palate. Acta Otolaryngologica 52:131–142, 1960.

Fahey D: Otologic care of cleft palate cases. Laryngoscope 75:570–587, 1965.

Fara M, Dvorak J: Abnormal anatomy of the muscles of palatopharyngeal closure in cleft palates. Plast Reconstr Surg 46:488–497, 1970.

Fara M, Weatherley-White R: Submucous cleft palate. In: Converse J (ed): "Reconstructive Plastic Surgery, Vol. 4: Cleft Lip and Palate, Craniofacial Deformities." Philadelphia: W.B. Saunders Co., 1977.

Fara M: Congenital defects in the hard palate: Observation of five cases. Plast Reconstr Surg 48, 1:44–47, 1971.

Fara M: Hrivnakova J, Sedlackova E: Submucous cleft palates. Acta Chirurgiae Plasticae, 13, 4:221–234, 1971.

Faure-Beaulieu (no initials given), Garcin R: Etude anatomique d'un cas de myoclonies velo-pharyngo-laryngees. Revue Neurologique 72:734–739, 1940.

Fletcher S: Hypernasal voice as an indication of regional growth and developmental disturbances. Logos 3, 1:3–12, 1960.

Foix C, Chavany J, Hillemand P: Les syndrome myoclonique de la calotte, étude anatomo-clinique due nystagmus, du voile, et des myoclonies rythmiques associees, oculaires, faciles. Revue Neurologique 33:942–956, 1926.

Foster H: Report of a case of bifid or double uvula. Med Herald 14:15–16, 1895.

Freeman W: Palatal myoclonus: Report on two cases with necropsy. Arch Neurol Psychiatr 29:742–755, 1933.

Freud E: The otolaryngologist and the symptom of hyper-rhinolalia. Arch Otolaryngol 70:32–41, 1959.

Fridenburg P: Congenital detachment of faucial pillars and isolation of palato-glossus muscle. Laryngoscope 18:567–571, 1908.

Gallet J: Le nystagmus du voile, Thesis. Paris, 1927.

Gaines F: Frequency and effect of hearing losses in cleft palate cases. J Speech Dis 5,2:141–149, 1940.

Garcin R, Chavany J, Kipfer M: Sur le cas de deux soeurs atteintes l'une de myoclonie isolée du voile du palais, l'autre de mouvements oscillatoires rythmes des orteils. Revue Neurologique 77:135–138, 1945.

Gavron G: The impact of cleft lip and palate deformity on the nasopharyngeal airway. J Dent Assoc of South Africa 36:747–750, 1981.

Gibb A: Hypernasality (rhinolalia aperta) following tonsil and adenoid removal. J Laryngol Otol 72:433–451, 1958.

Gibb A: Unusual complications of tonsil and adenoid removal. J Laryngol 83:1159–1174, 1969.

Gibb A, Stewart I: Hypernasality following tonsil dissection—hysterical aetiology. J Laryngol Otol 89:779–781, 1975.

Glover D: A long range evaluation of cleft palate repair. Plast Reconstr Surg 27, 1:19–30, 1961.

Goldstone A, Horton C: Should adenotonsillectomy be done in the cleft palate patient? Virginia Med Monthly 98:133–138, 1971.

Goode R, Ross J: Velopharyngeal insufficiency after adenoidectomy. Arch Otolaryngol 96:223–226, 1972.
Graham M: A longitudinal study of ear disease and hearing loss in patients with cleft lips and palates. Transactions of the Am Acad Ophthalmol Otolaryngol March–April, 1963, pp 213–222.
Graham M, Lierle D: Posterior pharyngeal flap palatoplasty and its relationship to ear disease and hearing loss. Laryngoscope 72:1750–1755, 1962.
Graham M: Otologic assessment and management of the cleft palate individual. In: Graham M (ed): "Cleft Palate: Middle Ear Disease and Hearing Loss." Springfield, IL: C.C. Thomas, 1978.
Greene M: Speech of children before and after removal of tonsils and adenoids. J Speech Hear Dis 22:361–370, 1957.
Guillain G, Mollaret P: Deux cas du myoclonies synchrones et rythmees velo-pharyngo-laryngo-oculo-diaphragmatiques. Revue Neurologique 23:545–566, 1931.
Guillain G, Mollaret P, Bertrand I: Sur la lesion responsable du syndrome myoclonique du tronc cerebral. Revue Neurologique 2: 666–675, 1933.
Guillain G: The syndrome of synchronous and rhythmic palato-pharyngo-laryngo-oculo-diaphragmatic myoclonus. Proc R Soc Med 31:1031–1038, 1938.
Guillain G, Thurel R, Bertrand I: Examen anatomo-pathologique d'us cas de myoclonies velo-pharyngo-oculo-diaphragmatiques associees a des myoclonies squelettiques synchrones. Revue Neurologique 2:801–812, 1933.
Gutzmann H: Ueber die angeborene Insufficienz des Gaumensegels. Berlin, Klin, Woch. 37:809–813, 1899.
Gylling U, Soivio A: Submucous cleft palates. Acta Chiurgiae Scandinavia 129:282–287, 1965.
Halfond M, Ballenger J: An audiologic and otorhinologic study of cleft-lip and cleft-palate cases. AMA Arch Otolaryngol 64:335–340, 1956.
Handelman C, Osborne G: Growth of the nasopharynx and adenoid development from one to eighteen years. Angle Orthodont 46, 3:243–259, 1976.
Hardy J, Netsell R, Schweiger J, Morris H: Management of velopharyngeal dysfunction in cerebral palsy. J Speech Hear Dis 34, 2:123–127, 1969.
Hardy J, Rembolt R, Spriestersbach D, Jayapathy B: Surgical management of palatal paresis and speech problems in cerebral palsy: A preliminary report. J Speech Hear Dis 26, 4:320–325, 1961.
Hegarty I: Case study of velar and facial paralysis. J Speech Hear Dis 25:409–411, 1960.
Heller J, Gens G, Moe D, Lewin M: Velopharyngeal insufficiency in patients with neurologic, emotional and mental disorders. J Speech Hear Dis 39:350–359, 1974.
Henderson J: The congenital facial diplegia syndrome: Clinical features, pathology and etiology. Brain 62:381–403, 1939.
Herrmann C, Crandall P, Fang H: Palatal myoclonus: A new approach to the understanding of its production. Neurology 7, 1:37–51, 1957.
Hillemand P, Chavany J, Trelles O: Le problem anatomique du nystagmus du voile, du palais. Revue Neurologique 64:1–17, 1935.
Hirose H, Kiritani S, Sawashima M: Patterns of dysarthric movement in patients with amyotrophic lateral sclerosis and pseudobulbar palsy. Folia Phoniatrica 34:106–112, 1982.
Hoffman R: Persistant pharyngeal membrane. Arch Otolaryngol 105:286–287, 1979.
Holborow C: Conductive deafness associated with the cleft-palate deformity. Proc R Soc Med 55:305–307, 1962.
Holmes E, Reed G: Hearing and deafness in cleft-palate patients. AMA Arch Otolaryngol 62:620–624, 1955.
Honjow I, Isshiki N, Kitajima K: Congenital and acquired hypernasalities. Folia Phoniatrica 21:266–276, 1969.
Hoopes J, Dellon A, Fabrikant J, Edgerton M, Soliman A: Cineradiographic definition of the functional anatomy and pathophysiology of the velopharynx. Cleft Palate J 7:443–454, 1970.
Hoopes J, Dellon A, Fabrikant J, Soliman A: Idiopathic hypernasality: Cineradiographic evaluation and etiologic considerations. J Speech Hear Dis 35:44–50, 1970.
Hub M, Jirasek J: Perzistence stredni casti membrane buccopharynicae. Cas Lek Cesk 99:1297–1299, 1961.
Itoh M, Sasanuma S, Ushijima T: Velar movements during speech in a patient with apraxia of speech. Annu Bull Res Inst Logoped Phoniatr University of Tokyo, 11:67–75, 1977.
Itoh M, Sasanuma S, Hirose H: Articulatory dynamics in a patient with apraxia of speech. Presented before the Academy of Aphasia, Chicago, 1978.

Jackson I, McGlynn M, Huskie C: Velopharyngeal incompetence in the absence of cleft palate: Results of treatment in 20 cases. Plast Reconstr Surg 66, 2:211–213, 1980.

Jacobson M, Gorman W: Palatal myoclonus and primary nystagmus following trauma. Arch Neurol Psychiatr 62:798–801, 1949.

Jafek B, Balkany T, Wong M, Bryant K: Surgical management of the hypodynamic palate. Arch Otolaryngol 105:347–350, 1979.

Johns D, Salyer K: Surgical and prosthetic management of neurogenic speech disorders. In: Johns D (ed): "Clinical Management of Neurogenic Communicative Disorders." Boston: Little, Brown and Co., 1978.

Jonesco-Sisesti N, Hornet T: Le problème du nystagmus velo-palato-oculaire. Les degenerescences hypertrophiques systematisees du complexe olivaire bulbaire consecutive aux lesions due noyau duetele du cervelet. Rev d'Oto-Neuro-Ophthalmologie 17:418, 1949.

Kaplan E: The occult submucous cleft palate. Cleft Palate J 12:356–368, 1975.

Kelly AB: Congenital insufficiency of the palate. J Laryngol Rhinol Otol 25:281–358, 1910.

Kent R, Netsell R: Articulatory abnormalities in athetoid cerebral palsy. J Speech Hear Dis 43, 3:353–373, 1978.

Keogh C: Paralysis of the pharynx. J Laryngol Otol 70:344–351, 1956.

Kono D, Young L, Holtmann B: The association of submucous cleft palate and clefting of the primary palate. Cleft Palate J 18, 3:207–209, 1981.

Kouyoumdjian A, McDonald J: Association of congenital adrenal neuroblastoma with multiple anomalies including an unusual oropharyngeal cavity (imperforate buccopharyngeal membrane?). Cancer 14:784–788, 1951.

Kriens O: An anatomical approach to veloplasty. Plastic Reconstr Surg 43:29–41, 1969.

Kriens O: Anatomy of the velopharyngeal area in cleft palate. Clin Plast Surg 2:261–283, 1975.

Kruk J, Troncynska J: Velopharyngeal insufficiency in children with Sedlackova's syndrome. Acta Chirurgiae Plasticae 20:13–17, 1978.

Languth P: Speech with palatal dysfunction. Proc R Soc Med (Section of Laryngology) 65:413–416, 1972.

Langworthy O, Grimmer R: A physiological study of the movements in palatal myoclonus. Johns Hopkins Hosp Bull 65:101–111, 1939.

Lawshe B, Hardy J, Schweigher J, VanAllen J: Management of a patient with velopharyngeal incompetency of undetermined origin: A clinical report. J Speech Hear Dis 36, 4:547–555, 1971.

Lawson L, Chierici G, Castro A, Harvold E, Miller E, Owsley J: Effects of adenoidectomy on the speech of children with potential velopharyngeal dysfunction. J Speech Hear Dis 37, 3:390–402, 1972.

Leach W: Generalized muscular diseases presenting as pharyngeal dysphagia. J Laryngol Otol 76 (Jan–June):237–240, 1962.

Lermoyez M: L'insuffisance velo-palatine. Ann Maladies l'Orielle Larynx 18, 3:161–205, 1892.

Leshin N, Stone T: Continuous rhythmic movements of the palate, pharynx and larynx. Arch Neurol Psychiatr 26:1236–1250, 1931.

Leung V: Tonsils and adenoids—current thinking. J Nebraska Dent Assoc 58, 2:9–12, 1981.

Lewin M, Croft C, Shprintzen R: Velopharyngeal insufficiency due to hypoplasia of the musculus uvulae and occult submucous cleft palate. Plast Reconstr Surg 65, 5:585–591, 1980.

Lhermitte J, Sigwald J: Myoclonies rythmees du voile, du pharynx, du larynx et du membre superieur gauche au cours d'un syndrome lateral du bule. Revue Neurologique 73:81–86, 1941.

Linder-Aronson S: Adenoids: Their effect on mode of breathing and airflow and their relation to characteristics of facial skeleton and the dentition. Acta Oto-Laryngologica [Suppl] 265:1–132, 1970.

Linder-Aronson S, Backstrom A: A comparison between mouth and nose breathers with respect to occlusion and facial dimensions. Odontologisk Revy 11:343–376, 1960.

Linder-Aronson S: Dimensions of face and palate in nose breathers habitual mouth breathers. Odontologisk Revy 14:187–200, 1963.

Linder-Aronson S: Respiratory function in relation to facial morphology and the dentition. Br J Orthodont 6:59–71, 1979.

Linthicum H, Boyd H, Keaster J: Incidence of middle ear disease in children with cleft palate. Cleft Palate Bull 9:23–25, 1959.

Loeb W: Speech, hearing, and the cleft palate. Arch Otolaryngol 79:4–14, 1964.

Longacre J: Congenital atresia of the oropharynx. Plast Reconstr Surg 8:341–348, 1951.

Lowry R, Courtemanche A, MacDonald C: Submucous cleft palate and the general practitioner. Can Med Assoc J 109:995–997, 1973.

Lubit D: Before an adenoidectomy: Stop! Look! Listen! N Y State J Med 67:681–685, 1967.

Luce E, McGibbon B, Hoopes H: Velopharyngeal insufficiency in hemifacial microsomia. Plast Reconstr Surg 60:602–606, 1977.

MacKenzie J: Some remarks on anomalies of the uvula, with special reference to double uvula. Johns Hopkins Hosp Rep 2, 1:32–36, 1890.

Mason R, Warren D: Adenoid involution and developing hypernasality in cleft palate. J Speech Hear Dis 45:469–480, 1980.

Mason R: Preventing speech disorders following adenoidectomy by preoperative examination. Clin Pediatr 12:405–414, 1973.

Massengill R, Fetterolf J: A cleft palate condition not easily detected during routine examination. Folia Phoniatrica 20:7–12, 1968.

Massengill R, Quinn G: Adenoidal atrophy, velopharyngeal incompetence and sucking exercises: A two year follow-up case report. Cleft Palate J 11:196–199, 1974.

Massengill R, Pickrell K, Robinson M: Results of pushback operations in treatment of submucous cleft palate. Plast Reconstr Surg 51:432–435, 1973.

Mattucci K: Cleft palate patient: Otologic management. N Y State J Med 79:333–339, 1979.

Maue-Dickson W: Cleft lip and palate research: An updated state of the art. Section II. Anatomy and physiology. Cleft Palate J 14:270–287, 1977.

Maue-Dickson W: The craniofacial complex in cleft lip and palate: An updated review of anatomy and function. Cleft Palate J 16:291–317, 1979.

Maue-Dickson W, Dickson D: Anatomy and physiology related to cleft palate: Current research and clinical implications. Plast Reconstr Surg 65, 1:83–90, 1980.

Maue-Dickson W, Dickson D, Rood S: Anatomy of the eustachian tube and related structures in age-matched human fetuses with and without cleft palate. Trans Am Acad Ophthalmol Otolaryngol 82:159–163, 1976.

Mazaheri M, Millard R, Erickson D: Cineradiographic comparison of normal to noncleft subjects with velopharyngeal inadequacy. Cleft Palate J 1:199–209, 1964.

McCoy F, Zahorsky C: A new approach to the elusive dynamic pharyngeal flap. Plast Reconstr Surg 49, 2:160–164, 1972.

McNamara J: Influence of respiratory pattern on craniofacial growth. Angle Orthodont 51, 4:269–300, 1981.

McNamara J (ed): "Naso-respiratory Function and Craniofacial Growth." Monograph 9, Craniofacial Growth Series, Center for Human Growth and Development, University of Michigan, Ann Arbor, 1979.

McWilliams B, Musgrave R: Differential diagnosis and management of hypernasal voices in children. Trans Am Acad Ophthalmol Otolaryngol March–April, 1965, pp 322–331.

Means J: Clefts of the hard and soft palate. S Med Rec 24:24, 1894.

Meskin L, Gorlin R, Isaacson R: Abnormal morphology of the soft palate: I. The prevalence of cleft uvula. Cleft Palate J 1, 3:342–346, 1964.

Meskin L, Gorlin R, Isaacson R: Abnormal morphology of the soft palate: II. The genetics of cleft uvula. Cleft Palate J 2, 1:40–45, 1965.

Meskin L, Gorlin R, Isaacson J: Cleft uvula—A microform of cleft palate. Acta Chirurgiae Plasticae 8, 2:91–95, 1966.

Metcalf C: Two palatal anomalies. Boston Med Surg J 159:409–410, 1908.

Meyerson M, Foushee D: Speech, language and hearing in Moebius syndrome: A study of 22 patients. Dev Med Child Neurol 20:357–365, 1978.

Miller M: Hearing problems associated with cleft palate. Ann Otol Rhinol Laryngol 68:90–99, 1959.

Minami R, Kaplan E, Wu G, Jobe R: Velopharyngeal incompetence without overt cleft palate. Plast Reconstr Surg 55, 5:573–587, 1975.

Mitts T, Garrett W, Hurwitz D: Cleft of the hard palate with soft palate integrity. Cleft Palate J 18, 3:204–206, 1981.

Morris H, Krueger L, Bumsted R: Indications of congenital palatal incompetence before diagnosis. Ann Otol Rhinol Laryngol 91:115–118, 1982.

Morris H: The speech pathologist looks at the tonsils and the adenoids. Ann Otol Rhinol Laryngol Supplement 19, 84, 2:63–66, 1975.

Mullendore J, Stoudt R: Speech patterns of muscular dystrophic individuals. J Speech Hear Dis 26:252–257, 1961.

Nathanson M: Palatal myoclonus. Arch Neurol Psychiatry 75:285–296, 1956.

Neiman G, Simpson R: A roentgencephalometric investigation of the effect of adenoid removal upon selected measures of velopharyngeal function. Cleft Palate J 12:377–389, 1975.

Nelson F: Eustachian tube anatomy and physiology in cleft palate. In: Graham M (ed): "Cleft Palate: Middle Ear Disease and Hearing Loss." Springfield, IL: C.C. Thomas, 1978.

Netsell R: Evaluation of velopharyngeal function in dysarthria. J Speech Hear Dis 34, 2: 113–122, 1969.

Netsell R: The velopharynx in perspective. Symposium of Treatment of the Velopharynx for Individuals with Dysarthria. Boys Town National Institute, May, 1983.

Newcomb J: Anatomical defects in the faucial pillars. Laryngoscope 2:220–224, 1897.

Noll JD: Remediation of impaired resonance among patients with neuropathologies of speech. In: Lass N, McReynolds L, Northern J, Yoder D (eds): "Speech, Language and Hearing, Vol. II: Pathologies of Speech and Language." Philadelphia: W.B. Saunders, 1982, pp 556–571.

Ohmann-Dumesmil A: Congenital cleft uvula—report of a case. Laryngoscope 3:217–218, 1897.

Oldfield M, McNaughton I: Congenital abnormalities of the pillars of the fauces and the action of the posterior pillars and nasopharyngeal valve during speech. J Laryngol Otol 61:594–600, 1946.

O'Ryan F, Gallagher D, LeBanc J, Epker B: The relation between nasorespiratory function and dentofacial morphology: A review. Am J Orthodont 83, 5:403–410, 1982.

Owsley J, Chierici G, Miller E, Lawson L, Blackfield H: Cephalometric evaluation of palatal dysfunction in patients without overt cleft palate. Plast Reconstr Surg 39:562–568, 1967.

Panis R: Adenotonsillektomie bei Kindern mit Kippen-Kiefer-Gaumen-Spalte (LKS). Indikation, Ausfuhrung und Ergebnisse von 20 Operationen. Laryngologie, Rhinologie, Otologie 59/2:83–87, 1980.

Paradise J, Bluestone C: Toward rational indications for tonsil and adenoid surgery. Hosp Pract 11, 2:79–87, 1976.

Paradise J: Clinical trials of tonsillectomy and adenoidectomy: Limitations of existing studies and a current effort to evaluate efficacy. S Med J 69, 8:1049–1053, 1976.

Paradise J: Tonsillectomy and adenoidectomy. In: Bluestone C, Stool S (eds): "Pediatric Otolaryngology, Vol. II." Philadelphia: W.B. Saunders, 1983.

Paradise J: Why T&A remains moot. Pediatrics 49:648–651, 1972.

Parkins F, Barbero G: The oral cavity. In: Vaughan V, McKay R (eds): "Nelson's Textbook of Pediatrics." Philadelphia: W.B. Saunders Co., 1975.

Passavant G: Ueber die Beseitigung der naselnden Sprache bei angeborenen Spalten des harten und Weichen Gaumens. Archiv fuer Klinisch Chirurgie 6:333–349, 1865.

Passavant G: Zweiter Artikel uber die operation der angeborenen Spalten des harten Gaumens und der damit complicirten Hasenscharten. Archiv Heilkunde 3:305–338, 1862.

Peterson-Falzone S: Nasal distortions and compensatory articulations in velopharyngeal competent speakers. Presented before the 4th International Congress on Cleft Palate and Related Craniofacial Anomalies, Acapulco, May, 1981.

Peterson S: Nasal emission as a component of the misarticulation of sibilants and affricates. J Speech Hear Dis 40:106–114, 1975.

Pickrell K, Massengill R, Quinn G, Brooks R, Robinson M: The effect of adenoidectomy on velopharyngeal competence in cleft palate patients. Br J Plast Surg 29:134–136, 1976.

Pigott R: The nasendoscopic appearance of the normal palato-pharyngeal valve. Plast Reconstr Surg 43:19–24, 1969.

Pigott R, Benson J, White R: Nasendoscopy in the diagnosis of velo-pharyngeal incompetence. Plast Reconstr Surg 43:141–147, 1969.

Pitt M, Ingram T: The radiology of speech disorders in childhood: Part I: Disorders and their study. Radiography 41, 483:53–59, 1975.

Pitt M, Ingram T: The radiology of speech disorders in childhood: Part II: Radiology in the diagnosis of speech disorders. Radiography 41, 484, 1975:90–104.

Pollack M, Shprintzen R: Velopharyngeal insufficiency in neurofibromatosis. Int Pediatr Otorhinolaryngol 3:257–262, 1981.

Pollack M, Shprintzen R, Zimmerman-Manchester K: Velopharyngeal insufficiency: The neurological perspective. A report of 32 cases. Dev Med Child Neurol 21:194–201, 1979.

Porterfield H, Mohler S, Sandel A: Submucous cleft palate. Plast Reconstr Surg 58, 1:60–65, 1976.

Porterfield H, Trabue J, Terry J, Stimpert R: Hypernasality in noncleft palate patients. Plast Reconstr Surg 37, 3:216–220, 1966.

Pruzansky S: Congenital palatopharyngeal incompetence: Clinical, radiographic and genetic studies. J

Dent Res 47:1013, 1968.
Pruzansky S: Contributions of roentgenographic cephalometry to the study of congenital and acquired malformations of the face. Dent Clin N Am 1960, pp 395–417.
Pruzansky S: Peterson-Falzone S, Laffer J, Parris P: Hypernasality in the absence of overt cleft: Commentary on nomenclature, diagnosis, classification and research design. Presented before the 3rd International Congress on Cleft Palate and Related Craniofacial Anomalies, Toronto, 1977.
Pruzansky S: Roentgencephalometric studies of tonsils and adenoids in normal and pathologic states. Ann Otol Rhinol Laryngol [Suppl] 19, 84, 2:55–62, 1975.
Pruzansky S: The role of the orthodontist in a cleft palate team. Plast Reconstr Surg 14,1:10–29, 1954.
Quick C, Gundlach K: Adenoid facies. Laryngoscope 88:327–333, 1978.
Randall P, Bakes F, Kennedy C: Cleft palate-type speech in the absence of cleft palate. Plast Reconstr Surg 25, 2:484–495, 1960.
Rees T, Wood-Smith D, Swinyard C, Converse J: Electromyographic evaluation of submucous cleft palate: A possible aid to operative planning. Plast Reconstr Surg 50, 6:592–594, 1967.
Richstein A, Jonas I: Offenes Naseln nach operativen Eingriffen im Oro- und Nasopharynx. Arch Oto-Rhino-Laryngol 232:29–41, 1981.
Ricketts R: The cranial base and soft structures in cleft palate speech and breathing. Plast Reconstr Surg 14, 1:47–61, 1954.
Riley H, Brock S: Rhythmic myoclonus of the muscles of the palate, larynx and other regions: Clinical report of three cases. Arch Neurol Psychiatry 29:726–741, 1933.
Roberts W: Speech defects following adenotonsillectomy. Rocky Mountain Med J 56:67–69, 1959.
Rood S, Doyle W: The nasopharyngeal orifice of the auditory tube: Implications for tubal dynamics anatomy. Cleft Palate J 19, 2:119–128, 1982.
Rosenbek J, LaPointe L: The dysarthrias: Description, diagnosis and treatment. In: Johns D (ed): "Clinical Management of Neurogenic Communicative Disorders." Boston: Little, Brown, 1978.
Roux JP: Memoire sue la Staphylorraphie, ou Suture du Voile du Palais. J.S. Chaude, 1825.
Roux JP: (untitled) Lancet 1:694, 1835.
Rubin L: The Moebius syndrome: Bilateral facial diplegia. Clin Plast Surg 3, 4:625–636, 1976.
Saad E: The bifid uvula in ear, nose and throat practice. Laryngoscope 85, 4:734–737, 1975.
Saad E: The underdeveloped palate in ear, nose and throat practice. Laryngoscope 90:1371–1377, 1980.
Sataloff J, Fraser M: Hearing loss in children with cleft palates. AMA Arch Otolaryngol 55:61–64, 1952.
Scammon R, Harris J, Jackson C: "The Measurement of Man." Minneapolis: University of Minnesota Press, 1930.
Schweiger J, Netsell R, Sommerfeld R: Prosthetic management and speech improvement in individuals with dysarthria of the palate. J Am Dent Assoc 80:1348–1353, 1970.
Sedlackova E: Insufficiency of the palatolaryngeal passage disorder. Casopis Lekaru Ceskych (Prague) 94:1304–1307, 1955.
Sedlackova E, Lastova M, Sram R: Contribution to knowledge of soft palate innervation. Folia Phoniatrica 25:434–441, 1973.
Seemann M: Contribution a la pathogenic et la symptomatologie de la fissure sous-muqueuse du palais osseux. Archives Internationales de Laryngologie, 30:388–402, 1924.
Seghers M: Une malformation rare: L'imperforation oropharyngienne. Acta Paediatrica Belgique 20:130–137, 1966.
Seif S, Dellon A: Anatomic relationships between the human levator and tensor veli palatini and the eustachian tube. Cleft Palate J 15, 4:329–336, 1978.
Severeid L: Longitudinal study of the efficacy of adenoidectomy in children with cleft palate and secretory otitis media. Trans Am Acad Ophthalmol Otolaryngol 76:1319–1324, 1972.
Severeid L: Pharyngeal disease and velopharyngeal competency and their relationship to ear disease and hearing loss. In: Graham M (ed): "Cleft Palate: Middle Ear Disease and Hearing Loss." Springfield, IL: C.C. Thomas, 1978.
Shapiro B, Meskin L, Cervenka J, Pruzansky S: Cleft uvula: A microform of facial clefts and its genetic basis. Birth Defects: Original Article Series VII, 7:80–82, 1971.
Shapiro R: Velopharyngeal insufficiency starting at puberty without adenoidectomy. Int J Pediatr Otorhinolaryngol 2:255–260, 1980.
Shprintzen R, Croft C: Abnormalities of the eustachian tube orifice in individuals with cleft palate. Int J Pediatr Otorhinolaryngol 3:15–23, 1981.
Shprintzen R, Croft C, Berkman M, Rakoff S: Velo-pharyngeal insufficiency in the facio-auriculo-vertebral malformation complex. Cleft Palate J 18:132–143, 1980.

Shprintzen R, Goldberg R, Lewin M, Sidoti E, Berkman M, Argamaso R, Young D: A new syndrome involving cleft palate, cardiac anomalies, typical facies, and learning disabilities: Velo-cardio-facial syndrome. Cleft Palate J 15:56–62, 1978.

Shprintzen R, Rakoff S, Skolnick M, Lavorato A: Incongruous movements of the velum and lateral pharyngeal walls. Cleft Palate J 14, 2:148–157, 1977.

Shprintzen F, Schwartz R, Daniller A, Hoch L: The morphologic significance of bifid uvula: Is it a marker for submucous cleft palate? Presented before the American Cleft Palate Association, Indianapolis, May, 1983.

Shufeldt R: Two uvulae in a man. N Y Med J 41(June 27):723–724, 1885.

Shy G, Carmichael E: Persistent rhythmic contractions of the ipsilateral pharynx, larynx, vocal cord, face and arm following trauma. Proc R Soc Med 42:65–66, 1949.

Skolnik E: Otologic evaluation in cleft palate patients. Laryngoscope 68:1908–1949, 1958.

Smiley G: A possible genesis for cleft palate formation. Plast Reconstr Surg 50:930–393, 1972.

Somers L: Bifid uvula with degeneracy. N Y Med J 64(November 21):683–684, 1896.

Spencer H: Pharyngeal and laryngeal "nystagmus." Lancet 2:702, 1886.

Starr C, Meskin L, Shapiro B, Weist K: Nasality and cleft uvula. Cleft Palate J 8:189–195, 1971.

Stewart J, Ott J, LaGace R: Submucous cleft palate. Birth Defects: Original Article Series VII, 7:64–66, 1971.

Stimson G: Congenital insufficiency of the palate. JAMA February 13, 1909, p 559.

Stool S, Beery Q: Diagnosis and treatment of ear disease in cleft palate children. In: Bzoch K (ed): "Communicative Disorders Related to Cleft Lip and Palate." 2nd edition. Boston: Little, Brown, 1979.

Stueber K, Wilhelmsen H: Use of the pharyngeal flap in the treatment of congenital velopharyngeal incompetence. Plast Reconstr Surg 73, 2:219–222, 1984.

Sturim H, Jacob C: Teflon pharyngoplasty. Plast Reconstr Surg 49, 2:180–185, 1972.

Subtelny J, Koepp-Baker H: The significance of adenoid tissue in velopharyngeal function. Plast Reconstr Surg 17, 3:235–250, 1956.

Subtelny J: A cephalometric study of the growth of the soft palate. Plast Reconstr Surg 19, 1:49–62, 1957.

Swanson P, Luttrell C, Magladery J: Myoclonus: A report of 67 cases and review of the literature. Medicine 41:339–356, 1962.

Szabo S, Rehak G, Hirschberg J: Phoniatrische und kieferothopadische Untersuchungen in Fallen mit kongenital verkurztem Gaumensegel. XVIth Int Congr Logoped Phoniatr Interlaken, 1974, pp 478–482 (published by Karger, Basel, 1976).

Thaler S, Smith H: Submucous cleft palate. Arch Otolaryngol 88:184–189, 1968.

Tolarova M, Havlova Z, Ruzickova J: Distribution of signs considered as microforms of lip and/or palate clefts in normal population of 3 to 6 year old individuals. Acta Chirurgiae Plasticae 9:184–194, 1967.

Tolarova M, Havlova Z, Ruzickova J: The distribution of characters considered to be microforms of cleft lip and/or palate in a population of normal 18–21-year-old subjects. Acta Chirurgiae Plasticae 91:1–14, 1967b.

Trelat U: Imperfect intonation and its cause. Lancet I:553, 1870a.

Trelat U: Malformation de la voute et la voile du palais. Circonstances exceptionelles. Bull Soc Chir Paris 8:450, 1868. Also appeared in Am J Dent Sci 1:608, 1867.

Trelat U: Vice de conformation du voile dupalais—etiologie rapport entre la brievete de la voute palatine et la cacophonie special. Bull Soc Chir Paris 10:1870b. (Also appeared in Dental Cosmos 12:329, 1870.)

Trier W: Velopharngeal incompetency in the absence of overt cleft palate: Anatomic and surgical considerations. Cleft Palate J 20, 3:209–217, 1983.

Trost J: Articulatory additions to the classical description of the speech of persons with cleft palate. Cleft Palate Journal 18, 3:193–203, 1981a.

Trost J: Differential diagnosis of velopharyngeal disorders. Commun Dis 6, 7(July):1981b.

van Bogaert L, Bertrand I: Sur les myoclonies associees synchrones et rythmiques par lesions enfoyer du trone cerebral. Revue Neurologique 1:203–214, 1928.

Van Gelder L: Open nasal speech following adenoidectomy and tonsillectomy. J Commun Dis 7:263–267, 1974.

Veau V: "Division Palatine." Paris: Masson et Cie, 1931.

Vinicoff A: Clinical evaluation of cleft palate patients and their speech. Plast Reconstr Surg 25, 5:496–502, 1960.

Vrticka K: La fermeture velo-pharingee avant et apres la tonsillectomie et l'adenoidectomie. Bull Audimophonol 7, 3:95–106, 1977.

Wallner L, Hill B, Waldrop W, Monroe C: Voice changes following adenotonsillectomy: A study of velar function by cinefluorography and video tape. Laryngoscope 8: 1410–1418, 1968.

Warren D, Bevin A, Winslow R: Posterior pillar webbing and palatopharyngeus displacement: Possible causes of congenital incompetence. Cleft Palate J 15, 1:68–72, 1978.

Warren D, Duany I, Fischer N: Nasal pathway resistance in normal and cleft lip and palate subjects. Cleft Palate J 6:134–140, 1969.

Weatherley-White RCA, Sakura C, Brenner L, Stewart J, Ott J: Submucous cleft palate: Its incidence, natural history and indications for treatment. Plast Reconstr Surg 49:297–304, 1972.

Weatherley-White RCA: Submucous cleft palate. In: Calana J (ed): "Recent Advances in Plastic Surgery, I." Edinburgh: Churchill Livingstone, 1976.

Weber J, Chase R: Stress velopharyngeal incompetence in an oboe player. Cleft Palate J 7:858–861, 1970.

Weinberg B, Bosma J, Shanks J, DeMyer W: Mytonic dystrophy initially manifested by speech disability. J Speech Hear Dis 33:51–59, 1968.

Wertz R: Neuropathologies of speech and language: An introduction to patient management. In: John D (ed): "Clinical Management of Neurogenic Communicative Disorders." Boston: Little, Brown, 1978.

Whaley J: The otolaryngologist's role in the case of the cleft palate patient. J Can Dent Assoc 23:547–575, 1957.

Winters H: "Congenital Short Palate." Lochem, 1975.

Winters H: Some historical remarks on congenital short palate. Br J Plast Surg 19, 4:308–312, 1966.

Wolski W: Hypernasality as the presenting symptom of myasthenia gravis. J Speech Hear Dis 32, 1:36–38, 1967.

Worster-Drought C: Congenital suprabulbar paresis. J Laryngol Otol 70:453–463, 1956.

Worster-Drought C: Speech disorders in children. Dev Med Child Neurol 10:427–440, 1968.

IV. CEPHALOMETRIC STUDIES

Contrasting Mandibular Growth and Facial Development In Long Face Syndrome, Juvenile Rheumatoid Polyarthritis, and Mandibulofacial Dysostosis

Arne Björk and Vibeke Skieller
Institute of Orthodontics, Royal Dental College, Copenhagen, Denmark

The complex rotation process of the mandible during growth is elucidated by longitudinal roentgencephalometric analyses, using metallic implants as fixed references. Contrasting development of face and mandibular shape is described in three subjects. In the so-called long face syndrome, development is characterized by increasing inclination of the mandible during growth with only moderate remodeling. In the subjects with juvenile rheumatoid polyarthritis and mandibulofacial dysostosis, the increase in mandibular inclination is moderate. However, the mandibular corpus rotates backward to an extreme extent within the more stable soft tissue matrix, giving rise to the characteristic development of angular notching with an extended angular process at the lower border.

Key words: roentgencephalometry, growth analysis, long face syndrome, juvenile rheumatoid polyarthritis, mandibulofacial dysostosis

INTRODUCTION

With the introduction of the metallic implant technique, where small tantalum pins are inserted into the jaws as fixed reference points, more precise information of facial growth in humans could be obtained from longitudinal cephalometric radiographs [Björk, 1968]. The most striking feature of facial development, as seen from profile radiographs, is the considerable rotary movement of the bony jaws during growth, forward or backward, within the soft tissue matrix and that the shape of the jaws normally is kept stable by the associated substantial surface remodeling [Björk and Skieller, 1972, 1976]. The rotation of the maxillary and of the mandibular corpus inside the soft tissue matrix is termed intramatrix rotation [Björk and Skieller, 1983].

The present paper describes complex facial development in three cases of backward rotation, where two different types of facial development were distinguished.

COMPONENTS OF MANDIBULAR ROTATION

Backward growth rotation of the face has generally been considered simply to be backward rotation of the mandible with the center of rotation at the condyles.

Address reprint requests to Arne Björk, Professor, Odont. Dr., Institute of Orthodontics, Royal Dental College, Jagtvej 160, DK - 2100 Copenhagen, Denmark.

However, facial development in backward-rotating cases often does not show a single growth pattern, but is in fact composed of a wide variety of complex maxillary and mandibular rotations.

The complex rotation processes are more readily understood if the bony mandibular corpus and its soft tissue covering—the matrix—are regarded as two independent systems capable of independent rotary movements during growth. In order to understand the different patterns of mandibular rotation, the rotation has been divided into three components.

Matrix rotation refers to the rotation of the soft tissue matrix of the mandible relative to the anterior cranial base. On profile radiographs the soft tissue matrix is defined by a tangential line to the lower border of the mandible [Björk, 1947]. A backward change in inclination of the tangential line relative to the anterior cranial base is designated as positive. The matrix rotation is sometimes forward and sometimes backward in the same subject during the growth period with the condyles as the center of rotation and can thus be described as a pendulum movement. This is schematically illustrated in Figure 1a.

Intramatrix rotation expresses the growth rotation of the mandibular corpus within its soft tissue matrix and can be measured by the changing inclination of the implant line in the mandibular corpus relative to the tangential mandibular line. Backward intramatrix rotation is designated as positive when the implant line rotates backward relative to the tangential mandibular line.

The center of backward intramatrix rotation is situated somewhere in the corpus, possibly at the most posterior occluding molars, and not at the condyles. When the mandibular corpus rotates backward within the matrix, the anterior part of the corpus is pressed downward into the soft tissue matrix, resulting in resorption at the lower

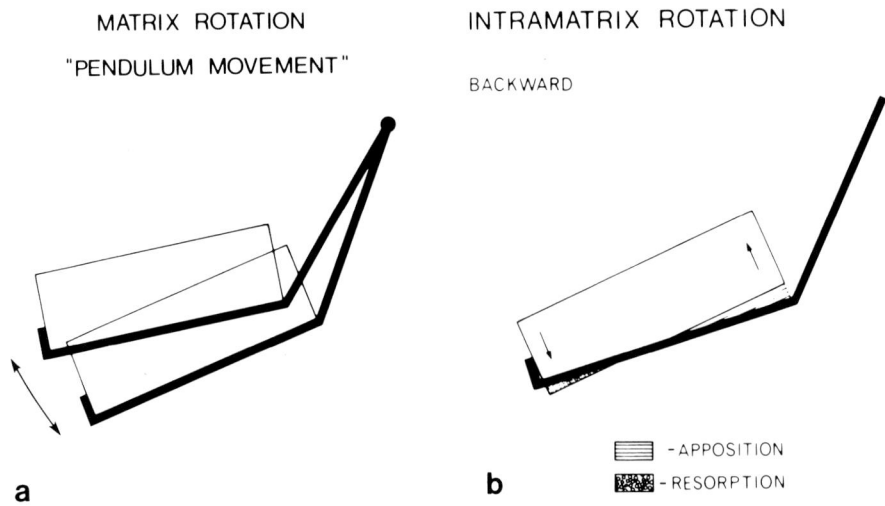

Fig. 1. a. Changes in inclination of the lower border of the mandible in the face during growth express a rotation of the soft tissue matrix. The matrix rotation often shows a pendulum movement with the center at the condyles. b. Intramatrix rotation represents a rotation of the mandibular corpus within its matrix. Backward intramatrix rotation results in resorption below the symphysis and apposition below the angle. Apposition may occur at the chin point. The center of rotation is situated in the corpus.

surface of the symphysis. The posterior part of the corpus is lifted up from its soft tissue matrix, stretching the periosteum, with which apposition takes place below the mandibular angle. The angular notching and the extended angular process is thus an expression of the remodeling processes associating intramatrix rotation, schematically illustrated in Figure 1b.

Usually, the *intramatrix rotation* is considerable, while the matrix rotation is moderate and may even be in the opposite direction.

Total rotation is defined as change in inclination of the implant line in the mandibular corpus relative to the anterior cranial base during growth. Backward rotation of the implant line is designated as positive. Total rotation is the sum of matrix and intramatrix rotations. The total rotation is dependent on a combination of the rotation centers of its two components.

FACIAL DEVELOPMENT IN BACKWARD-ROTATING CASES

Two distinct types of facial development will be described in three cases.

Long Face Syndrome (Case 7176)

This girl shown in Figure 2 represents what has been called a high-angle case or long face syndrome. Metallic implants were inserted in both jaws at the age of 9 years, and facial development was followed yearly. At the age of 17 years, facial growth was completed, and orthodontic treatment of the open bite was instituted with extraction of all first permanent molars. Treatment was finished at the age of 20 years and the last examination took place at 30 years of age.

In the facial tracing (Fig. 3a), the inclination of the implant line at three stages indicates a marked backward total rotation of the mandibular corpus relative to the anterior cranial base. There is virtually no change in the position of the temporomandibular fossae in the cranial base. The symphysis moved forward and was lowered in

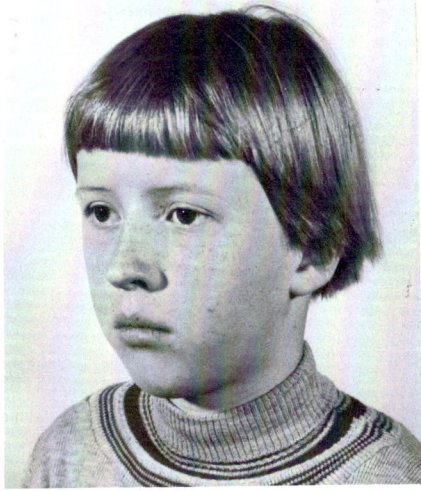 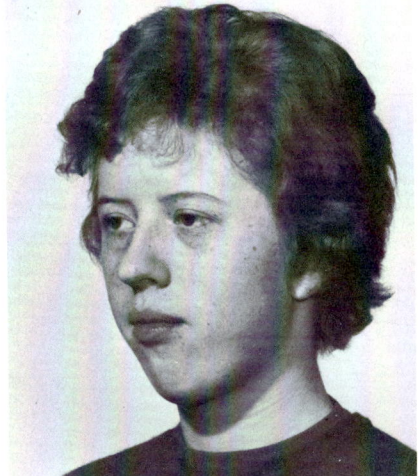

Fig. 2. Case 7176: Photographs at 9 years, 3 months, and at 24 years, 6 months, of a girl with long face syndrome.

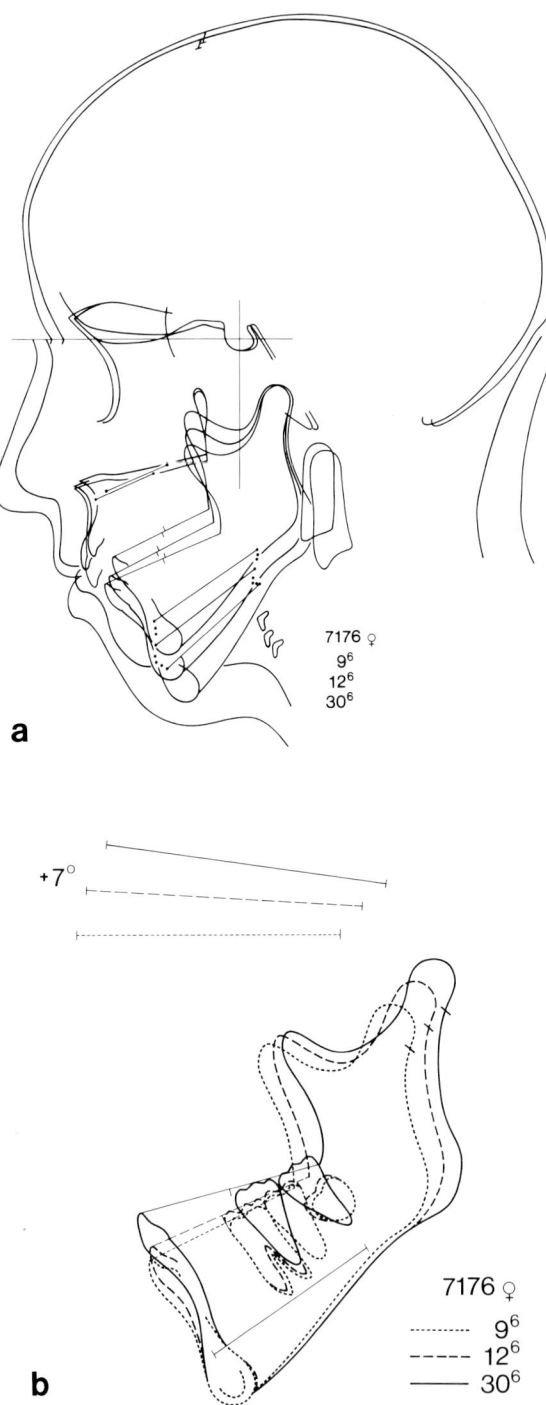

Fig. 3. Case 7176: a. Craniofacial tracing with the implant line at three stages. Dots indicate the yearly position of the implants. b. Mandibular tracing from three stages superimposed on the implant line.

the face while condylar growth was taking place. During the treatment period the symphysis did not move forward but continued to be lowered.

During the observation period the total backward rotation of the mandible was +7 degrees, expressed by the rotation of the implant line relative to the anterior cranial base. The dominating component was a backward matrix rotation of +5 degrees. Added to this, an intramatrix rotation of the mandibular corpus within its matrix occurred by +2 degrees.

In the mandibular tracing (Fig. 3b), the nasion-sella line at the three stages illustrate the total rotation of + 7 degrees backward. Considerable backward-directed growth took place at the condyles associated with marked apposition along the entire posterior border of the ramus and marked resorption at the anterior border. The apposition below the angular region is a result of the moderate backward intramatrix rotation, which lifted up the posterior part of the corpus from its matrix. As is often the case in backward-rotating subjects of the matrix-rotation type, the symphysis was slender and of considerable height. The alveolar prognathism decreased during the growth period.

The backward rotation comprises the entire skull (Fig. 3a). Determined from the implant line in the maxilla, the maxillary corpus rotated backward +1 degree and the calvaria was raised with an increase in height of 5 mm from bregma to the odontoid process of the epistropheus.

Facial growth in this case represents an extreme example of normal variation in facial physiognomy and illustrates facial development in which the dominating factor was backward matrix rotation, with only a small amount of backward intramatrix rotation.

Juvenile Rheumatoid Polyarthritis (Case 1988)

A different type of backward rotating face is seen with hypoplastic growth at the mandibular condyles in Stills' disease. The facial development in a girl with juvenile rheumatoid polyarthritis was followed annually from 8 to 17 years of age. Both mandibular condyles were affected with increasing restriction of jaw movements. Assimilation of the atlas and fusion of the upper vertebrae limited movements of the head. The skeleton as a whole was seriously affected, gradually making walking impossible.

The face was malformed (Fig. 4) and the mandible was extremely retrognathic and inclined backward. Metallic implants were inserted in both maxilla and mandible. In the facial profile tracing (Fig. 5a) the implant line is shown at first and last stage. The tracing gives the impression that only a minor positional change of the mandible took place. This relative stability, however, only concerns the soft tissue matrix, represented by the mandibular outline. As determined from the implants, forward movement of the mandible in the face was due mainly to lowering of the condylar fossae in the cranial base and only to a small extent to condylar growth. The prominence of the symphysis in the face increased further by apposition at the chin point, which is not seen in normal cases.

Marked resorption at the condylar head may occur in juvenile rheumatoid arthritis, as shown in longitudinal studies by Rönning and Väliaho [1981]. In the present case, only a small amount of condylar growth took place during the first half of the observation period, followed by resorption at the condyles in the second half. The symphysis changed its forward course in the face during the later observation period and was carried backwards, as seen from the implants in the facial tracing.

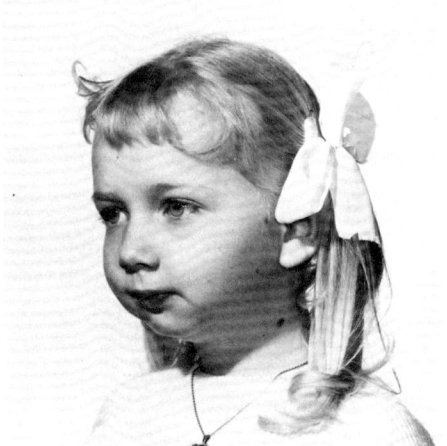 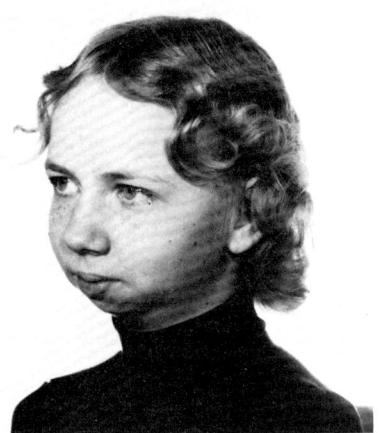

Fig. 4. Case 1988: Photographs at 8 years, 3 months, and at 17 years, 3 months, of a girl with juvenile rheumatoid polyarthritis.

The vertical development was even more dramatically seen from backward rotation of the implant line in the facial tracing. The posterior implant was raised, indicating an upward movement of the posterior part of the corpus relative to the matrix. As the implant lines from the two stages intersect in the corpus, the center of total rotation cannot be in the condyles and is dependent on a combination of the position of both matrix and intramatrix rotation centers.

The mandibular tracing, orientated on the implant line (Fig. 5b), shows remodeling of the entire mandible during rotation of the corpus within its matrix. The intramatrix rotation evidently has its center of rotation at the occlusal surface of the lower molars, which resulted in a downward movement of the symphysis into the soft tissue matrix with resorption at its lower border. At the chin point the symphysis was drawn backward from its matrix, resulting in apposition anteriorly at the chin. The photographs show that the rotation has led to a soft-tissue double chin typical of backward intramatrix rotation. Also as a result of the position of the intramatrix rotation center, the angular process is lifted out of its matrix, leading to apposition at the lower border in this area. There was considerable remodeling of the ramus with marked apposition along the entire posterior border, including the neck of the condylar process, and with extreme resorption anteriorly at the ramus, including the muscular process.

The eruption of the lower molars was hindered by the abnormal growth pattern, not allowing sufficient uprighting of the teeth to compensate for the rotation. The intermolar angle was acute, characteristic of backward rotation. There was compensatory increased eruption of the lower incisors and they became retroclined.

During the growth period, the matrix rotation was somewhat forward, returning to its original inclination at adult age (Fig. 5a). In contrast, the intramatrix rotation was directed continuously backward to an extreme value of +16 degrees at adult age. The total rotation thus amounted to +16 degrees at this age.

It is not known to what extent maxillary growth is primarily affected in this disease. The facial tracing shows a fairly normal amount of forward growth of the maxilla, more so than that of the mandible. From the maxillary implants and from

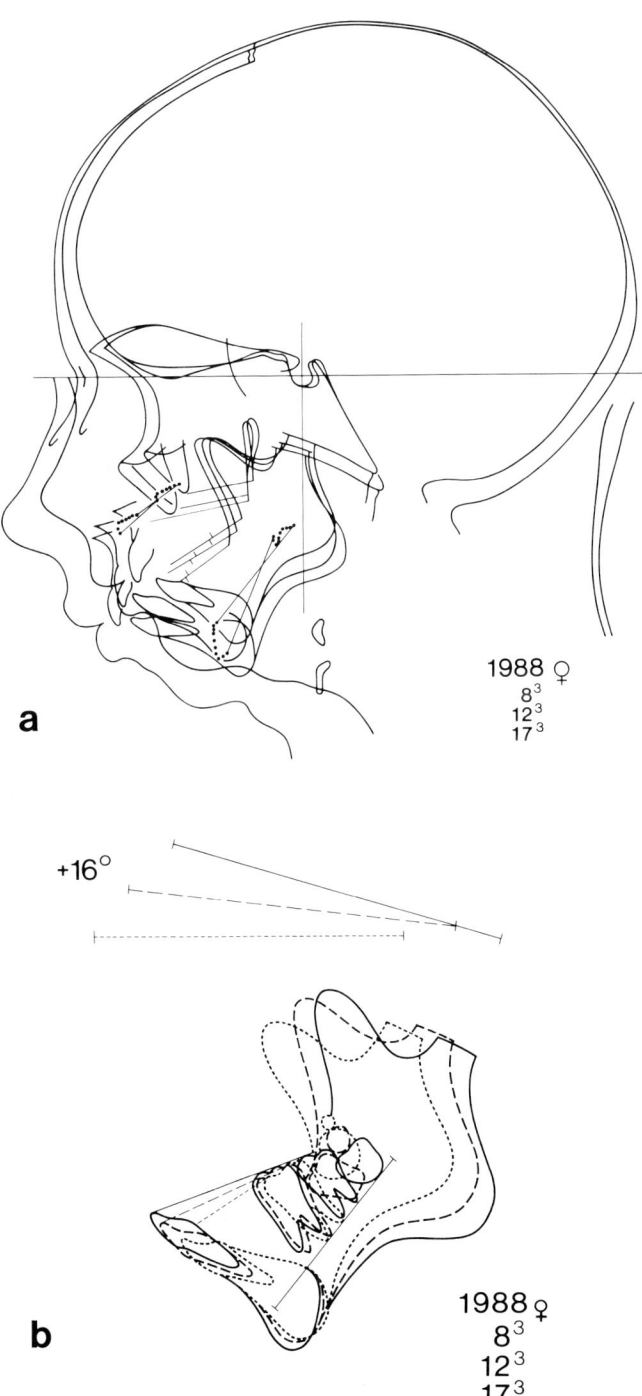

Fig. 5. Case 1988: a. Craniofacial tracing with implant line at three stages. Dots indicate the yearly position of the implant. b. Mandibular tracing from three stages superimposed on the implant line.

the inclination of the anterior surface of the zygomatic process, it is obvious that increasing backward rotation of the maxillary corpus took place, probably secondary to the rotation of the mandible.

Engel and Brodie [1947] pointed out the characteristic shape of the lower border of the mandible with angular notching in juvenile rheumatoid polyarthritis. Odenrick [1977] noted a general tendency for increased backward inclination of the mandible. The extreme extent to which the mandibular corpus could rotate backward within its matrix in this disease was first realized with the use of metallic implants [Björk, 1962].

Mandibulofacial Dysostosis (Case 2138)

Mandibular hypoplasia in a genetically transmitted craniofacial deformity is now discussed. Facial development in a boy with mandibulofacial dysostosis was followed yearly from 10 to 20 years of age with metallic implants in both jaws. Examination, including radiographs, showed the physical and skeletal symptoms characterizing this syndrome. The physiognomy is shown in Figure 6.

The mandibular condyles were small and ball-shaped. In contrast to the mandibular hypoplasia in juvenile polyarthritis, the condylar cartilage in this case retained its growing capacity although to a somewhat reduced degree. Movements of the mandible were unrestricted.

The profile radiographs show that the face is retrognathic with an extreme backward-inclined mandible (Fig. 7). The facial tracing (Fig. 8a) shows little change in the facial outline from the age of 10 years. The mandible appears to have been lowered in the face with little change in inclination as assessed from its lower border.

The protrusion of the mandible in the face during growth was due to three factors: lowering of the condylar fossae in the markedly bent cranial base, growth at the condyles, and marked apposition at the chin point. The vertical development of the mandible, as determined from the implant line, was complicated and was characterized by extreme backward total rotation of the corpus relative to the anterior cranial base. The anterior implant was continuously lowered in the face in a somewhat

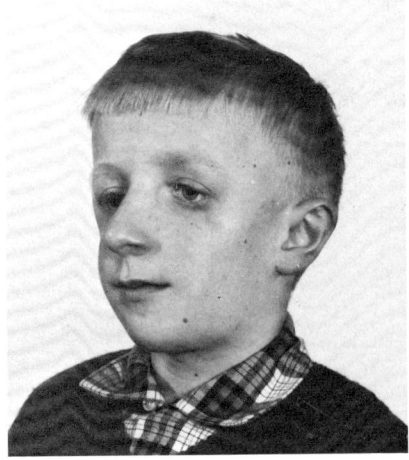
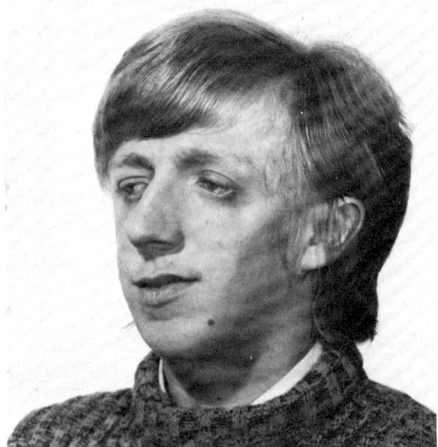

Fig. 6. Case 2138: Photographs at 10 years, 7 months, and at 20 years, 7 months, of a boy with mandibulofacial dysostosis.

Mandibular Growth in Three Syndromes 135

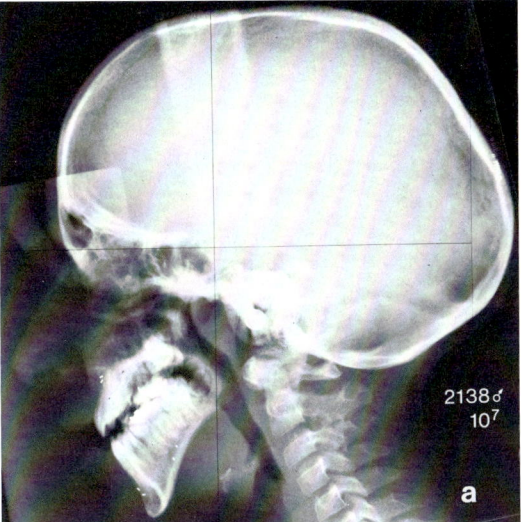

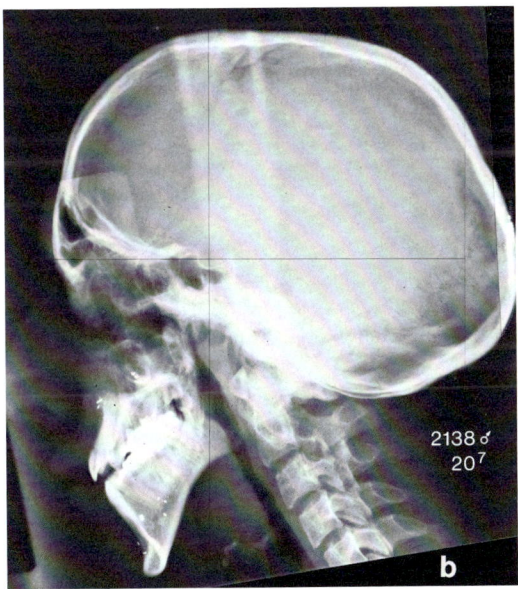

Fig. 7. Case 2138: Profile radiographs at a. 10 years, 7 months, and b. 20 years, 7 months.

backward direction. The lowering of the posterior implant followed an S-shaped course, at first forward, then forward and downward and finally slightly upward. On the facial tracing the implant lines from the three stages intersect, indicating that the backward intramatrix rotation constituted the greatest part of the total rotation, as in the case of juvenile polyarthritis.

The intramatrix rotation was directed backward by +13.5 degrees and the matrix rotation, also backward-directed, was only +2.5 degrees with a maximum at puberty. The small change in inclination of the lower border of the mandible is apparent from

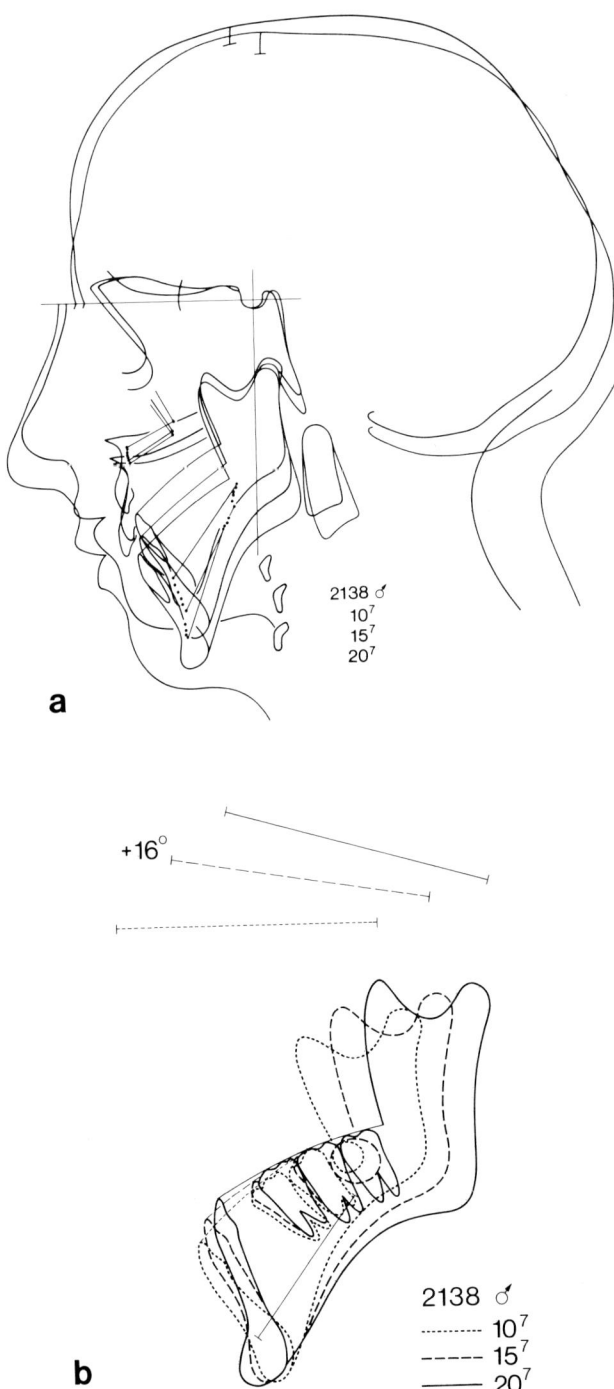

Fig. 8. Case 2138: a. Craniofacial tracing with the implant line at three stages. Dots indicate the yearly position of the implants. b. Mandibular tracing from three stages superimposed on the implant line.

the facial tracing. The total rotation, the sum of these components, increased to +16 degrees backward.

With the marked intramatrix rotation, considerable remodeling of the whole mandible took place. The mandibular corpus was rolled backward against the upper teeth (Fig. 8b). Thus, the intramatrix rotation had its center at the occlusal surface of the lower first molars and subsequently at the occlusal surface of the second molars.

Because of the short radius of rotation, the bony symphysis was pressed downward into the soft tissue matrix and somewhat retracted from the matrix at the chin point, resulting in resorption at the lower and posterior surface of the symphysis, while apposition took place at the anterior surface of the chin. Change in shape of the anterior surface of the symphysis can be seen in the profile radiographs.

The backward intramatrix rotation of the corpus lifted up the posterior part from its matrix, resulting in apposition posteriorly below the angular process.

The ramus was rotated forward and remodeled, with increased anterior resorption and marked posterior apposition by the intramatrix rotation. It is important to note that the remodeling affected the whole ramus, including the hypoplastic condylar heads. The limited cartilaginous growth at the condyles could not account for the large backward displacement seen in the mandibular tracing. As the condylar growth was reduced, the lack of cartilaginous growth was compensated by periosteal bone production.

The facial tracing shows a short upper face sagitally with a large anterior height. From the implant line it is seen that sutural growth in sagittal length of the maxilla was restricted and the maxillary corpus rotated markedly backward, as was also determined from the change in inclination of the anterior surface of the zygomatic process.The nasal floor was maintained parallel by compensatory remodeling. The typical shape of the nasal floor can, as described by Delaire [1974], be called a downward deflection of the maxillary base, a shape that seems to characterize the more pronounced backward rotating facial growth pattern.

From the mandibular tracing it is seen that the molars, secondary to the rotation, were forced distally with some uprighting. The compensatory eruption of the incisors was quite marked and also directed distally. The curve of Spee retained its characteristic reverse shape. The abnormal condylar growth hindered the eruption of the molars, and their roots consequently had to grow downward in the bone, which is not seen in normal development.

During development the calvaria seems to have been depressed downward-backward over the spinal column (Fig. 8a) with a diminishing height of 5 mm from bregma to the odontoid process of the epistropheus, a deformation that hypothetically could be related to the neck muscle system.

The shape of the lower border of the mandible during development in mandibulofacial dysostosis has been described by Roberts et al, [1975]. The anatomical aberration in this condition has been further studied on dry skulls from our collection [Dahl et al, 1975; Dahl and Björk, 1981].

The dominating factor in facial development in this and in the previous case of mandibular hypoplasia is an extreme intramatrix rotation of the mandibular corpus within the soft tissue matrix, leading to the characteristic shape of the lower border.

CONCLUSION

The aberrant growth pattern in craniofacial deformities can best be detected roentgencephalometrically by using metallic implants as references, which justifies their use in pathological cases. It is obvious that orthodontic or surgical treatment must be planned with due consideration of the specific growth patterns.

ACKNOWLEDGMENTS

This study was supported in part by grants from the Danish Medical Research Foundation and the Danish Dental Association.

REFERENCES

Björk A: The face in profile. An anthropological x-ray investigation in Swedish children and conscripts. Sven Tandlak Tidskr 40 [suppl]: 1947, 2nd printing, Odont. Bookshop, Copenhagen, 1972.

Björk A: Facial growth in bilateral hypoplasia of the mandibular condyles. A radiographic, cephalometric study of a case, using metallic implants. In Kraus BS, Riedel RA (eds): "Vistas in Orthodontics." Philadelphia: Lea & Febiger, 1962, pp 347–358.

Björk A: The use of metallic implants in the study of facial growth in children: Method and application. Am J Phys Anthropol 29:243–254, 1968.

Björk A, Skieller V: Facial development and tooth eruption. An implant study at the age of puberty. Am J Orthod 62:339–383, 1972.

Björk A, Skieller V: Postnatal growth and development of the maxillary complex. In McNamara Jr JA (ed): "Factors Affecting the Growth of the Midface." Ann Arbor, MI: Monograph Number 6, Craniofacial Growth Series, Center for Human Growth and Development, The University of Michigan, 1976, pp 61-99.

Björk A, Skieller V: Normal and abnormal growth of the mandible. A synthesis of longitudinal cephalometric implant studies over a period of 25 years. Eur J Orthod 5:1–46, 1983.

Dahl E, Björk A: Ossification defects and craniofacial morphology in incomplete forms of mandibulofacial dysostosis. A description of two dry skills. Cleft Palate J 18:83–89, 1981.

Dahl E, Kreiborg S, Björk A: A morphologic description of a dry skull with mandibulofacial dysostosis. Scand J Dent Res 83:257–266, 1975.

Delaire J: Considération sur l'accroissement du pré-maxillaire chez l'homme. Rev Stomatol 75:951–969, 1974.

Engel MB, Brodie AG: Condylar growth and mandibular deformities. Surgery 22:976–992, 1947.

Odenrich L: Potential micrognathia in children with juvenile rheumatoid arthritis. Trans Eur Orthod Soc 53:207–216, 1977.

Roberts FG, Pruzansky S, Aduss H: An X-radiocephalometric study of mandibulofacial dysostosis in man. Arch Oral Biol 20:265–281, 1975.

Rönning O, Väliaho M-L: Progress of mandibular condyle lesions in juvenile rheumatoid arthritis. Proc Finn Dent Soc 77:151–157, 1981.

A Morphometric Analysis of the Craniofacial Configuration in Achondroplasia

M. Michael Cohen, Jr, Geoffrey F. Walker, and Ceib Phillips

Dalhousie University, Halifax, Nova Scotia, Canada (M.M.C.), School of Dentistry, University of Michigan, Ann Arbor, (G.F.W.), and School of Dentistry, University of North Carolina, Chapel Hill, (C.P.)

Human achondroplasia can be viewed as an experimental model for studying the effects of abnormal endochondral bone formation on the development of the skull as a whole. In this study, lateral cephalograms of 25 adult males and 26 adult females with achondroplasia were converted to a two-dimensional coordinate model of craniofacial morphology and analyzed using 66 linear, angular, and area variables. Lateral cephalograms of 951 normal adults were used for comparison.

Two sample t-tests were used to compare achondroplastic cephalograms with normal cephalograms. Multivariate statistical analysis included Hotelling's T^2 and discriminant function analysis. Selected variables were graphed as profile patterns in which mean values were expressed as standard deviation units (Z scores) relative to the norm. Finally, Calcomp plots were used for visual inspection and for comparison of the average cephalometric tracings of male and female achondroplastic subjects with normal male and female subjects, respectively.

Significant findings in achondroplasia included enlarged calvaria, frontal bossing, large frontal sinuses, occipital prominence, normal anterior cranial base length, strikingly shortened posterior cranial base length, an acute cranial base angle, a short nasal bone that was deformed and depressed, short upper facial height, recessed maxilla, posterior tilt of the nasal floor, and a prognathic mandible that was anteriorly displaced but of normal size with a normal gonial angle and a high coronoid process.

The finding of normal anterior cranial base length in achondroplastic subjects was surprising since the cranial base is preformed in cartilage and hypoplasia and shortening would be expected. Since the brain is enlarged in achondroplasia, the expanding frontal lobes may possibly influence the growth of the anterior cranial base, since it is known to follow a neural pattern of growth.

Cribriform plate length was strikingly reduced, but anterior sphenoidal length was strikingly increased, compensating for the shortened cribriform plate length and suggesting that growth in the length of the anterior cranial base takes place primarily by adaptation at one site—namely, the sphenoethmoidal synchondrosis.

Strikingly short posterior cranial base length was interpreted as resulting from hypoplasia of bone that is preformed in cartilage with possible early closure of the spheno-occipital synchondrosis. The exaggerated closure of the cranial base angle in achondroplasia may be related to an increased brain size and possibly earlier than normal closure of the intersphenoidal synchondrosis.

The acute cranial base angle strongly suggests that the natural balance of the achondroplastic head on the spinal column tilts the face downward. The finding of an exaggerated

---

Address reprint requests to M. Michael Cohen, Jr., DMD, PhD, Dalhousie University, Halifax, Nova Scotia, Canada B3H 3J5.

© 1985 Alan R. Liss, Inc.

external bony protuberance on the occipital bone may also be related to head balance. The protuberance corresponds to the areas of muscle attachment of the rectus capitis posterior minor and rectus capitis posterior major muscles. These muscles aid in holding the head upright and in extension against resistance or gravity. With the heavy head load in achondroplastic subjects and the tendency of the face to tilt downward, increased neck muscle use may be responsible for the exaggerated bony occipital convexity. Since achondroplastic adults must hyperextend the head when interacting with normal adults throughout their lives, the increased muscle use may possibly explain why the bony protuberance reaches statistical significance only in achondroplastic adults.

Shortened maxillary length and upper facial height are probably related to hypoplastic growth of the nasal capsule, which is preformed in cartilage and would be expected to be affected in achondroplasia. The shortened, deformed, and depressed nasal bones are membranous in origin and would not be anticipated to be affected. The configuration of the nasal bone in achondroplasia probably results secondarily from two opposing tendencies—to dip in superiorly because of the hypoplastic nasal septum and to pull out inferiorly to uplift the nose. The posterior tilting of the nasal floor suggests an adaptation to a narrow nasopharyngeal airway. Since the acute cranial base angle constricts the nasopharynx, the posterior tilt allows a wider opening of the nasopharynx.

The normal mandibular length in achondroplasia can probably be related to the condylar cartilage that grows appositionally instead of interstitially, as the chondrocranium does. The mandibular prognathism found in achondroplasia, in spite of the finding of normal mandibular size, can be related to the more acute cranial base flexure. Thus, the mandible, of normal dimensions, is more anteriorly positioned than usual. The large coronoid process may be related to increased muscle stretch of the temporalis from an anteriorly placed mandible. It is also possible that the hyperextension of the achondroplastic head, necessary for interaction with other adults, results in a natural opening of the jaws, which is counteracted by increased use of the temporalis muscles among others.

Sex differences in the measurements of adult achondroplastic subjects were different than sex differences in the same measurements of normal subjects. Because of this finding, the data were subjected to multivariate analysis. Using Hotelling's T^2 as an indication of overall measurement differences between groups, there was good separation between normal male and female subjects, but poor separation between achondroplastic male and female subjects. Thus, the measurement differences produced by the pathologic conditions of achondroplasia totally override the normal male and female differences that are expected to occur.

Profile patterning of selected measurements showed that female achondroplastic subjects had more extreme values for several variables than male achondroplastic subjects. The reasons for the more extreme values and greater variability of female achondroplastic measurements in this study are obscure.

The biological interpretation of the differences between achondroplastic and normal subjects was consistent with the results of a stepwise discriminant function analysis. For example, the most discriminating variable with respect to achondroplastic males was the measurement from basion to the anterior nasal spine. In achondroplastic subjects, this dimension crosses a shortened maxilla, a hypoplastic cranial base, and an acutely flexed cranial base angle, all of which are strikingly abnormal and involved by the pathologic process.

Key words: achondroplasia, chondrodysplasia, cephalometric study, morphometric analysis

INTRODUCTION

The craniofacial configuration in achondroplasia is the subject of this investigation. Pruzansky has written:

> The skull is a community of bones and organ systems of diverse phylogenetic origin and variable patterns of development, altogether relating to several functions vital to the life and well-being of the

> organism. If in the course of development one
> member of this community is affected adversely,
> inevitably other parts will suffer [Pruzansky, 1973].

Nowhere is this more true than in achondroplasia, the most common form of short-limbed dwarfism. The disorder can be viewed as an experimental model for studying the effects of abnormal endochondral bone formation on the development of the skull as a whole.

METHODS

Achondroplastic Subjects

For the purposes of this study, achondroplastic dwarfs were recruited from Little People of America, a national organization of dwarfs. Lateral cephalograms were obtained for analysis at the 1969 national meeting in Minneapolis, Minnesota, and the 1970 national meeting in Portland, Oregon. A total of 104 cephalometric radiographs were taken on 93 chondrodysplastic subjects, the overwhelming majority of whom were achondroplastic dwarfs. In this paper, the adult achondroplastic sample (over age 20), consisting of 25 males and 26 females, is analyzed.

Cephalograms were obtained on all subjects with the head oriented in the Frankfurt plane by a cephalostat. A fixed x-ray source was used with the central ray perpendicular to the film. The focus-object distance was 152.4 cm. The cephalometric technique used for adult male achondroplasts was a static adaptation of the cephalometric laminagraphic apparatus at the University of Minnesota [Speidel, 1967]. Broadbent-Bolton apparatus [Broadbent, 1931, 1937] was used to obtain cephalograms of adult female achondroplasts. The use of different cephalostats and different techniques resulted in different magnifications of the cephalograms. By adjusting for the percent magnification of each cephalogram, the data were made comparable for analysis. A lateral cephalogram of an achondroplastic dwarf is illustrated in Figure 1.

Sources of Sample Bias

When studying morphological variability, it is ideal for the condition under study to be ascertained independently of the phenotype, as is possible, for example, with trisomy 21 syndrome [Cohen, 1981]. Since there is no way to define achondroplasia independently of the phenotype, the intrasyndrome population variability of morphometric traits might be reduced.

There are several possible sources of bias in the sample of achondroplasts chosen for this study. Some dwarfs do not join Little People of America because they do not wish to acknowledge their position psychologically [Weingberg, 1968]. It is theoretically possible that such disavowal may be correlated with the severity of craniofacial malformation. It is known that facial appearance can affect self-image [Goffman, 1963; MacGregor, 1970]. If achondroplastic dwarfs with severe craniofacial malformation were less likely to join Little People of America, the sample would be truncated toward the less severe end of the phenotypic spectrum. On the other hand, it also seems theoretically possible that achondroplastic dwarfs with only mild craniofacial malformation might refrain from joining Little People of America because their self-image permitted greater acceptance in the outside world, and, hence, they would have less need to identify with an organization. This would tend to truncate the sample towards the more severe end of the phenotypic spectrum. It is probable that

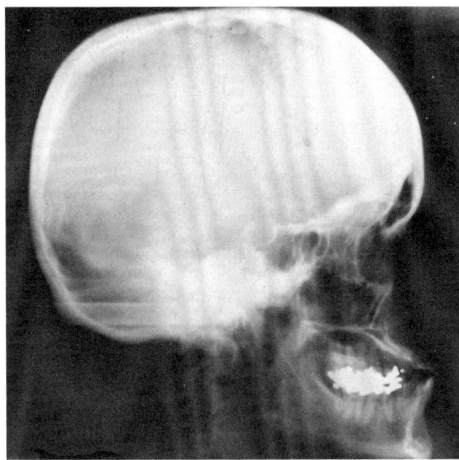

Fig. 1. Lateral cephalogram of a subject with achondroplasia.

the psychosocial effects of disproportionate short stature, a feature of all achondroplastic dwarfs, tend to override the effects of various degrees of craniofacial malformation.

Ruling Out Conditions That Simulate Achondroplasia

A number of conditions simulate achondroplasia and have been confused with it in the past. Obviously, it is essential to exclude such conditions from the achondroplastic sample. At the present time, achondroplasia is differentiated from pseudoachondroplastic conditions on the basis of clinical criteria, radiologic criteria [Langer et al, 1967, 1968], or a combination of both. Such criteria were sufficient to assure diagnostic homogeneity in this sample.

Normal Subjects for Comparison

The normal subjects used for comparison were 951 healthy white individuals from five areas in Philadelphia. The population is divided into 444 males and 507 females. The cephalograms were taken between 1948 and 1968 as part of a growth study at the University of Pennsylvania directed by Wilton M. Krogman. Each cephalogram was taken using the Broadbent-Bolton cephalostat. This particular population was selected to be the control sample because the cephalograms had previously been digitized and the information was conveniently stored in numerical form in the data bank at the University of Michigan.

Computer Morphometric Model

Cephalograms were converted to the two-dimensional coordinate model of craniofacial morphology described by Walker [1969, 1972; Walker and Kowalski, 1971, 1972, 1974]. An electronic tracing of an achondroplastic cephalogram (Calcomp plot) is illustrated in Figure 2.

All cephalograms were traced on sheets of transparent matte acetate. Sagittal projections of the parietal, occipital, frontal, sphenoid, nasal bones, maxilla, and mandible were included in the tracing. One hundred seventy-seven anatomical and derived coordinate points, which compose the mathematical model, were marked on

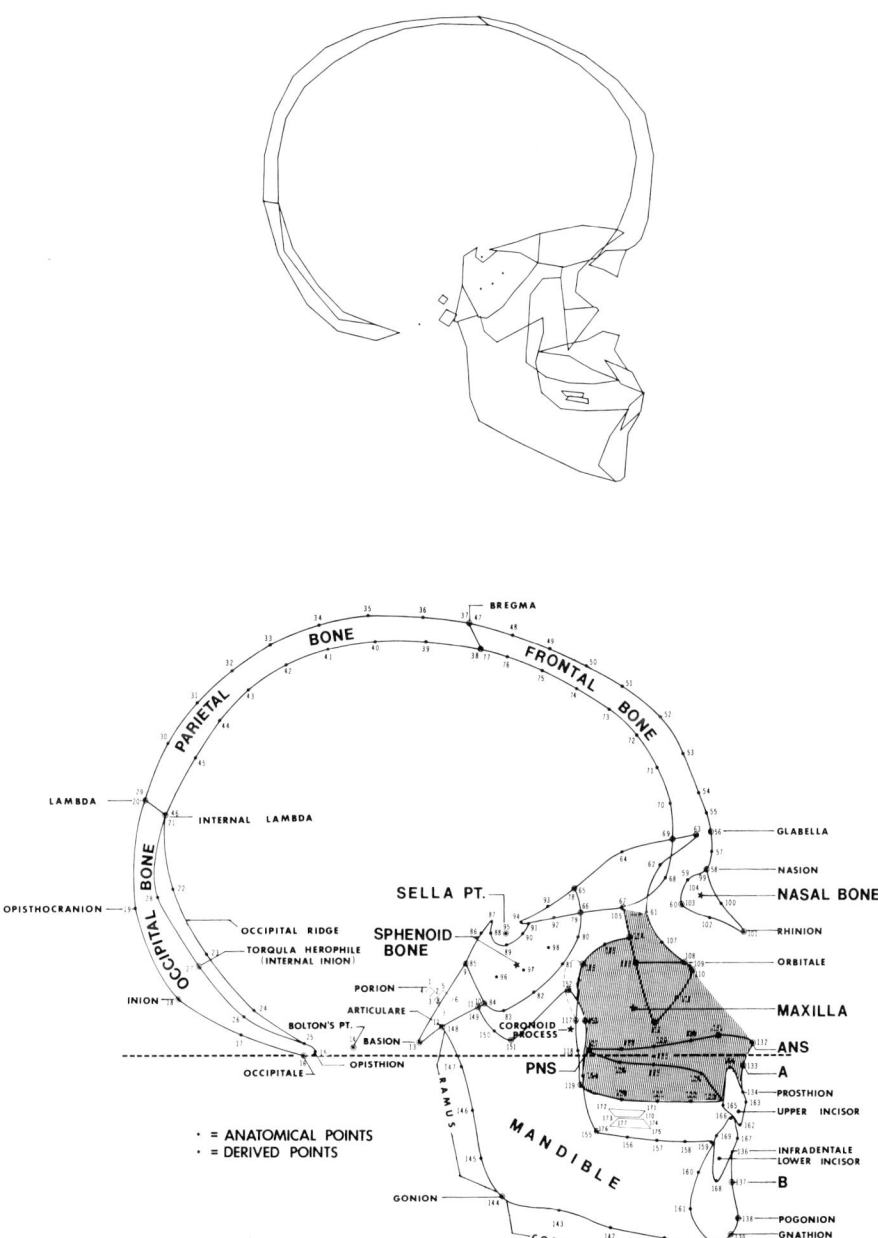

Fig. 3. Two-dimensional model with 177 coordinate points used to describe craniofacial morphology [from Walker and Kowalski, 1971].

the tracings (Fig. 3). Each marked tracing was placed on an electronic scanning device, and the machine was set so that the coordinate axes were centered at a convenient origin and in a convenient orientation. Point No. 1 was recorded and continued in an unbroken sequence through point No. 177, so that the coordinates of all the points were recorded consecutively. The digital information was fed to a key

TABLE I. Cephalometric Measurements

Measurements	Defined cephalometric points
General linear (Fig. 4)	
Maxillary length	127,132
Total mandibular length	139,148
Mandibular body length	138,144
Nasal bone length	99,101
Basion-nasion	13,99
Basion-anterior nasal spine	13,132
Basion-gnathion	13,139
Posterior cranial base length	13,95
Basisphenoid length	85,95
Anterior sphenoidal length	66,95
Cribriform plate length	66,68
Frontal bone width	58,68
Anterior cranial base length	58,95
Anterior facial height	58,140
Upper facial height	58,132
Lower facial height	132,140
Posterior facial height	95,144
Foramen magnum length	13,15
Head height (porion)	1,36
Head height (basion)	13,37
Head length	19,56
Orbital height	63,108
Three-point angular (Fig. 5)	
Articulare-gonion-gnathion angle	148-144-139
Nasion-sella-basion angle	58- 95-13
Sella-nasion-point A	95- 58-133
Sella-nasion-point B	95- 58-137
Point A-nasion-point B	133- 58-137
Facial convexity	58-133-138
Nasal angle	99-100-101
Frontal convexity	47- 51- 56
Occipital convexity	20- 18- 16
Foramen magnum angle	15- 13- 86
Orbital roof angle	64- 94- 67
Four-point angular (Fig. 5)	
Anterior cranial base plane/maxillary plane	58- 95/127-132
Anterior cranial base plane/mandibular plane	58- 95/139-144
Walker-Krogman line/foramen magnum plane	16-135/ 13- 15
X absolute perpendicular to sella vertical (Fig. 6)	
Midfrontal point to sella vertical	95,51
Glabella to sella vertical	95,56
Nasion to sella vertical	95,58
Rhinion to sella vertical	95,101
Malar prominence	95,110
Anterior nasal spine to sella vertical	95,132
Maxillary alveolar prognathism	95,134
Mandibular alveolar prognathism	95,136
Pogonion to sella vertical	95,138
Area (Figs. 7,8)	

(continued)

TABLE I. Cephalometric Measurements (continued)

Measurements	Defined cephalometric points
Area (Figs. 7,8)	
Posterior endocranial area	87,13,15,27,28, 46,44,42,40
Anterior endocranial area	87,40,38,74,72, 70,69,68,67
Mandibular ramus area	144,148,149,151, 152,153,154,155
Mandibular body area	144,155,157,136, 137,138,140,143
Basi-occipital area	9,10,11,12,13
Anterior sphenoidal area	82,89,90,91,92, 79,80,81
Posterior sphenoidal area	85,86,87,88,89, 82,83,84
Maxillary area	134,123,121,116 117,105,58,101,132
Frontal sinus area	54,55,56,57,58, 59,68,70
Nasal bone area	103,104,99,100, 101,102
Hypophyseal fossa area	87,91,90,89,88
Ratio (Fig. 9)	
$\dfrac{\text{Anterior cranial base length}}{\text{Mandibular body length}}$	$\dfrac{58\text{-}95}{139\text{-}144}$
$\dfrac{\text{Anterior cranial base length}}{\text{Maxillary length}}$	$\dfrac{58\text{-}95}{127\text{-}132}$
$\dfrac{\text{Posterior cranial base length}}{\text{Anterior cranial base length}}$	$\dfrac{13\text{-}95}{58\text{-}95}$
$\dfrac{\text{Mandibular ramus length}}{\text{Mandibular body length}}$	$\dfrac{144\text{-}148}{139\text{-}144}$
$\dfrac{\text{Upper facial height}}{\text{Lower facial height}}$	$\dfrac{58\text{-}132}{132\text{-}140}$
$\dfrac{\text{Anterior facial height}}{\text{Posterior facial height}}$	$\dfrac{58\text{-}140}{95\text{-}144}$
$\dfrac{\text{Head height (from porion)}}{\text{Head length}}$	$\dfrac{1\text{-}36}{19\text{-}56}$
$\dfrac{\text{Head height (from basion)}}{\text{Head length}}$	$\dfrac{13\text{-}37}{19\text{-}56}$

punch machine, which automatically punched the required coordinate values on cards. Values were also converted to magnetic tape for processing on a digital computer.

Selection of Cephalometric Measurements

Cephalometric measurements were specifically selected to be in accord with the purpose of this investigation, namely, to study the effects of abnormal endochondral bone formation on the development of the achondroplastic skull as a whole. Linear measurements are defined in Table I and illustrated in Figure 4. Angular measure-

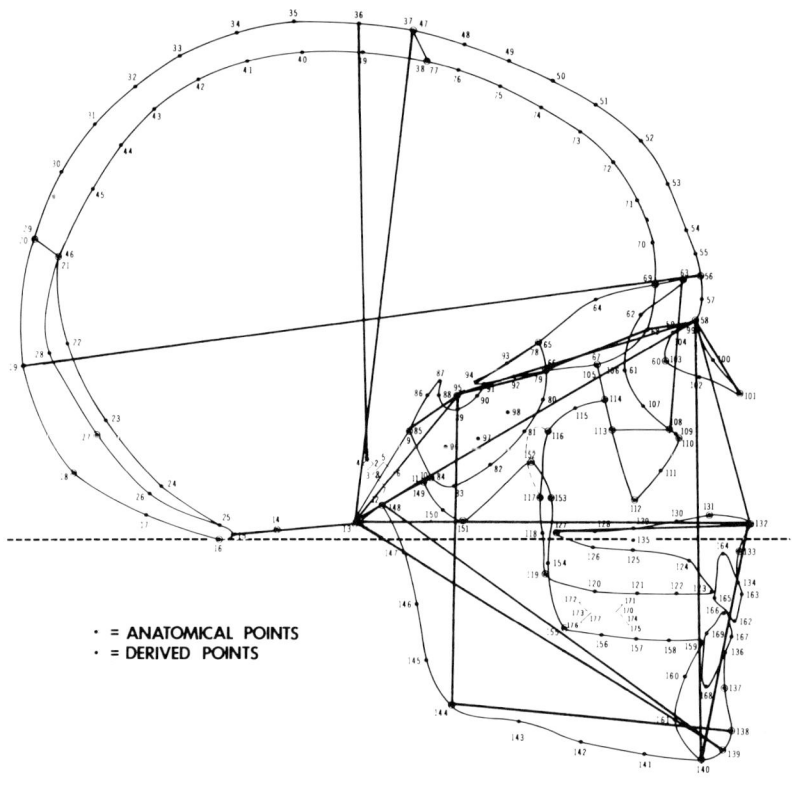
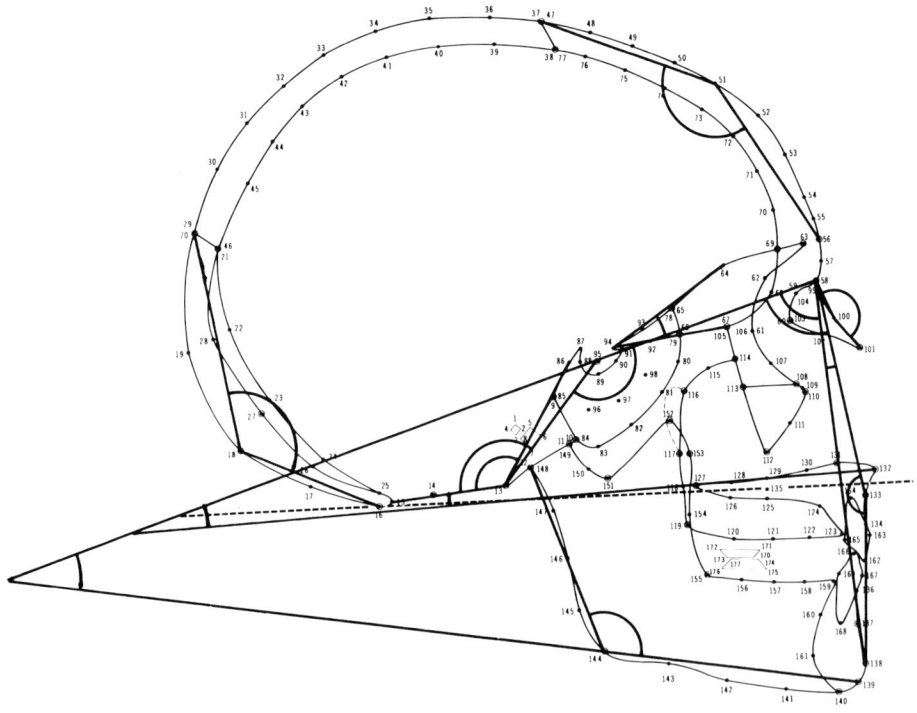

Fig. 5. Angular measurements. See Table I.

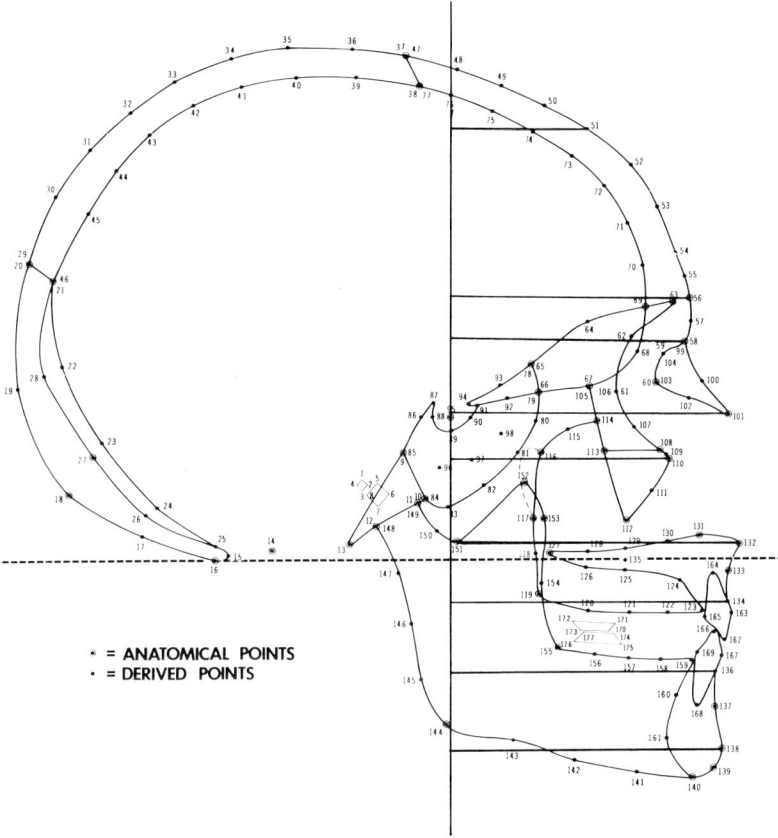

Fig. 6. Linear measurements perpendicular to sella vertical. See Table I.

ments are defined in Table I and illustrated in Figure 5. A second group of linear measurements is defined in Table I and illustrated in Figure 6. In this set of measurements, a vertical line was constructed through sella point perpendicular to the Walker-Krogman line, allowing various linear measurements of the bony facial profile. Areas are defined in Table I and illustrated in Figures 7 and 8. An area is calculated by dividing it into triangles. The computer calculates the area of each triangle and sums the triangles for each defined area. For example, the endocranial area (which reflects cranial volume) is divided into triangles in Figure 7. The computer then calculates the area of each triangle and adds all the triangles together to give the endocranial area. In practice, because there are so many perimeter defining points, the computer does not give all the triangular areas on one line of the printout; two lines are required. Thus, the endocranial area must be listed as two separate variables—the "posterior endocranial area" and the "anterior endocranial area." Together they make up the "total endocranial area." Two variables are also necessary to define the sphenoidal area and the mandibular area. Finally, a series of craniofacial ratios is defined in Table 1 and illustrated in Figure 9.

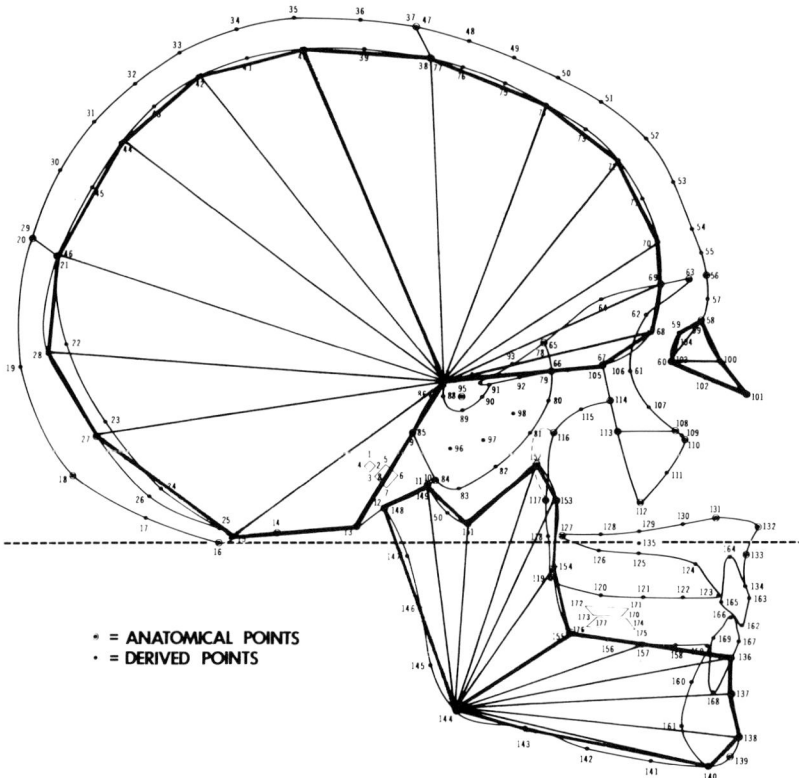

Fig. 7. Area measurements (endocranial, nasal, and mandibular). See Table I.

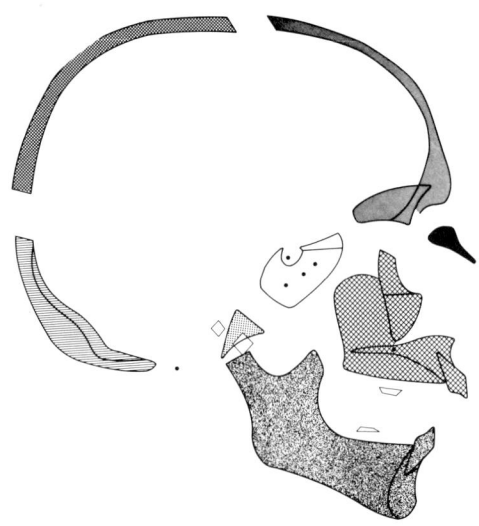

Fig. 8. Morphological structures disarticulated to show area measurements. See Table I [from Walker and Kowalski, 1972].

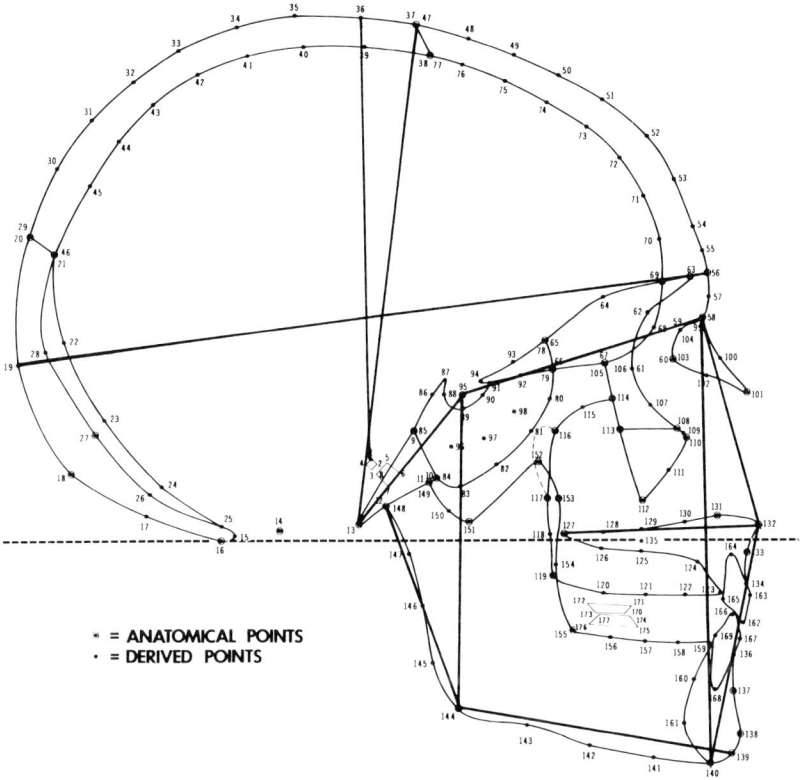

Fig. 9. Ratio measurements. See Table I.

In all, linear measurements, angular measurements, areas, and ratios comprise 66 variables. Some deliberate redundancy was built into the variables to allow maximum selection of the best variables. For example, of two slightly different measurements of the same phenomenon, one might turn out to be better than the other because point location is more accurate for one than for the other. Since this only becomes apparent after the analysis of data, it seemed reasonable to select more variables rather than less, and to discard poor variables when they became apparent.

Analysis of Data

Analysis of data included (1) various statistical methods, (2) profile pattern analysis, and (3) visual comparison of cephalometric tracings. Statistical analysis was performed at the University of Michigan Computing Center on the MTS (Michigan Terminal System). The computer was an IBM system/360 Model 67 full-duplex system. Statistical packages from MIDAS (Michigan Interactive Data Analysis System) were used in the analysis of data [Ericson, 1975].

Descriptive measures for each of the 66 variables included means, standard deviations, maximum values, and minimum values. Histograms were generated for each variable as a check on the normality of each distribution. Correlation coefficients were determined between each variable and every other variable. Two-sample t-tests were used to compare achondroplastic cephalograms with normal cephalograms. Multivariate statistical analysis included Hotelling's T^2 and discriminant function analysis [Marriott, 1974; Kowalski, 1972b]. Selected variables were graphed as profile patterns in which mean values were expressed as standard deviation units (Z scores) relative to the norm [Garn, 1955]. Finally, Calcomp plots [Walker and Kowalski, 1972] were used for visual inspection (Fig. 2) and for comparison of the average cephalometric tracings of male and female achondroplastic subjects with normal male and female subjects respectively.

RESULTS

In the interest of conserving space, histograms showing the distribution of each variable; unscaled raw data; scaled raw data transformed by the proper enlargement factor to make data comparable; correlation coefficients between each variable and every other variable; and descriptive measures including means, standard deviations, and maximum and minimum values are omitted from this paper.

In general, histograms showing the distributions of the 66 variables did not reveal any radical departures from normality for either the achondroplastic or normal samples, although slight departures from normality were observed in a few of the variables. Because some deliberate redundancy was built into the variables to allow maximum selection of the best variables, correlation coefficients were inspected when slightly different measurements of essentially the same phenomenon were utilized. Correlation coefficients were also inspected whenever there was any other reason to believe that two measurements might be correlated. It was arbitrarily decided to choose $r = .6$ as being significant since 36% (r^2) of the variability can be explained.

The results of two-sample t-tests are summarized in Tables II–V:

   Table II: Achondroplastic males vs. normal males
   Table III: Achondroplastic females vs. normal females
   Table IV: Achondroplastic males vs. achondroplastic females
   Table V: Normal males vs. normal females

Only statistically significant comparisons are presented. Type I errors are compounded by multiple comparisons. Therefore, the .001 level of significance was chosen so that only 1 in 1,000 t-tests would be judged to be significant by chance. Although radical departures from normality were not observed for any variable, it has already been mentioned that mild departures were occasionally noted. The t-test is a particularly robust statistical procedure with respect to both departures from normality and homoscedasticity [Kowalski, 1972a].

Profile patterns are illustrated in Figures 10–13:

   Selected linear measurements (Fig. 10, 11)
   Selected angular measurements (Fig. 12)
   Selected area measurements (Fig. 13)

The details of the stepwise discriminant function analysis are omitted from this paper. However, the results showed that the measurements most useful for discrimi-

TABLE II. Adult Achondroplastic Males vs Adult Normal Males

Measurement	Significant differences for t-tests[1]
Nasal bone length	N > A
Basion-nasion length	N > A
Basion-anterior nasal spine length	N > A
Posterior cranial base length	N > A
Anterior sphenoidal length	A > N
Cribriform plate length	N > A
Upper facial height	N > A
Posterior facial height	A > N
Head height (porion)	A > N
Nasion-sella-basion angle	N > A
Sella-nasion-point B	A > N
Point A-nasion-point B	A > N
Facial convexity	A > N
Nasal angle	N > A
Frontal convexity	N > A
Occipital convexity	N > A
Foramen magnum angle	N > A
Anterior cranial base plane/maxillary plane	A > N
Walker-Krogman line/foramen magnum plane	A > N
Midfrontal to sella vertical	A > N
Glabella to sella vertical	A > N
Rhinion to sella vertical	N > A
Anterior nasal spine to sella vertical	N > A
Endocranial area continued	A > N
Basi-occipital area	N > A
Sphenoidal area	A > N
Frontal sinus area	A > N
Anterior cranial base length/mandibular body length	N > A
Posterior cranial base length/anterior cranial base length	N > A
Mandibular ramus length/mandibular body length	A > N
Upper facial height/lower facial height	N > A
Anterior facial height/posterior facial height	N > A
Head height (porion)/head length	A > N

[1]N, normal; A, achondroplastic; $p < .001$.

nating between male achondroplastic subjects and normal subjects, in order, are as follows:

1. Distance from basion to anterior nasal spine
2. Mandibular alveolar prognathism
3. Frontal sinus area

The details of Hotelling's T^2 are omitted from this paper. However, the results showed that by using T^2 as an indication of the overall measurement differences between groups, there was good separation between achondroplastic male and normal male subjects, between achondroplastic female and normal female subjects, and

TABLE III. Adult Achondroplastic Females vs Adult Normal Females

Measurement	Significant differences for t-tests[1]
Maxillary length	N > A
Mandibular body length	A > N
Nasal bone length	N > A
Basion-nasion length	N > A
Basion-anterior nasal spine length	N > A
Posterior cranial base length	N > A
Basisphenoid length	N > A
Anterior sphenoidal length	A > N
Cribriform plate length	N > A
Upper face height	N > A
Head height (porion)	A > N
Head length	N > A
Nasion-sella-basion angle	N > A
Sella-nasion-point A	N > A
Point A-nasion-point B	A > N
Facial convexity	A > N
Nasal angle	N > A
Frontal convexity	N > A
Walker-Krogman line/foramen magnum plane	A > N
Midfrontal to sella vertical	A > N
Glabella to sella vertical	A > N
Rhinion to sella vertical	N > A
Anterior nasal spine to sella vertical	N > A
Endocranial area continued	A > N
Basi-occipital area	N > A
Sphenoidal area	A > N
Frontal sinus area	A > N
Anterior cranial base length/mandibular body length	N > A
Anterior cranial base length/maxillary length	A > N
Posterior cranial base length/anterior cranial base length	N > A
Mandibular ramus length/mandibular body length	A > N
Upper facial height/lower facial height	N > A
Head height (porion)/head length	A > N

[1]N, normal; A, achondroplastic. p < .001.

between normal male and female subjects. Achondroplastic male and female subjects could not be separated by Hotelling's T^2.

Visual inspection of Calcomp points (see Fig. 2) revealed striking differences between achondroplastic and normal subjects. The calvaria was enlarged in achondroplastic subjects. Furthermore, achondroplastic subjects had more frontal and occipital prominence than normal subjects. The anterior cranial base length was similar in both, but the posterior cranial base was dramatically shortened and the cranial base angle was more acute in achondroplastic subjects. There was no apparent difference in foramen magnum size. The nasal bone was short, deformed, and depressed in the achondroplastic subjects. The upper facial height was short, the maxilla was recessed,

TABLE IV. Adult Achondroplastic Males vs Adult Achondroplastic Females

Measurement	Significant differences for t tests[1]
Total mandibular length	M > F
Posterior cranial base length	M > F
Basisphenoid length	M > F
Posterior facial height	M > F
Head height (basion)	M > F
Frontal convexity	M > F
Head length	M > F
Anterior cranial base plane/maxillary plane	M > F
Anterior cranial base plane/mandibular plane	M > F
Walker-Krogman line/foramen magnum plane	F > M
Glabella to sella vertical	M > F
Endocranial area	M > F
Mandibular area	M > F
Posterior cranial base length/anterior cranial base length	M > F

[1]M, males; F, females. $p < .001$.

TABLE V. Adult Normal Males vs Adult Normal Females

Measurement	Significant differences for t-tests[1]
Total mandibular length	M > F
Mandibular body length	M > F*
Basion-nasion length	M > F
Basion-gnathion length	M > F
Anterior cranial base length	M > F
Total facial height	M > F
Posterior facial height	M > F
Foramen magnum length	M > F
Head length	M > F
Glabella to sella vertical	M > F
Nasion to sella vertical	M > F
Rhinion to sella vertical	M > F
Anterior nasal spine to sella vertical	M > F
Mandibular area	M > F
Mandibular area continued	M > F
Maxillary area	M > F

[1]M, males; F, females. $p < .001$. *Borderline significance.

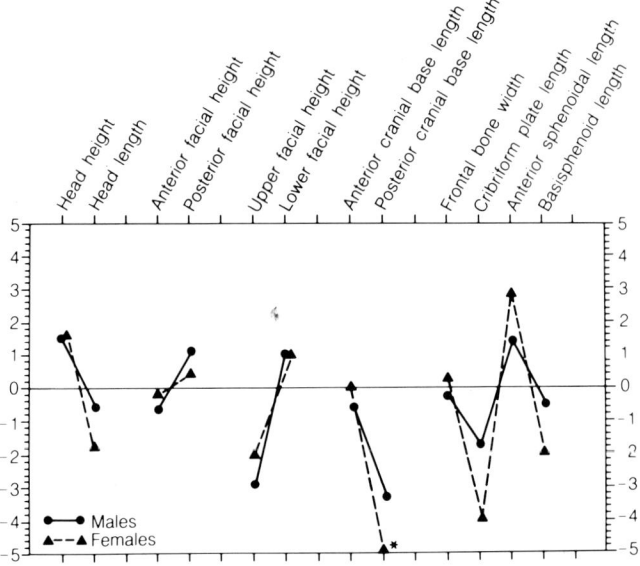

Fig. 10. Profile pattern of selected linear measurements of adult male and female achondroplasts graphed as standard deviations from the norm. Asterisk means actually −5.8 standard deviations. Zero line indicates normal mean values for each measurement. Numbers indicate standard deviations, plus and minus, from mean values.

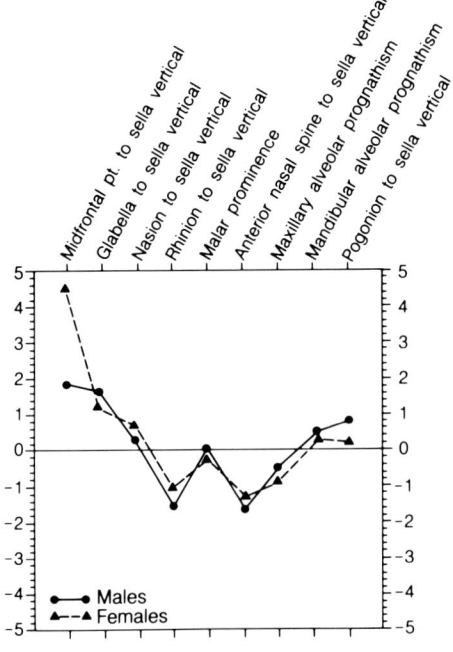

Fig. 11. Profile pattern of selected linear measurements of adult male and female achondroplasts graphed as standard deviations from the norm. All measurements shown are perpendicular to sella vertical. Zero line indicates normal mean values for each measurement. Numbers indicate standard deviations, plus and minus, from mean values.

Morphometric Analysis of Achondroplasia 155

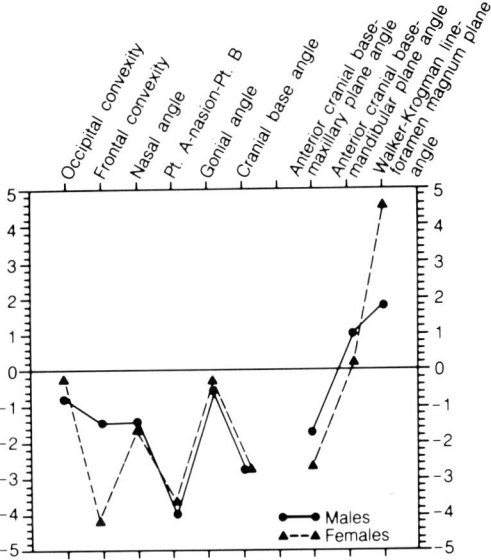

Fig. 12. Profile pattern of selected angular measurements of adult male and female achondroplasts graphed as standard deviations from the norm. Zero line indicates normal mean values for each measurement. Numbers indicate standard deviations, plus and minus, from mean values.

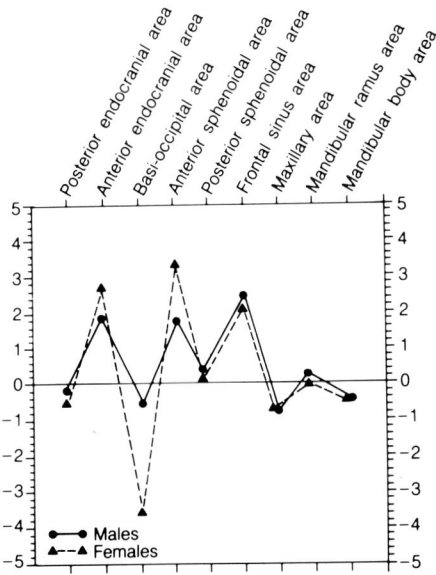

Fig. 13. Profile pattern of selected area measurements of adult male and female achondroplasts graphed as standard deviations from the norm. Zero line indicates normal mean values for each measurement. Numbers indicate standard deviations, plus and minus, from mean values.

and the nasal floor was tilted posteriorly in achondroplastic subjects compared to normal subjects. The mandible was anteriorly displaced in achondroplastic subjects, but the size, shape, and gonial angle of the mandible were normal. However, the coronoid process was higher in achondroplastic subjects.

DISCUSSION

This section discusses and interprets the findings in the cranial base, calvaria and face of achondroplastic subjects. Comments are also made on sex differences, variability of measurements, and discriminant function analysis.

Cranial Base

In achondroplasia, the anterior cranial base length from nasion to sella turcica was found to be normal in length. The posterior cranial base length was strikingly shortened, and the cranial base angle was much more acute than in normal subjects (Tables II, III, Figs. 10,12). These findings are consistent with the preliminary studies of Bjork [1955] and Pedersen [1970].

Since endochondral bone formation is known to be affected in achondroplasia [Rimoin, 1975; Rimoin and Silberberg, 1971; Rimoin et al, 1976] and since the cranial base is preformed in cartilage, hypoplasia and shortening of the cranial base would be expected. Therefore, the finding of a normal anterior cranial base length in achondroplastic subjects is surprising. In order to attempt to understand this phenomenon, a brief summary of the extensive literature on the growth and development of the anterior cranial base will be presented. Normal growth sites along the midline of the anterior cranial base include the external surface of the frontal bone, the frontoethmoidal suture, the sphenoethmoidal synchondrosis, and the intersphenoidal synchondrosis [Scott, 1958]. The cephalometric anterior cranial base (nasion to sella turcica) can be divided into frontal bone width, cribriform plate length, and anterior sphenoidal length (Table I, Fig. 4). Frontal bone width follows the general skeletal growth curve. That portion of the anterior cranial base from sella turcica to the foramen caecum follows a neural pattern of growth [Ford, 1958]. Frontal bone thickness grows in linear fashion between 3 years of age and adulthood. According to Ford [1958], cribriform plate length has ceased increasing by 2 years of age and linear growth from the sphenoethmoidal synchondrosis to sella turcica is complete by approximately 7 years of age. Hoyte [1975], in comparing the anterior cranial base length measurements of various authors, observed a discrepancy of 16% in the estimated cribriform plate length, suggesting one of two possible conclusions. Either the cribriform plate length increases after 2 years of age, in which case Ford [1958] was mistaken in his observation of its cessation of growth after 2 years of age, or Brodie's [1955] percentage attributions for the anterior cranial base were incorrect. It is possible that unilateral growth at the sphenoidal side of the sphenoethmoidal synchondrosis may take place after cessation of ethmoidal growth [Hoyte, 1975].

The normal anterior cranial base length in achondroplasia is understandable, in part, by applying Moss's functional matrix theory [1962, 1968, 1971]. According to this theory, the brain furnishes the primary growth and bones of the cranial base and calvaria respond secondarily to this force. Since the brain is enlarged in achondroplasia, the expanding frontal lobes may possibly influence the growth of the anterior cranial base, especially since the base is known to follow a neural pattern of growth in normal subjects [Ford, 1958].

Weinman and Sicher [1955] observed that trunk length in achondroplasia is nearly normal. Although the vertebrae are preformed in cartilage and would therefore be expected to be hypoplastic, the essentially normal trunk length was attributed to the numerous growth centers that are available in the vertebral column, which allow more adequate growth to take place. Pedersen [1970] suggested that the larger number of growth sites along the anterior cranial base compared with the small number available along the posterior cranial base might play a role similar to that of the vertebral column by allowing more adequate bone growth response to the growing brain in the anterior cranial fossa.

The results of this study suggest a different explanation than the one proposed by Pedersen [1970] for the normal anterior cranial base length observed in achondroplasia. The use of the computer morphometric model in this study permitted subdivision of the cephalometric anterior cranial base length into its component lengths, namely, frontal bone width, cribriform plate length, and anterior sphenoidal length. A profile pattern of these measurements appears in Figure 10. It will be observed that there are no significant differences in frontal bone width between achondroplastic and normal subjects. This result is anticipated because the frontal bone is membranous rather than endochondral in origin. Hence, it would not be expected to be subject to the growth deficiency that characterizes bones preformed in cartilage in achondroplasia. Frontal bone width in normal subjects grows by expansion of the frontal sinuses and by external apposition of bone [Scott, 1958; Bjork, 1955]. Apparently, the same is true of achondroplastic subjects.

Cribriform plate length in achondroplasia is strikingly reduced (Fig. 10). This result is also expected because the ethmoid bone is preformed in cartilage.

Anterior sphenoidal length, however, is strikingly increased in achondroplastic subjects (Fig. 10). This result is unexpected since the sphenoid bone is preformed in cartilage. The increased anterior sphenoidal length compensates for the shortened cribriform plate length, resulting in an anterior cranial base length that approximates the norm. Thus, the findings in this study suggest that growth in the length of the anterior cranial base, directed by brain growth, takes place primarily by adaptation at one site rather than among the many sites available along the anterior cranial base as suggested by Pedersen [1970]. The two growth sites along the anterior sphenoidal area are the intersphenoidal synchondrosis and the sphenoethmoidal synchondrosis. Since the intersphenoidal synchondrosis closes shortly after birth [Scott, 1958], the most compensatory postnatal growth site along the anterior cranial base in achondroplasia is apparently the sphenoethmoidal synchondrosis. Recalling that Hoyte [1975] found some disparity in how different authors estimated cribriform plate length of normal subjects, he suggested that one possibility might be more growth than suspected at the sphenoethmoidal synchondrosis entirely on the sphenoidal side of the synchondrosis, since presumably growth in the length of the cribriform plate is completed by 2 years of age. He further noted that presumed unilateral growth at a bicameral growth disc would be a phenomenon equal to the disproportionate growth typical of beveled sutures in the cranial vault. Further studies, especially histologic, are necessary to resolve this issue. However, if the disparity that Hoyte [1975] observed is resolved by proof that more growth occurs at the sphenoethmoidal synchondrosis than previously realized in normal subjects, then the interpretation of compensatory adaptation at this site in achondroplasia takes on more significance.

The finding of a strikingly short posterior cranial base (sella turcica to basion) in achondroplasia (Fig. 10) makes good biological sense because, as previously mentioned, the cranial base is preformed in cartilage and it is endochondral bone formation that is affected in achondroplasia. Although difficulty in point location of basion was a factor in failure to ascertain small foramen magnum size (vide infra), it is probably not a significant factor in determining posterior cranial base length since the order of magnitude of the latter measurement is so much greater on the one hand and the degree of reduction of the measurement in achondroplasia is so great on the other.

Growth in length of the normal posterior base takes place primarily at the spheno-occipital synchondrosis with some bony apposition occurring at the anterior lip of the foramen magnum [Enlow, 1969, 1975]. Most of the growth deficiency in the length of the posterior cranial base in achondroplasia results from lack of growth at the spheno-occipital synchondrosis. Normally, closure of the spheno-occipital synchondrosis occurs between 11 and 16 years of age [Irwin, 1960; Powell and Brodie, 1963; Ingervall and Thilander, 1972]. In the present study, three midline sagittal laminagraphs of young achondroplastic subjects indicated that closure probably occurred prior to 8 or 9 years of age. Pedersen [1970] reported similar findings. Thus, hypoplasia of the posterior cranial base may result from earlier closure of the spheno-occipital synchondrosis in achondroplastic subjects than in normal subjects.

The cranial base angle is much more acute in achondroplastic subjects than in normal subjects. Thus, the clivus has an almost vertical orientation. Changes in the flexure of the normal cranial base both prenatally and postnatally have been discussed elsewhere [Bjork, 1947, 1955; Brodie, 1941, 1955; Ford, 1958; Kvinnsland, 1973; Ortiz-Monasterio and Brodie, 1949; Scott, 1958; Zuckerman, 1955]. It is known that the degree of cranial base flexure in man is greater than in other primates because of an increase in brain size [Zuckerman, 1955] and because of earlier closure of the intersphenoidal synchondrosis [Scott, 1958]. The exaggerated closure of the cranial base angle in achondroplasia may be related to an increased brain size and possibly earlier than normal closure of the intersphenoidal and spheno-occipital synchondroses.

The finding of no significant difference in foramen magnum size in achondroplastic and normal subjects in the present study is clearly at variance with the findings of other authors [Langer et al, 1967, 1968; Brash, 1956; Crawford et al, 1976]. The studies of Langer et al [1967, 1968] are based on diagnostic radiographs, and in their judgment, the foramen magnum in achondroplastic dwarfs is small. Crawford et al [1976] made the same judgment of small foramen magnum size in their study, which was based on both diagnostic radiographs and tomograms. Brash [1956] shows a picture of an achondroplastic skull in basilar view; the foramen magnum appears significantly smaller than normal. Our conclusion is that errors were made in the location of point basion in this study (foramen magnum length is measured from basion to opisthion) and that the foramen magnum is indeed smaller than normal. Difficulty in locating basion can be attributed to the superimposition of the mastoids on the posterior cranial base [Langer et al, 1967]. In the present study, midline sagittal laminagraphs in three achondroplastic subjects confirmed small foramen magnum size.

The angle made by the foramen magnum plane and the Walker-Krogman line is significantly increased in achondroplastic subjects (Fig. 12) and probably results from hypoplasia of the posterior cranial base. The degree to which this angle is increased probably cannot be determined with great accuracy because the points defining the plane are opisthion and basion (Table I, Fig. 5) and, as already noted, point basion was not located with great accuracy in achondroplastic subjects in this study.

The acute cranial base angle and the increase in the foramen magnum angle strongly suggest that the natural balance of the achondroplastic head on the spinal column tilts the face downward. The balance of the head is largely determined by the location of the foramen magnum, and Bjork [1955] has shown that the position of the foramen magnum is related to the degree of flexure of the cranial base. An obtuse cranial base angle produces posterior displacement of the foramen magnum and results in the face's tilting upward. An acute cranial base angle produces anterior displacement of the foramen magnum and results in the face's tilting downward. Since the cranial base angle in achondroplasia is much more acute than normal, the foramen magnum is anteriorly displaced and the natural head balance favors the downward tilt of the face. The increase in the foramen magnum plane contributes to this tendency.

The finding of an exaggerated external bony protuberance on the occipital bone in achondroplastic subjects can also be interpreted as being related to head balance. Radiographically, the protuberance seems to correspond to the areas of muscle attachment of the rectus capitis posterior minor and rectus capitis posterior major muscles. These muscles aid in holding the head upright and in extension against resistance or gravity. With the heavy head load in achondroplastic subjects and the tendency of the face to tilt downward, increased neck muscle use may be responsible for the exaggerated bony protuberance. Occipital convexity reaches statistical significance, however, only in the adult male achondroplastic sample (Table II).

The bony protuberance reflecting increased muscle use is probably related to two factors. First, the extensor muscles of the neck are probably used more commonly in achondroplasts to counteract the natural tendency of the head to tilt downward and forward. Exaggerated use of the neck extensor muscles would be necessary simply to hold the head erect. Second, normal children hyperextend the head when talking to adults. Once they grow up this is not necessary. However, achondroplastic adults must continue to hyperextend the head throughout their lives when talking to others. This fact may possibly explain why the bony protuberance on the occipital bone reaches statistical significance only in achondroplastic adults.

Other changes in the cranial base have been reported by Crawford et al [1976]. Using laminagraphic studies, they found that the petrous portion of the temporal bone was most distorted with a strikingly abnormal orientation of the internal and external acoustic meatuses and the labyrinth. Despite the abnormal orientation of the vestibular apparatus, achondroplastic dwarfs are known to have a normal sense of balance. The eustachian tubes are abnormally oriented and abnormally wide. These changes are probably causative of the frequent bouts of otitis media to which achondroplastic children are subject. Thus, mastoid air cell development is minimal in achondroplasia.

Calvaria

The endocranial area is significantly larger in achondroplastic subjects than in normal subjects (Tables II, III; Fig. 13). The findings of significantly increased frontal bossing (Tables II, III; Figs. 11, 12), enlarged frontal sinus area (Tables II, III; Fig. 13), and head height (Tables II, III) are consistent with this. The endocranial area reflects brain size and can be considered a measure of it. In achondroplasia, most of the brain enlargement occurs in the anterior half of the endocranial area (Fig. 13).

These findings confirm those of other authors. Pedersen [1970], using a cephalometric adaptation of the Lee-Pearson formula for cranial capacity, found a mean cranial capacity of 1,552 cubic centimeters compared to 1,259 cubic centimeters for normal subjects. Horton et al [1977, 1978] and Shepard and Graham [1967] found a larger-than-average head circumference in achondroplastic subjects. Enlarged calvaria was found to be characteristic of achondroplasia in the studies of Langer et al [1967, 1968]. They noted that newborns with achondroplasia may or may not have enlarged heads, that disproportionate growth of the head occurred compared to the rest of the body, and that enlargement of the calvaria eventually ensued in achondroplasts whose head sizes were normal at birth.

It is commonly known that achondroplastic dwarfs are slow in the development of motor milestones and are hypotonic during the first few months of life. Head control may not occur until 3–4 months of age [Maroteaux and Lamy, 1964]. Although late head control can be related to early hypotonia, the enlarged head in achondroplasia is probably the major factor. Siebens et al [1978] have postulated that because the heads of achondroplastic children are enlarged, loading of the vertical spine is increased. The lax ligaments and misshapen vertebrae predispose the spine to yielding under vertical stress, resulting in abnormal spinal curvature, especially an accentuated lumbosacral lordosis. Langer et al [1967, 1968] and Scott [1972], among others, have observed that mild thoracolumbar kyphosis is characteristic of achondroplastic infants before they begin to walk. With weight bearing and ambulation, the exaggerated lordosis develops. Thus, Siebens et al [1978] concluded that the achondroplastic spine was acquired rather than being a constitutional feature of the condition. They calculated that, on the average, the achondroplastic head would load the spine by approximately 47% more than the normal head.

Enlargement of the calvaria in achondroplasia has been attributed to true megaloencephaly [Dennis et al, 1961] and hydrocephalus [Langer et al, 1967; Cohen et al, 1967; Dandy, 1921; James et al, 1972; Mueller et al, 1977; Pierre-Kahn et al, 1980; Wise et al, 1971]. True megaloencephaly is a less attractive hypothesis to account for the enlarged calvaria because a second mechanism must be postulated to explain the enlarged brain. Clearly, genes are known to have pleiotropic effects, and this could be true of achondroplasia, an autosomal dominant disorder. However, hydrocephalus is a more frugal hypothesis because it can be explained on the basis of the bony abnormalities in the cranial base. Most authors favor enlargement on this basis.

Dennis et al [1961] described five cases of achondroplasia that were autopsied and concluded that enlargement of the head represented true megaloencephaly. However, all of their patients died of respiratory and/or cardiac failure. Cerebral edema caused by agonal ataxia may have produced the increase in brain weight noted in these patients. Furthermore, three of the five patients were noted to have had ventricular dilatation.

Ventricular dilatation has been reported by several authors [James et al, 1972; Mueller et al, 1977; Wise et al, 1971]. Most evidence to date seems to favor communicating hydrocephalus. James et al [1972] demonstrated communicating hydrocephalus in two achondroplastic children with cisternography. Mueller et al [1977] postulated two possibilities. First, early hydrocephalus may be caused by cerebrospinal fluid outlet obstruction resulting from a small posterior fossa which becomes compensated later in life secondary to bony structural maturation. Second, achondroplasts may have obstruction of cerebrospinal fluid flow at the subarachnoid villi or in the venous sinuses secondary to retrograde pressure from marginal jugular veins. These could be compensated in size secondary to small jugular foramina that resulted from faulty endochondral ossification in the posterior fossa.

Pierre-Kahn et al [1980] studied hydrocephalus in 25 achondroplastic patients. They suggested that the hydrocephalus was related to constriction of the sigmoid sinus at the level of narrowed jugular foramina, resulting in a rise in intracranial venous pressure. They further noted that, in most instances, the hydrocephalus stabilized spontaneously in early life. Further studies are necessary to determine if the jugular foramina are small or if their emissary vein foramina are enlarged in achondroplasia.

Face

Facial profile measurements in achondroplasia are graphed as standard deviations from the norm in Figure 11. Frontal bossing has already been discussed as an adaptation to increased brain size in achondroplasia. The frontal sinuses are significantly larger in achondroplastic subjects than in normal subjects (Tables II, III; Fig. 13). Mueller et al [1977] have observed that the sphenoidal sinus is also enlarged.

Maxillary length was shorter than normal in achondroplastic subjects, and this was statistically significant at the .01 level of confidence, but not at the .001 level, which was chosen in this study to reduce the number of type I errors. Upper facial height was strikingly shorter in the achondroplastic sample (Tables II, III; Fig. 10). These findings agree with those of Pedersen [1970]. Short maxillary length and upper facial height in this study are probably related to hypoplastic growth of the nasal capsule, which is preformed in cartilage and would be expected to be affected in achondroplasia.

Although cartilage of the face participates in the development of the face, the exact role has been debated [Koski, 1968, 1975, 1977; Babula et al, 1970]. Some have considered cartilage of the face as a primary growth effector that is intrinsically regulated. Others view cartilage of the face as being totally passive and adaptive. Both views are equally one-sided and probably erroneous [Koski, 1975]. The finding of a retrusive midface in achondroplastic subjects in this study supports an intrinsic role for cartilage of the face since bone preformed in cartilage is known to be hypoplastic in achondroplasia.

The nasal bone has already been noted to be shortened, deformed, and depressed (Tables II, III; Fig. 2). The nasal bones are membranous in origin and therefore would not be anticipated to be affected. However, bones are known to be adaptive. The configuration of the nasal bone in achondroplasia probably results secondarily from two opposing tendencies—to dip in superiorly because of the hypoplastic nasal septum and to pull out inferiorly to uplift the nose.

An unusual finding in this study was the tilting of the nasal floor posteriorly in achondroplastic subjects (Fig. 2). This is statistically significant as the anterior cranial base-maxillary plane angle (Tables II, III; Fig. 12). The tilting of the nasal floor suggests an adaptation to a narrow nasopharyngeal airway. Since the acute cranial base angle constricts the nasopharynx, the posterior tilt allows a wider opening of the nasopharynx. It is conceivable that eustachian tube infection and achondroplastic speech may be affected by posterior tilting of the nasal floor.

Mandibular size was the same in achondroplastic and normal subjects. There were no significant differences in mandibular length or mandibular ramus or body area (Tables II, III; Fig. 13). Pedersen's results [1970] were similar. No significant differences were observed in the gonial angle between achondroplastic and normal subjects, although in viewing some cephalograms of growing achondroplasts, the gonial angle decreased with age as it does in the general population [Jensen and Palling, 1954]. Pedersen [1970] found a significant difference between the gonial angle of achondroplastic and normal subjects, but this may be due to small sample size.

The normal-sized mandible in achondroplasia makes good biological sense. Although Meckel's cartilage determines the shape of the developing mandible as the cartilaginous core of the first branchial arch, resorption of Meckel's cartilage is already proceeding at 55 mm crown–rump length, and it disappears from the mandible before birth [Koski, 1975]. Most of the mandible develops in membrane bone and would therefore not be anticipated to be affected in achondroplasia. The condylar cartilage of the mandible arises from a mesenchymal cell condensation as secondary cartilage close to the ossifying condylar process which it joins. It is totally separate from Meckel's cartilage. The histologic organization and biochemical composition of condylar cartilage is clearly different from growth plate-type of cartilage [Koski, 1975]. Weinman and Sicher [1955] suggested that the normal size of the mandible in achondroplasia may be a function of the different type of cartilage at the head of the condyle, which grows appositionally instead of interstitially, as the chondrocranium does. If the achondroplasia gene only produces an effect on interstitially growing cartilage, then it does not affect the mandible.

Although the mandible was observed to be no larger in achondroplastic subjects than in normal subjects, mandibular prognathism was noted to be pronounced. This reached statistical significance in variables sella turcica-nasion-point B and point A-nasion-point B (Tables II, III). This finding can be related to the more acute cranial base flexure in achondroplasia. Thus, the mandible, of normal dimensions, is more anteriorly positioned than normal.

The coronoid process is related to the temporalis muscle that attaches to it. The process depends upon muscle function. If the temporalis muscle is severed experimentally in animals, the coronoid process does not develop properly [Washburn, 1951, 1962]. Increased muscle use would result in enlargment of the coronoid process. It is possible that the large coronoid process in achondroplasia may be related to increased muscle stretch from an anteriorly placed mandible. It is also possible that the hyperextension of the achondroplastic head, necessary for interaction with other adults, results in a natural opening of the jaws that is counteracted by increased use of the temporalis muscles, among others.

Sex differences in the measurements of adult achondroplastic subjects (Table IV) were different than sex differences in the same measurements of normal subjects (Table V). Achondroplasts and normal subjects were only congruent for 5 of 16 significantly different measurements between the sexes. Using Hotelling's T^2 as an indication of overall measurement differences between groups, there was good separation between normal male and female subjects, but poor separation between achondroplastic male and female subjects. Thus, measurement differences produced by the pathologic condition of achondroplasia totally override normal male and female differences that are expected to occur.

Profile patterning of selected measurements (Figs. 10–13) showed that female achondroplastic subjects had more extreme values for several variables than male achondroplastic subjects. Nehne et al [1976], in their general anthropometric study, found that in all parameters except femoral length, female achondroplastic dwarfs compared to normal females of the same age were more severely affected than achondroplastic males compared to normal males of the same age. The reasons for the more extreme values and greater variability of female achondroplastic measurements in this study are obscure.

The biological intepretation of the difference between achondroplastic and normal subjects was consistent with the results of a stepwise discriminant function anlaysis. For example, the most discriminating variable with respect to achondroplastic males was the measurement from basion to the anterior nasal spine. In achondroplastic subjects, this dimension crosses a shortened maxilla, a hypoplastic cranial base, and an acutely flexed cranial base angle, all of which are strikingly abnormal and involved by the pathologic process.

REFERENCES

Babula WJ, Smiley GR, Dixon AD: The role of the cartilaginous nasal septum in midfacial growth. Am J Orthod 58:250–263, 1970.
Bjork A: "The Face in Profile." Lund: Berlingska Boktryckeriet, 1947.
Bjork A: Cranial base development. Am J Orthod 41:198–225, 1955.
Brash JC, McKeag, HTA, Scott, JH: "The Aetiology of Irregularity and Malocclusion of the Teeth." London: Spottiswoode, Ballantyne, and Co., 1956.
Broadbent BH: A new x-ray technique and its application to orthodontia. Angle Orthod 1:45–66, 1931.
Broadbent BH: Bolton standards and technique in orthodontic practice. Angle Orthod 7:209–233, 1937.
Brodie AG: On the growth pattern of the human head from the third month to the eighth year of life. Am J Anat 58:209–262, 1941.
Brodie AG: The behavior of the cranial base and its components as revealed by serial cephalometric roentgenograms. Angle Orthod 25:148–161,1955.
Cohen ME, Rosenthal AD, Matson DD: Neurological abnormalities in achondroplastic children. J Pediatr 71:367–376, 1967.
Cohen MM Jr: A critical review of cephalometric studies of dysmorphic syndromes. Koski Festschrift. Proc Finn Dent Soc 77:17–25, 1981.
Crawford DB, Ensor RE, Dorst JP: The chondrocranium in achondroplasia. In: Bosma JF (ed): "Development of the Basicranium." Bethesda: US Department of Health, Education, and Welfare Publication No. (NIH) 76-989,1976, pp 301–318.
Dandy WE: Hydrocephalus in chondrodystrophy. Johns Hopkins Hosp Bull 32:5–10, 1921.
Dennis JP, Rosenberg HS, Alvord EC Jr: Megalencephaly, internal hydrocephalus and other neurological aspects of achondroplasia. Brain 84:427–445, 1961.
Enlow DH: "The Human Face." New York: Harper and Row, 1969.
Enlow DH: "Handbook of Facial Growth." Philadelphia: WB Saunders, 1975.
Ericson WA: "A Manual of Elementary Statistics Using MIDAS." Ann Arbor: University of Michigan Press, 1975.
Ford EHR: Growth of the human cranial base. Am J Orthod 44:498–506, 1958.
Garn SM: Applications of pattern analysis to anthropometric data. Ann NY Acad Sci 63:537–552, 1955.
Goffman E: "Stigma—Notes on the Management of Spoiled Identity." Englewood Cliffs, NJ: Prentice-Hall, 1963.
Horton WA, Rotter JI, Kaitila I, Gursky J, Hall JG, Shepard TH, Rimoin DL: Growth curves in achondroplasia. Birth Defects 13(3C):101–107, 1977.

Horton WA, Rotter JI, Rimoin DL, Scott Cl, Hall JG. Standard growth curves for achondroplasia. J Pediatr 93:435–438, 1978.
Hoyte DAN: Critical analysis of the growth and length of the cranial base. Birth Defects 11(7):255–282, 1975.
Ingervall B, Thilander B: The human spheno-occipital synchondrosis. I. The time of closure appraised macroscopically. Acta Odont Scand 30:349–356, 1972.
Irwin GL: Roentgen determination of the time of closure of the spheno-occipital synchondrosis. Radiology 75:450–452, 1960.
James AE, Dorst JP, Methews ES, McKusick VA: Hydrocephalus in achondroplasia studied by cisternography. Pediatrics 49:46–49, 1972.
Jensen E, Palling M: The gonial angle, a survey. Am J Orthod 40:120–133, 1954.
Koski K: Cranial growth centers: Facts or fallacies. Am J Orthod 54:566–580, 1968.
Koski K: Cartilage in the face. Birth Defects 11(7):231–254, 1975.
Koski K. The role of the craniofacial cartilages in postnatal growth of the craniofacial skeleton. In: Dalberg AH, Graber, TM (eds): "Orofacial Growth and Development." The Hague: Mouton, 1977.
Kowalski CJ: "Statistical Aspects of Cephalometry, Vol 1. Univariate Problems." Ann Arbor: University of Michigan Press, 1972a.
Kowalski CJ: A commentary on the use of multivariate statistical methods in anthropometric research. Am J Phys Anthropol 36:119–132, 1972b.
Kvinnsland S: Changes in the foramen magnum axis during human foetal development. Acta Odont Scand 31:175–178, 1973.
Langer LO, Baumann PA, Gorlin RJ: Achondroplasia. Am J Roentgen Rad Therapy Nuc Med 100:12–26, 1967.
Langer LO, Baumann PA, Gorlin RJ: Achondroplasia: Clinical radiologic features with comments on genetic implications. Clin Pediatr 7:474–485, 1968.
MacGregor FC: Social and psychological implications of dentofacial disfigurement. Angle Orthod 40:231–233, 1970.
Maroteaux P, Lamy M: Achondroplasia in man and animals. Clin Orthop 33:91–103, 1964.
Marriott FHC: "The Interpretation of Multiple Observations." New York: Academic Press, 1974.
Moss ML: The functional matrix. In: Kraus BS, Riedel RA (eds): "Vistas in Orthodontics." Philadelphia: Lea and Febiger, 1962, pp 85–98.
Moss ML: Primacy of functional matrices in orofacial growth. Dent Pract 19:65–73, 1968.
Moss ML: Functional cranial analysis and functional matrix. ASHA Report 9:5–18, 1971.
Mueller SM, Bell W, Cornell S, Des Hamsher K, Dolan K: Achondroplasia and hydrocephalus. Neurology 27:430–434, 1977.
Nehne A-M, Riseborough EJ, Tredwell FJ: Skeletal growth and development of the achondroplastic dwarf. Clin Orthop 116:8–23, 1976.
Ortiz-Monasterio F, Brodie AG: On the growth of the human head from birth to the third month of life. Anat Rec 103:311–333, 1949.
Pedersen RV: A roentgenographic cephalometric survey of cranial and facial structures in the human achondroplastic dwarf. University of Washington, Master of Science Thesis, 1970.
Pierre-Kahn A, Hirsch JF, Renier D, Metzger J, Maroteaux P: Hydrocephalus and achondroplasia. Child's Brain 7:205–219, 1980.
Powell TV, Brodie AG: Closure of the spheno-occipital synchondrosis. Anat Rec 147:15–23, 1963.
Pruzansky S: Clinical investigation of the experiments of nature. ASHA Report 8:62–94, 1973.
Rimoin DL: The chondrodystrophies. In: Harris H, Hirschhorn K (eds): "Advances in Human Genetics." New York: Plenum Press, 1975, pp 1–118.
Rimoin DL, Silberberg R: Study of bone growth. N Engl J Med 284:111, 1971.
Rimoin DL, Silberberg R, Hollister DW: Chondro-osseous pathology in the chondrodystrophies. Clin Orthop Related Res 114:137–152, 1976.
Scott CI: The genetics of short stature. In: Steinberg AG, Bearn AG (eds): "Progress in Medical Genetics," Vol 8. New York: Grune and Stratton 1972, pp 243–299.
Scott JH: The cranial base. Am J Phys Anthropol 16:319–348, 1958.
Shepard TH, Graham BC: Achondroplastic dwarfism: Diagnosis and management. NW Med 66:451–456, 1967.

Siebens AA, Hungerford DS, Kirby NA: Curves of the achondroplastic spine: A new hypothesis. Johns Hopkins Med J 142:205-210, 1978.

Speidel TM: A method of adapting laminagraphy to cephalometric radiography. Master's Thesis, University of Minnesota, 1967.

Walker GF: Analysis of skull shape using mathematical models and a digital computer. Philadelphia Center for Research and Child Growth Report. University of Pennsylvania, Philadelphia, Pennsylvania, 1969.

Walker GF: A new approach to the analysis of craniofacial morphology and growth. Am J Orthod 51:221-230, 1972.

Walker GF, Kowalski CJ: A two-dimensional coordinate model for the qualification, description, analysis prediction, and simulation of craniofacial growth. Growth 35:191-211, 1971.

Walker GF, Kowalski CJ: Computer morphometries in craniofacial biology. Comput Biol Med 2:235-249, 1972.

Walker GF, Kowalski CJ: Computer-aided diagnosis of craniofacial abnormalities. Med Info 553-557, 1974.

Washburn SL: The new physical anthropology. Trans NY Acad Sci (Series 11) 13:298-304, 1951.

Washburn SL: The strategy of physical anthropology. In: Tax, S (ed): "Anthropology Today." Chicago: University of Chicago Press, 1-14, 1962.

Weinberg MS: The problems of midgets and dwarfs and organizational remedies: A study of the little people of America. J Health Soc Behav 9:65-71, 1968.

Weinman JP, Sicher H: "Bone and Bones." St. Louis: CV Mosby, 1955.

Wise BL, Sondheimer F, Kaufman S: Achondroplasia and hydrocephalus. Neuropadiatrie 3:106-113, 1971.

Zuckerman S: Age changes in the basicranial access of the human skull. Am J Phys Anthropol 13:521-539, 1955.

Craniovertebral Malformations in Hemifacial Microsomia

Alvaro A. Figueroa and Hans Friede
Center for Craniofacial Anomalies, University of Illinois College of Medicine, Chicago

>There is increasing evidence that hemifacial microsomia (HFM), Goldenhar syndrome (GS), and oculoauriculovertebral dysplasia (OAV) are part of a spectrum within a single entity. In support of this thesis are the family studies that have suggested that isolated microtia (M) may represent the mildest form of the condition [Kaye et al, 1979; Rollnick and Kaye, 1983].
>
>Vertebral malformations are pathognomonic of OAV, but they have also been described in HFM and GS. In this investigation we studied the frequency and type of cervical spine malformations in HFM, GS, OAV, and M. Our findings show that the frequency of cervical spine malformations in HFM and M was greater than values for a normal population. This further supports the probable association between HFM, GS, OAV, and M. Fusions were the most prevalent cervical spine malformation encountered. The study also included analysis of the cranial base and craniovertebral junction.

Key words: hemifacial microsomia, Goldenhar syndrome, oculoauriculovertebral dysplasia, microtia, craniovertebral malformations

INTRODUCTION

There is increasing evidence that hemifacial microsomia[1] (HFM), Goldenhar syndrome (GS), and oculoauriculovertebral dysplasia (OAV) are variants of the same condition with a phenotypic spectrum of severity [Gorlin et al, 1976; Kaye et al, 1979]. Malformations of the external ear (microtia [M]) of varying severity are a common feature in these entities [Pruzansky, 1969, 1973; Figueroa and Pruzansky, 1982]. External ear malformations may also occur in isolation with no associated anomalies [Aase, 1980; Melnick, 1980]. It has been suggested that in some families M may represent the mildest form of HFM, GS, or OAV [Rollnick and Kaye, 1983].

Malformations of the cervical vertebrae are one of the pathognomonic characteristics of OAV [Gorlin, 1963]. Malformations of the cervical spine have also been reported in some cases of HFM [Grabb, 1965; Ross, 1975]. The purpose of this paper was to investigate whether cervicovertebral malformations are not only limited to

---

EDITORS' NOTE: Dr. Pruzansky contributed to the research reported in this paper and was listed as a co-author prior to his death.

[1]In this paper, *hemifacial microsomia* is used as a general term and includes hemifacial microsomia (microtia and malformed mandible); Goldenhar syndrome (microtia, malformed mandible, and epibulbar dermoids/lipodermoids); and oculoauriculovertebral dysplasia (microtia, malformed mandible, epibulbar dermoids/lipodermoids, and vertebral anomalies).

Address reprint requests to Alvaro A. Figueroa, D.D.S., Center for Craniofacial Anomalies, University of Illinois, College of Medicine, P.O. Box 6998, Chicago, IL 60680.

© 1985 Alan R. Liss, Inc.

OAV, but also occur with greater than expected frequency in the other related entities (HFM and GS), including isolated M. In addition, malformations in the cervical spine might occur together with defects in the craniovertebral junction and cranial base [Schmidt et al, 1978]. Therefore, this area was also analyzed for malformations.

From the onset of this study, we recognized certain limitations that would result in under-reporting of the true occurrence of craniovertebral malformations. Since cephalometric radiographs would be used, the study was limited to the cervical region. Further, the whole cervical spine could not be visualized in every film and where there was superimposition of other skeletal structures, certain vertebral malformations would be difficult to recognize.

MATERIALS AND METHODS

The data base at the Center for Craniofacial Anomalies of the University of Illinois included 406 patients coded to have external ear malformations. Patients with known syndromes or associations such as mandibulofacial dysostosis, Nager syndrome, branchio-oto-renal syndrome, VATER and CHARGE associations, paramedian facial cleft, microphthalmia and chromosome anomalies were excluded for the purpose of this study. The remaining patients (N = 204; 132 males and 72 females) comprised the sample for this study. The patients were grouped into four diagnostic categories: M, HFM, GS, and OAV (Table I). The HFM subgroup had the largest number of patients (144), followed by M (48). The GS and OAV subgroups were the smallest, with only six patients each.

Longitudinal lateral and posteroanterior cephalometric radiographs were used in this study. Availability of serial records on the same individual permitted verification of findings observed in a single film as well as demonstration of the natural history of the malformation. When available, other radiographic examinations such as tomograms, thorax radiographs, etc., as well as the radiologist's reports were used to complement our study.

The cephalometric radiographs were examined for the following malformations in the cranial base, craniovertebral junction, and cervical spine.

Cranial Base Malformations

1. Kyphosis: cranial base angulation (Nasion-Sella-Basion) 2 SD below the norm ($\bar{X} = 130 \pm 5.0$ SD)[Riolo et al, 1974; Schmidt et al, 1978] (Fig. 1).
2. Platybasia: cranial base angulation (Nasion-Sella-Basion) 2 SD above the norm ($\bar{X} = 130 \pm 5.0$ SD) [Riolo et al, 1974; Schmidt et al, 1978] (Fig. 2).

TABLE I. Number and Distribution of Patients in the Four Diagnostic Categories Studied

Diagnostic categories	N	♂	♀
Isolated microtia (M)	48	34	14
Hemifacial microsomia (HFM)	144	94	50
Goldenhar syndrome (GS)	6	3	3
Oculoauriculovertebral dysplasia (OAV)	6	1	5
Total patients	204	132	72

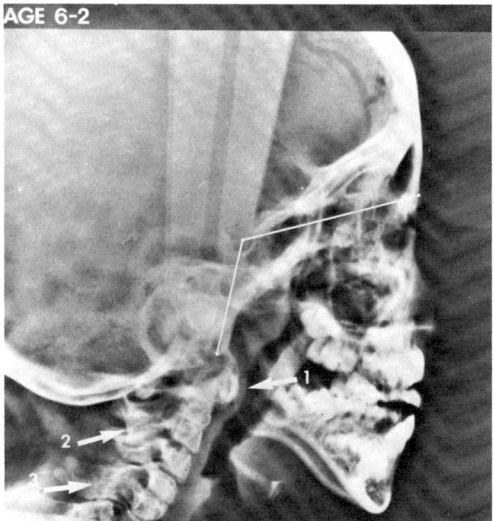

Fig. 1. CCFA #5718: female, age 6 years 2 months, left HFM. Basilar kyphosis (Nasion-Sella-Basion angle: 117°). Note the forward displacement of the atlas (C-1), with impingement on the airway (arrow 1) and fusion between C-2 and C-3 (arrow 2) as well as between C-4 and C-5 (arrow 3).

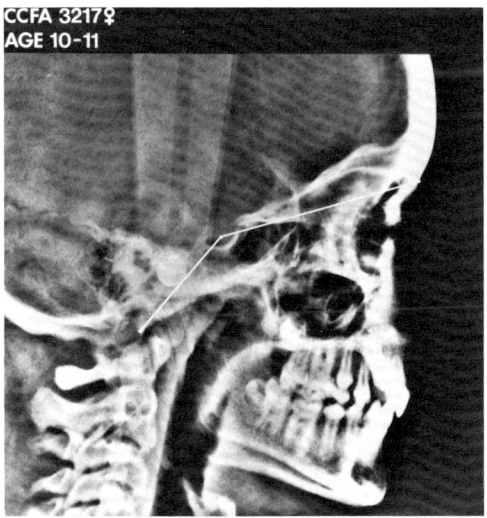

Fig. 2. CCFA #3217: female, age 10 years 11 months, right HFM. Platybasia (Nasion-Sella-Basion angle: 146°).

3. Occipitalization of the atlas (C-1): close approximation or contact with partial or complete fusion of the atlas to the occiput [Schmidt et al, 1978; Hensinger and MacEwen, 1982] (Figs. 3,4).

4. Basilar invagination or impression: cephalad position of the tip of the odontoid process of the axis with possible protrusion into foramen magnum [Chamberlain, 1939; McGregor, 1948; Hensinger and MacEwen, 1982] (Fig. 4; see also Fig. 8A).

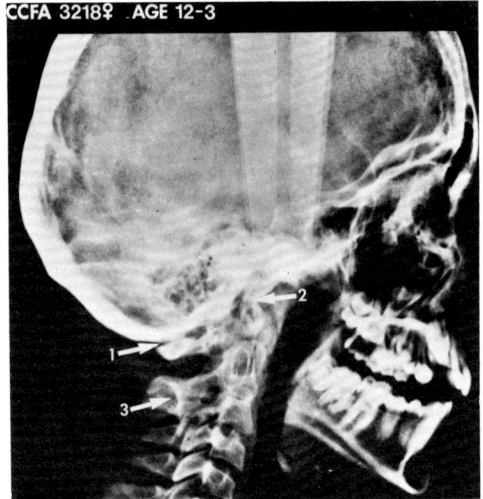

Fig. 3. CCFA #3218: female, age 12 years 3 months, bilateral M. Note the close approximation of the atlas to the occiput (arrow 1) and basion (anterior border of foramen magnum) (arrow 2). Fusion of the spinous processes of C-2 with C-3 is also shown (arrow 3).

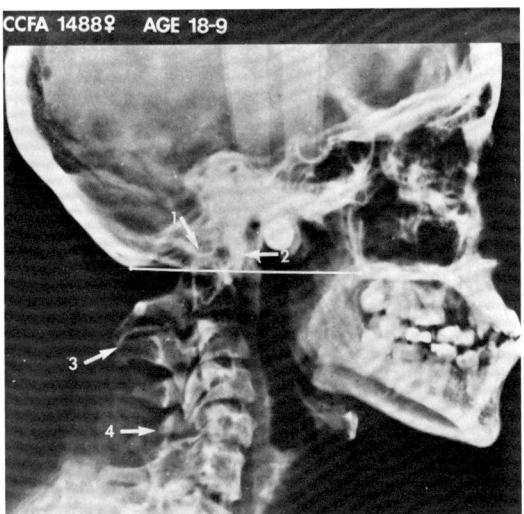

Fig. 4. CCFA #1488: female, age 18 years 9 months, right HFM. Multiple craniovertebral malformations: basilar invagination with tip of odontoid process (arrow 1); above McGregor's line (posterior nasal spine to occiput); occipitalization of the atlas, posterior arch of atlas is not distinguishable, the anterior tubercule is observed (arrow 2); fusion of spinous processes of C-2 with C-3 (arrow 3); spinous process of C-5 is hypoplastic (arrow 4).

Cervicovertebral Malformations

1. Fusion: failure of segmentation between two or more vertebrae. It may be partial (Fig. 5A) or total (Fig. 5B) [Shands and Bundens, 1956; Dolan, 1977].

2. Spina bifida: failure of fusion in the vertebral midline posteriorly or anteriorly [Pendergrass et al, 1956; Ruge and Wiltse, 1977; Caffey, 1978] (Fig. 6; see also Fig. 10).

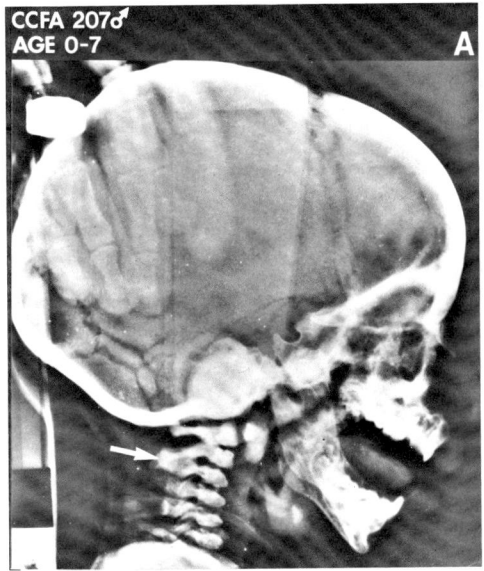
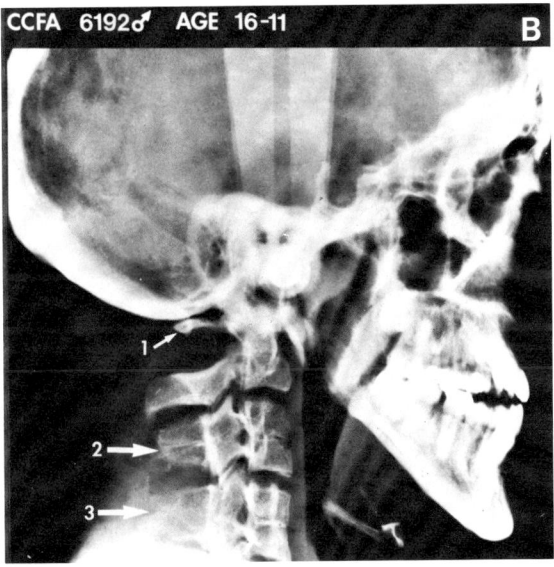

Fig.5. A) CCFA #207: male, age 7 months, right HFM. Note the early onset and partial vertebral fusion affecting the spinous process of C2 and C3 (arrow). B) CCFA #6192: male, age 16 years 11 months, bilateral M. Note the hypoplastic posterior arch of the atlas (arrrow 1) and its close approximation to the occiput. Fusion of the vertebral bodies and spinous processes of C-3 with C-4 (arrow 2) and C-5 with C-6 (arrow 3).

3. Accessory vertebra: presence of an additional vertebra [Caffey, 1978] (Fig. 7).
4. Hypoplastic vertebra: anomalous reduction in size of the whole vertebra or its parts (Figs. 4, 5B, 8).
5. Displaced vertebra: forward or backward displacement of the whole vertebra in relation to the occiput and the rest of the cervical column (Figs. 1, 9).
6. Scoliosis: abnormal lateral deviation of the cervical spine (Figs. 6A, 10).

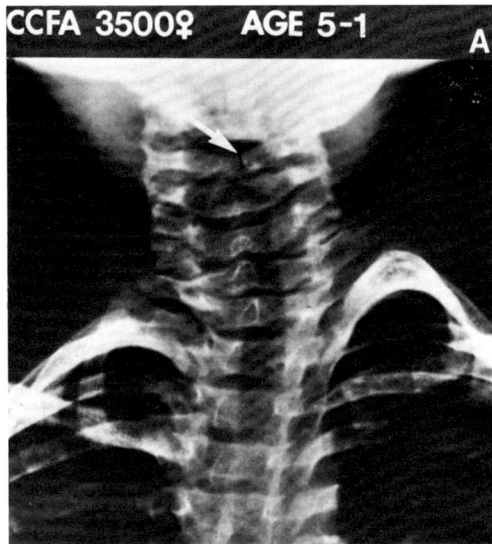

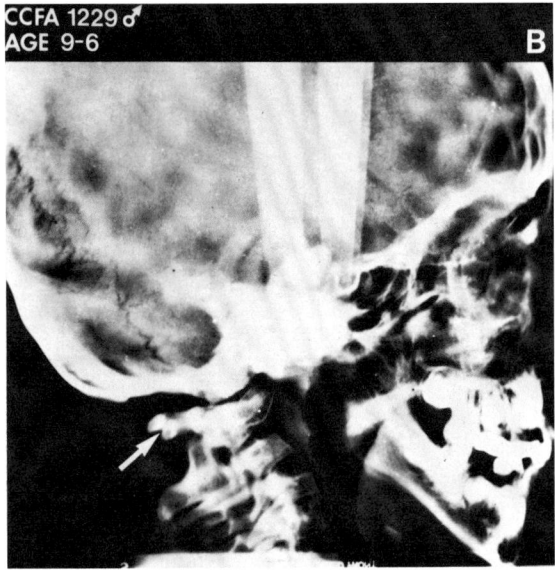

Fig.6. A) CCFA #3500: female, age 5 years 1 month, GS. Note spina bifida of C-3 (arrow) and scoliosis of the cervical spine. B) CCFA #1229: male, age 9 years 6 months, bilateral M. Spina bifida posterior (arrow).

RESULTS

Malformations of the cranial base and/or cervical spine were found in 57 (28%) of the total number of patients studied (Table II). Cervicovertebral malformations occurred more frequently than anomalies of the cranial base. The frequency of patients in each subgroup affected with malformations of the cranial base and/or cervical spine was about one fourth of those with M (29%) and essentially the same

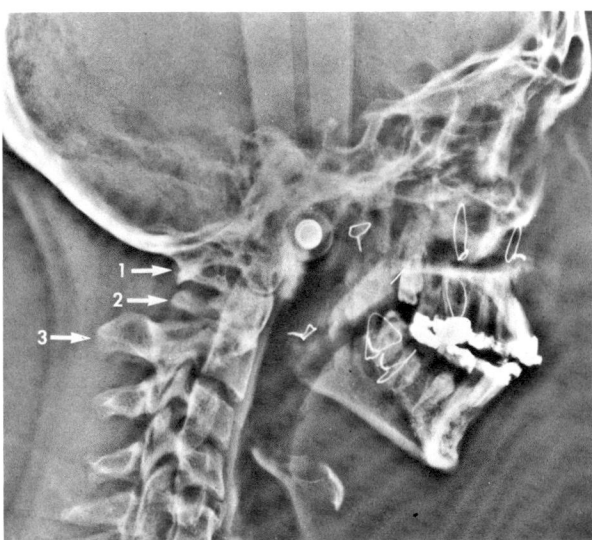

Fig. 7. CCFA #4803: male, age 20 years, left HFM. Extra or accessory vertebra (arrow 2) between the atlas (arrow 1) and the axis (arrow 3). Note hypoplastic posterior arch of the atlas and its close approximation to the occiput (occipitalization).

for HFM (24%). Three of the six patients with GS, and, by definition, all (six of six) of the OAV patients were affected.

The frequency of the different craniovertebral malformations is shown in Tables III and IV. In 18 patients more than one malformation was diagnosed. Platybasia (9/25) and occipitalization of the atlas (C-1) (9/25) were the most common malformations of the cranial base, each accounting for about one third of the instances. Of the 64 spinal anomalies, 47 (73%) were vertebral fusions, making this anomaly the most common of all the craniovertebral malformations. Only one case of accessory vertebra was recorded. The HFM subgroup was the only one that demonstrated examples of all the different types of cranial base and cervicovertebral malformations.

In the total sample studied there were four patients with the associated diagnosis of Klippel-Feil syndrome; three were in the HFM subgroup and one in the OAV subgroup. Of the three HFM patients two had malformations of both the cranial base and cervical spine: one was male with platybasia, basilar invagination, and block cervical fusions; the other was a female with basilar kyphosis, occipitalization of the atlas (C-1), and block cervical fusions. The third HFM patient had only spinal fusions. The remaining Klippel-Feil patient was a female in the OAV category with both cranial base and cervical malformations (basilar kyphosis and cervical block fusions).

DISCUSSION

Variants within a clinical entity are recognized by the presence of common or overlapping phenotypic traits. Demonstration of a new phenotypic feature shared by all the variants may add support to their association. The phenotypic characteristic shared by HFM, GS, and OAV is unilateral or bilateral malformation of the external

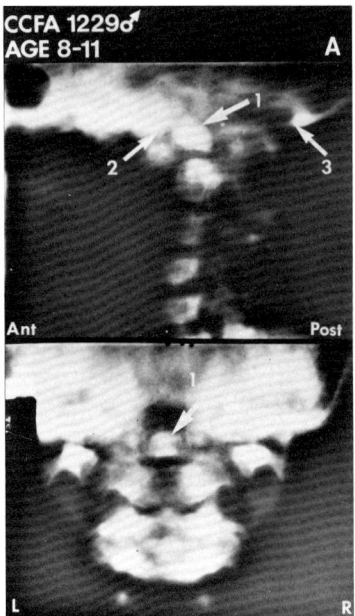
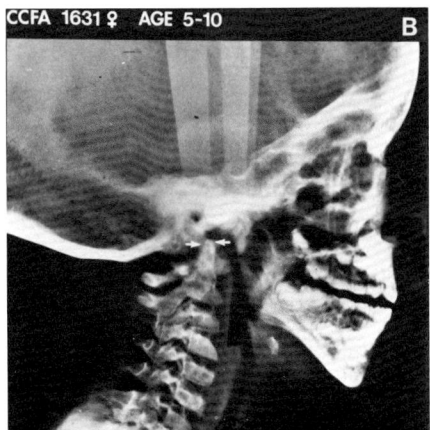
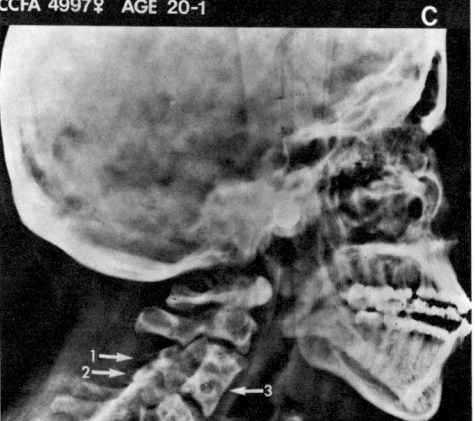

Fig. 8. A) CCFA #1229: male, age 8 years 11 months, bilateral M. Sagittal (top) and coronal (bottom) tomograms demonstrating hypoplasia of the odontoid process with nonfusion of its tip (arrow 1 top and bottom) to the rest of the process. The tip of the odontoid process is high into foramen magnum (basilar invagination). The anterior (arrow 2) and posterior (arrow 3) borders of foramen magnum are seen. B) CCFA #1631: female, age 5 years 10 months, right M. Note the thin tip of the odontoid process (arrows) as well as its unusual superior position in relation to the atlas. C) CCFA #4997: female, age 20 years 1 month, left HFM. Note the almost complete absent spinous process of C-3 and C-4 (arrows 1 and 2). The bodies of these vertebrae are also fused (arrow 3).

ear (microtia). Other phenotypic features such as mandibular malformations and epibulbar dermoids are common findings but not always present. Recent family studies [Kaye et al, 1979; Rollnick and Kaye, 1983] have suggested that isolated M may represent the mildest form of the phenotypic spectrum of *hemifacial microsomia*. This suggestion is supported by our finding of a similar frequency of craniovertebral

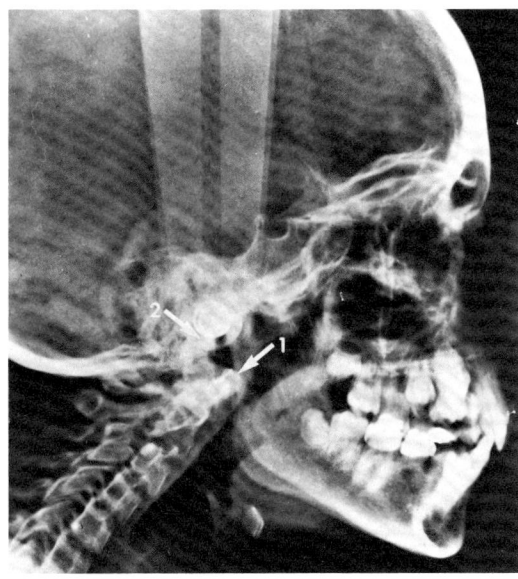

Fig. 9. CCFA #5249: female, age 11 years 9 months, right HFM. Forward displacement of the atlas (C-1) (arrow 1) in relation to basion (arrow 2) and the rest of the spine. Note the unusual angulation of the cervical spine.

malformations in M and HFM, the only subgroups where adequate sample sizes allowed for comparison.

The frequency of patients affected with cervical spine malformations in this study was slightly above 20% for both M and HFM. In a sample of 102 patients with "first and second branchial syndrome" Grabb [1965] found a frequency of malformation of 11% in the vertebrae and ribs. Ross [1975] mentioned an occurrence of cervical spine malformations of 20–30% in a sample of patients with HFM. Our frequency values as well as the ones reported by Grabb and Ross are clearly above those of the normal population, which range between 0.60 and 1.70% [Brown et al, 1964; Osborne et al, 1971].

Spinal malformations such as hemivertebra, fusions, spina bifida, scoliosis, supernumerary or accessory vertebra, and occipitalization of the atlas have been recognized previously in the diagnostic categories studied herein, although without giving occurrence rates [Grabb, 1965; Gorlin et al, 1976]. In the present investigation vertebral fusions were found to be the main cervical spine malformation (73%).

In addition to cervical malformations, anomalies of the cranial base were recognized in all the diagnostic categories although less frequently. The similar occurrence of cranial base malformations in the M and HFM subgroups also lends support to the association between M and *hemifacial microsomia*. In the normal population the incidence for some of these cranial base malformations is very low. For instance, Gunderson et al [1967] reported values of 0.5% for occipitalization of the atlas and 0.03% for basilar impression.

The four cases with the combined diagnosis of both HFM and OAV with Klippel-Feil syndrome were of interest. We also noted other cases that had radiologic as well

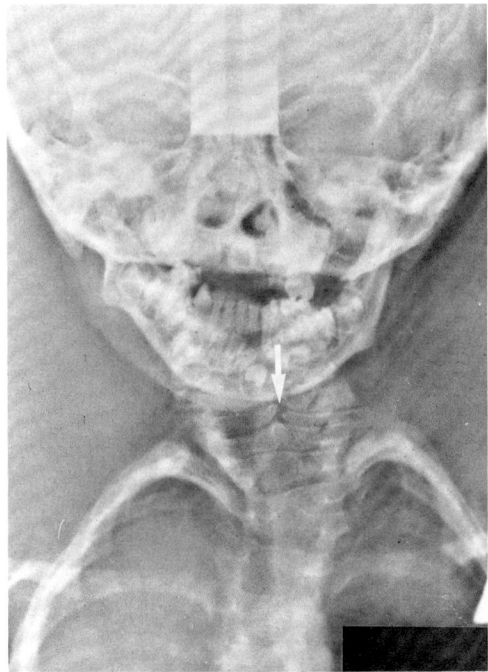

Fig. 10. CCFA #5036: male, age 4 years 9 months, right HFM. Cervical scoliosis. Note spine bifida in lower cervical vertebra (C-6) (arrow).

TABLE II. Number (N) and Percentage (%) of Patients Affected With Malformations of the Cranial Base (A), Cervical Vertebrae (B), and With Both Malformations (C) and Patients Without Craniovertebral Malformations

	Diagnostic category								Total	
	M		HFM		GS		OAV			
Malformation	N	%	N	%	N	%	N	%	N	%
Cranial base	3	6	4	3	1	16	—	—	8	4
Cervical vertebrae	9	19	22	15	2	34	5	84	38	19
Both A and B	2	4	8	6	—	—	1	16	11	5
Affected patients	14	29	34	24	3	50	6	100	57	28
Nonaffected patients	34	71	110	76	3	50	—	—	147	72
Total patients	48	100	144	100	6	100	6	100	204	100

as some clinical characteristics of this syndrome. The association between Klippel-Feil syndrome, HFM, and M has been noted previously [Helmi and Pruzansky, 1980], and Gellis and Feingold [1971] have speculated that GS, OAV, and Klippel-Feil syndrome are part of a spectrum of the same entity.

The high frequency of craniovertebral malformations in patients with *hemifacial microsomia*, and especially in the patients with the associated diagnosis of Klippel-Feil syndrome, is not easily explained on the basis of Poswillo's "hematoma formation theory" [1973] as the prime etiologic factor in the otomandibular malformations. Similar concerns have been expressed by Cohen [1982] in cases where HFM is

TABLE III. Number and Distribution of the Different Cranial Base Malformations in the Four Diagnostic Categories

Malformation	M ♂	M ♀	HFM ♂	HFM ♀	GS ♀	GS ♂	OAV ♂	OAV ♀	Total
Kyphosis	—	—	2	2	—	—	—	1	5
Platybasia	4	1	2	1	1	—	—	—	9
Occipitalization (C1)	2	—	4	3	—	—	—	—	9
Basilar invagination	—	—	2	—	—	—	—	—	2
Subtotal	6	1	10	6	1	—	—	1	
Total	7		16		1		1		25

TABLE IV. Numbers and Distribution of the Different Cervicovertebral Malformations in the Four Diagnostic Categories[1]

Malformation	M ♂	M ♀	HFM ♂	HFM ♀	GS ♂	GS ♀	OAV ♂	OAV ♀	Total
Fusion	5	5	20	10	1	—	1	5	47
Spina bifida	—	—	3	—	—	1	—	—	4
Accessory vertebra	—	—	1	—	—	—	—	—	1
Hypoplastic vertebra	1	1	—	3	—	—	—	—	5
Displaced vertebra	—	—	1	2	—	—	—	—	3
Scoliosis	—	—	—	2	—	1	—	1	4
Subtotal	6	6	25	17	1	2	1	6	
Total	12		42		3		7		64

[1]Note the large number (47) of fusions compared to the number of other malformations.

associated with malformations in other organ systems. These observations as well as the increased frequency of craniovertebral malformations found in *hemifacial microsomia* suggest a more generalized etiopathogenetic mechanism. The findings further support the thesis that M, HFM, GS, and OAV may all be part of the same broad, phenotypic spectrum.

ACKNOWLEDGMENTS

We want to take this opportunity to recognize the invaluable advice, support, and inspiration given to us by Dr. Samuel Pruzansky. Dr. Pruzansky introduced us to this area of clinical research. He was an integral part of this project and reviewed with one of us (A.A.F.), through many long nights and weekends, innumerable radiographs and clinical charts. At the same time, he shared his experience, vast knowledge, and personal ingenuity. To him we dedicate this work, and thank Drs. Cohen and Rollnick for providing us with the opportunity to do it.

Dr. Mahmood Mafee reviewed some of the radiographs, and Dr. Howard Aduss reviewed the manuscript and made helpful suggestions. Ms. Julie Jordan provided artistic assistance; Steven Schneider did the photography, and Joann Darrow typed the manuscript.

This study was supported in part by grants from the National Institutes of Health (DE 02872) and Maternal and Child Health Services, Department of Health and Human Services.

REFERENCES

Aase JM: Microtia—Clinical observations. Birth Defects XVI:289–297, 1980.
Brown MD, Templeton AW, Hodges III FJ: The incidence of acquired and congenital fusions in the cervical spine. AM J Roentgenol Radium Ther Nucl Med 92:1255–1259, 1964.
Caffey J: "Pediatric X-ray Diagnosis," Vol. 1, 7th ed. Chicago, London: Yearbook Medical Publishers Inc., 1978, pp 273–284.
Chamberlain WE: Basilar impression (platybasia). Yale J Biol Med 11:487–496, 1939.
Cohen JR MM: "The Child With Multiple Birth Defects." New York: Raven Press, 1982, 1982, pp 56–70.
Dolan KD: Developmental abnormalities of the cervical spine below the axis. Radiol Clin North Am 15:167–175, 1977.
Figueroa AA, Pruzansky S: The external ear, mandible and other components of hemifacial microsomia. J Maxillofac Surg 10:200–211, 1982.
Gellis SS, Feingold M: Congenital brevicollis (Klippel-Feil syndrome). Am J Dis Child 121:501–502, 1971.
Gorlin RJ: Oculoauriculovertebral syndrome. J Pediatr 63:991–999, 1963.
Gorlin RJ, Pindborg JJ, Cohen Jr, MM: "Syndromes of the Head and Neck." 2nd ed. New York: McGraw-Hill, 1976, pp 546–552.
Grabb WC: The first and second branchial arch syndrome. Plast Reconstr Surg 36:485–507, 1965.
Gunderson CH, Greenspan RH, Glaser GH, Lubs HA: The Klippel-Feil syndrome: genetic and clinical reevaluation of cervical fusion. Medicine 46:491–512, 1967.
Helmi C, Pruzansky S: Craniofacial and extracranial malformations in the Klippel-Feil syndrome. Cleft Palate J 17:65–88, 1980.
Hensinger RN, MacEwen GD: Congenital anomalies of the spine. In: Rothman RH, Simeone FA (eds): "The Spine," Philadelphia: W.B. Saunders Co., 1982, pp 188–239.
Kaye CI, Rollnick BR, Pruzansky S: Malformations of the auricle: Isolated and in syndromes. IV. Cumulative pedigree data. Birth Defects XV:163–169, 1979.
McGregor M: The significance of certain measurements of the skull in the diagnosis of basilar impression. Br J Radiol 21: 171–181, 1948.
Melnick, M: The etiology of external ear malformations and its relation to abnormalities of the middle ear, inner ear, and other organ systems. Birth Defects XVI:303–331, 1980.
Osborne GS, Pruzansky S, Koepp-Baker H: Upper cervical spine anomalies and osseous nasopharyngeal depth. J Speech Hearing Res 13:14–22, 1971.
Pendergrass EP, Schaeffer JP, Hodes PJ: "The Head and Neck in Roentgen Diagnosis," Vol II, 2nd ed. Springfield, Illinois: Charles C. Thomas, 1956, pp 1541–1558.
Poswillo D: The pathogenesis of the first and second branchial arch syndrome. Oral Surg 35:302–328, 1973.
Pruzansky S: Not all dwarfed mandibles are alike. Birth Defects V:120–129, 1969.
Pruzansky S: Clinical investigations of the experiments of nature. Am Speech Hearing Assoc Re 8:62–94, 1973.
Riolo SL, Moyers RE, McNamara Jr, JA, Hunter WS: "An Atlas of Craniofacial Growth and Development," Ann Arbor, Michigan: The University of Michigan, 1974.
Rollnick BR, Kaye CI: Hemifacial microsomia and variants: Pedigree data. Am J Med Genet 15:233–253, 1983.
Ross RB: Lateral facial dysplasia (first and second branchial arch syndrome, hemifacial microsomia). Birth Defects XI:51–59, 1975.
Ruge D, Wiltse LL: "Spinal Disorders: Diagnosis and Treatment." Philadelphia: Lea & Febiger, 1977, pp 239–245.
Schmidt H, Sartor K, Heckl RW: Bone malformations of the craniocervical region. In: Vinken PJ, Bruyn GW, Myrianthopoulos NC (eds): "Handbook of Clinical Neurology—Congenital Malformations of the Spine and Spinal Cord." Amsterdam: North-Holland Publishing Co., 1978, pp 1–98.
Shands AR, Bundens WD: Congenital deformities of the spine. An analysis of the roentgenograms of 700 children. Bull Hosp Dis 17:110–133, 1956.

The Beckwith-Wiedemann Syndrome: A Longitudinal Study of the Macroglossia and Dentofacial Complex

Hans Friede and Alvaro A. Figueroa

Center for Craniofacial Anomalies, University of Illinois College of Medicine, Chicago

Case reports provide insights into fundamental mechanisms and also assist clinicians in treatment of similarly affected patients [Pruzansky, 1976]. The present investigation examines the natural history of the macroglossia associated with a case of Beckwith-Wiedemann syndrome (BWS) and its influence on dentofacial development. Facial skeletal growth and tongue size were assessed by analyzing cephalometric radiographs from age 2 months to 7.5 years. The data were compared with cephalometric norms and new normative data derived from 13 patients with cleft lip. The major influence of the macroglossia was protrusion of dentoalveolar structures, particularly in the lower jaw. This resulted in an anterior cross-bite in the primary dentition. In addition, an abnormally obtuse gonial angle was observed increasing the effective length of the mandible. Tongue size in BWS was generally greater than the norm, but the increase with age paralleled the mean growth curve of the tongue in the control. Over time the base of the tongue became longer and the hyoid bone moved posteriorly and inferiorly, allowing for accomodation of the tongue within the oral cavity. The changes in tongue shape and dentofacial morphology support the position that early partial glossectomy should be delayed or abandoned. In cases where tongue reduction is considered necessary, the new cephalometric normative data on tongue size provided herein can be used to establish objective criteria for such surgery.

Key words: Beckwith-Wiedemann syndrome, cephalometry, dentofacial development, dentoalveolar protrusion, tongue, macroglossia

INTRODUCTION

The Beckwith-Wiedemann syndrome (BWS) was originally described in the 1960s, the cardinal characteristics being *e*xomphalos (omphalocele), *m*acroglossia, and *g*igantism (EMG syndrome) [Wiedemann, 1968]. A recent review of the literature on the syndrome indicated that the phenotypic traits had been substantially expanded [Sotelo-Avila et al, 1980]. In addition to the macroglossia, anomalies specifically related to the head region were facial flame nevus, ear lobe anomalies, mild microcephaly, prominent occiput, and maxillary hypoplasia with shortness of the orbital floor. However, none of the features constituting the syndrome should be considered obligatory [Cohen, 1971].

Macroglossia, together with defects of the abdominal wall (omphalocele, umbilical hernia, and diastasis recti), are the most constant signs of BWS [Cohen, 1971]. A survey by Filippi and McKusick [1970] showed that more than 95% of the patients

---

Address reprint requests to Hans Friede, Director, Center for Craniofacial Anomalies, University of Illinois College of Medicine, P.O. Box 6998, Chicago, IL 60680.

© 1985 Alan R. Liss, Inc.

displayed tongue enlargement and only two of their 45 studied subjects had normal tongue sizes as judged clinically. The degree of macroglossia varies and has been described as a general enlargement with difficulty in keeping the tongue within the oral cavity. In general, the macroglossia slowly regresses during the first years of life, although in some patients it may persist to adolescence. The mechanism for its resolution is not known, but both shrinkage of the tongue and catch-up growth of the structures that make up the oral cavity are suggested explanations [Cohen, 1969; Filippi and McKusick, 1970]. Some histological studies have revealed normal tongue tissue [Cohen, 1971; Irving, 1971], while others have shown mild hypertrophic changes of the muscle fibers [Schafer, 1968].

Difficulty in swallowing may occur at birth as well as later in the neonatal period. In extreme cases, surgical reduction of the tongue may be necessary to improve infant feeding [Irving, 1971]. For most patients, difficulties can be overcome by use of special nipples so that extraordinary measures such as tube feeding or surgery are rarely necessary. Another functional problem in early infancy is blockage of the airway by the enlarged tongue. Emergency situations due to sudden respiratory obstruction have been described [Filippi and McKusick, 1970]. If the airway is chronically restricted by the macroglossia, pulmonary hypertension and cor pulmonale may develop. Smith et al [1982] reported on a patient where tracheostomy was necessary to resolve the cardiomegaly and the increased pulmonary vascularity. The macroglossia may also limit tongue movements and thereby ffect speech [Abelson et al, 1941; Filippi and McKusick, 1970]. To prevent development of speech defects, it has been suggested that tongue size be reduced surgically during the first year of life [Schafer, 1968].

Several studies on BWS have reported an increased frequency of class III malocclusion due to mandibular prognathism [Abelson et al, 1941; Schafer, 1968; Cohen, 1969]. Irving [1971] stressed that in most cases this was not a true mandibular prognathism but was due to midfacial deficiency. This finding would account for the "family-likeness" of patients with BWS. Individuals with the syndrome were also judged to share other characteristics such as "bulging of the alveolus, retroclination of lower incisors and an anterior open bite." However, a roentgencephalometric study by Baer [1975] demonstrated that on the average, neither mandibular prognathism, maxillary hypoplasia, nor midfacial deficiency existed in a sample of 16 BWS patients. Yet the macroglossia was responsible for the anterior open bite, and the author speculated whether the enlarged tongue similarly had caused the increased effective length of the mandible and the abnormally obtuse gonial angle.

To obtain more precise data on the orofacial features in BWS, Cohen [1969] urged longitudinal roentgencephalometric studies. This information would help provide objective answers to many clinical questions. For example, should partial glossectomy be performed or will the macroglossia regress over time? Is the macroglossia responsible for the class III malocclusion by causing mandibular prognathism, or is the malocclusion due to hypoplasia of the midface? Answers to these questions would be of value in the planning of long-term patient care.

The purpose of this communication is to report the clinical and serial roentgencephalometric data on a patient with BWS from the age of 2 months to 7.5 years. Admittedly, the findings reported rely on only one case, but this pilot study, using long-term cephalometric data, may stimulate others to test specific findings on a larger group of patients with this syndrome.

CASE REPORT
Clinical Data

CCFA #4337 is a caucasian male born after a full-term uncomplicated pregnancy. He was the second child of nonconsanguineous parents. Birth weight was low (2.4 kg; below 5th percentile) as was height (49 cm; 10th percentile). Immediately after birth the tongue was recorded to be large and protrusive, but neither feeding nor respiration were affected. There were signs of flammeus nevi in the region of the nasal bridge.

At 2 months of age, the patient was referred to the Center for Craniofacial Anomalies with the chief parental complaint of macroglossia (Fig. 1). Facial characteristics included a wide head with frontal bossing and a depressed nasal bridge. Examination of the abdomen revealed diverticulation of the recti muscles and a small umbilical hernia (Fig. 2). Mild hepatosplenomegaly was diagnosed at the age of 16 months. At this time a remarkable gain in weight as well as length (above 95th percentile) was recorded but at later visits both of these parameters slowly returned to the low normal range.

At the initial 2-month examination, the macroglossia was clinically significant, but at 16 months of age the tongue was less protrusive. It was still carried between the separated lips, a habit persisting during most of the study period. The tongue also seemed very mobile and could be extended beyond the tip of the patient's nose (Fig. 3).

Speech evaluation at 3.5 years indicated some deficiencies in articulation with substitutions and omissions, which together with slow syllabic sequencing gave an

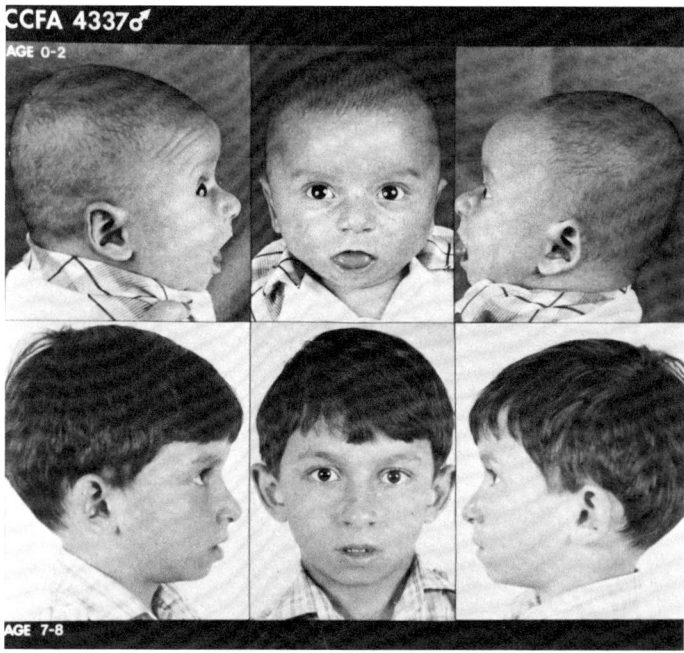

Fig. 1. CCFA #4337, Beckwith-Wiedemann syndrome. At age 2 months note protrusion of the tongue. At 7 years 8 months notice lip fullness due to compensatory dentoalveolar protrusion.

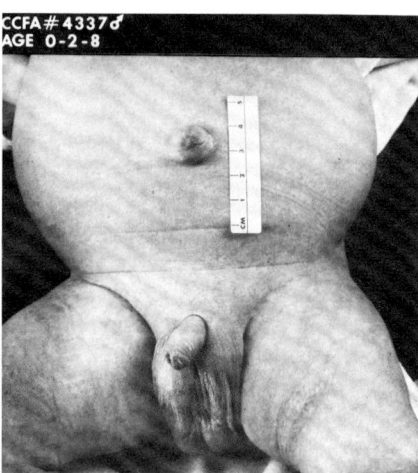

Fig. 2. CCFA #4337, age 2 months 8 days. Mild umbilical hernia.

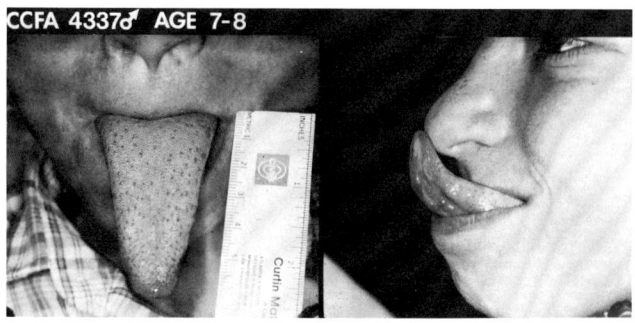

Fig. 3. CCFA #4337, age 7 years 8 months. Unusual ability for tongue extrusion.

overall intelligibility of about 50%. Prolonged speech therapy resulted in improvements, but at 7.5 years the patient still demonstrated subnormal speech for his age with an intelligibility of approximately 85%.

At 2 years of age, occlusion of the buccal segments was normal (Fig. 4). A mild functional anterior cross-bite of the primary dentition was corrected spontaneously when the permanent incisors erupted.

Roentgencephalometric data were obtained at approximately yearly intervals from age 2 months to 7 years 8 months (Fig. 5). Actual measurements and superimpositions of tracings of lateral roentgencephalometric films for comparison with normative values [Bolton Standards, Broadbent et al, 1975] were performed at ages 1, 4, and 7 years.

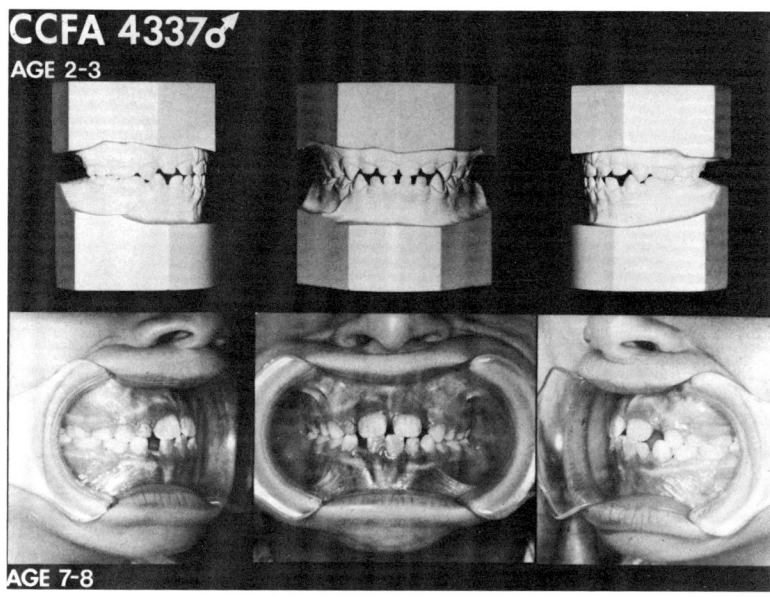

Fig. 4. Intraoral features of CCFA #4337 at age 2 years 3 months (top) and at 7 years 8 months (bottom). The early tendency to anterior cross-bite was corrected spontaneously when the permanent incisors erupted.

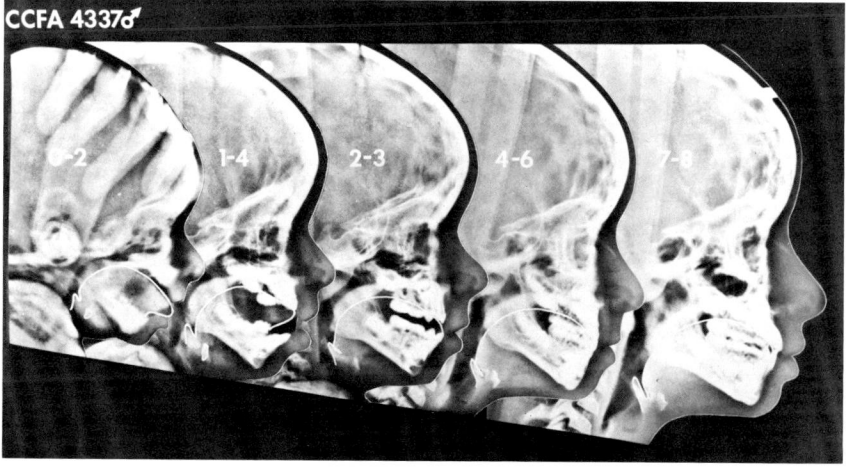

Fig. 5. CCFA #4337, composite of selected cephalometric radiographs demonstrating the change in position of the tongue with age and the correction of the anterior cross-bite.

184   Friede and Figueroa

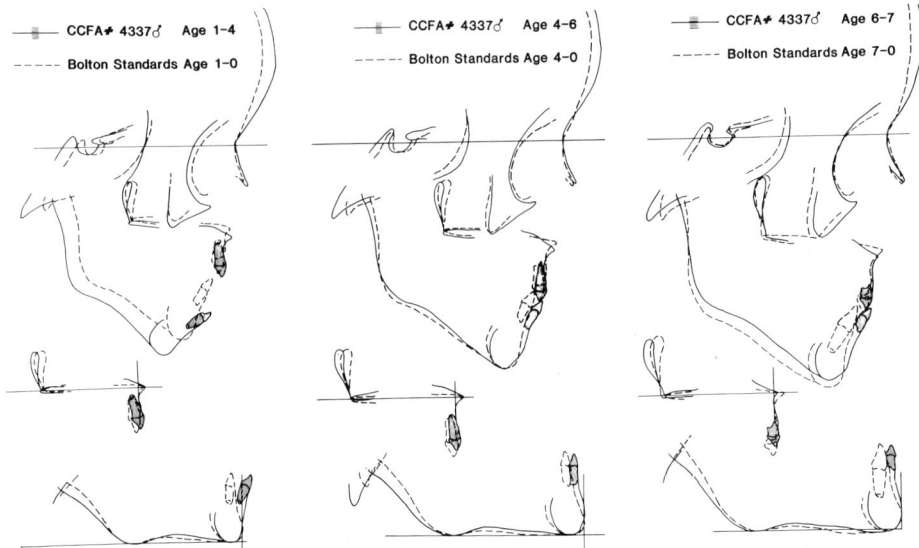

Fig. 6. Selected tracings of CCFA #4337 superimposed on norm tracings. The major difference is the dentoalveolar protrusion in the mandible. There is also an abnormally obtuse gonial angle and increased effective length of the mandible in the BWS patient.

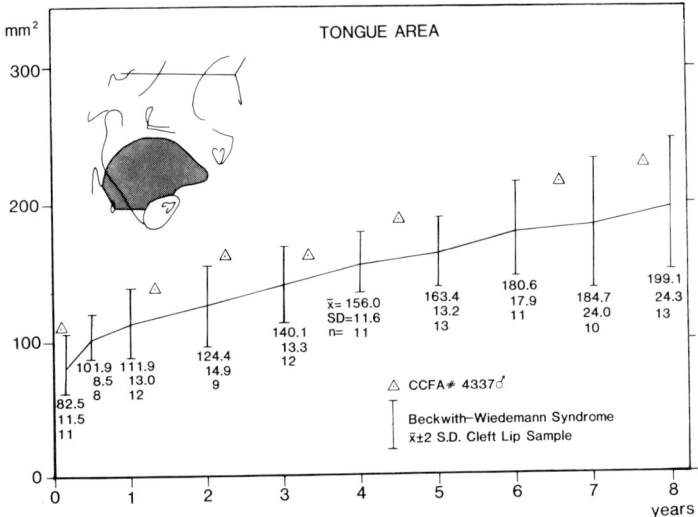

Fig. 7. Tongue size measurement of CCFA #4337 compared to normative data obtained from patients with cleft lip. The mean ($\bar{X}$), standard deviation (SD) and number of control patients (n) for each age group studied are indicated. Note the increased tongue size of CCFA #4337 and the growth rate paralleling the norm.

At the ages studied the maxillary and mandibular denture bases were in a normal position, relative to each other and in relation to the anterior cranial base (Fig. 6). The dentoalveolar area, especially in the lower jaw and at the earliest age, deviated from the norm. It was protrusive and there was proclination of the incisors. In addition, the angle between the body and ramus of the mandible (gonial angle) was more obtuse and the distance from the condyle to the chin (effective length of the mandible) was greater than the norm at all three ages when compared to the Bolton Standards. The neurocranium was of normal size but demonstrated a tendency to frontal bossing. The position of the infraorbital rim was normal.

The tongue, as seen in the lateral projection, was traced to analyze its size and shape and to evaluate how these parameters changed with growth. The base of the tongue was defined by two planes: one from the estimated point of attachment of the geniohyoid muscle at the symphysis to the most anterior point on the hyoid bone and the other by a plane from the hyoid bone to the vallecula at the root of the tongue (Fig. 7). The area bordered by these lines and the dorsum of the tongue was measured with a planimeter. Data for comparison were obtained from our longitudinal records of a sample of 13 patients with cleft lip who were of similar age, sex, and race. Craniofacial development in patients with this cleft type is considered to be the same as that of nonclefts [Hunter, 1981], and tongue development can be expected to be normal.

The area of the tongue in our patient with BWS was larger than in the control subjects during the entire study period. At an early age, some measurements were more than 2 SD greater than the mean values of the control. However, growth in size of the tongue with age did not differ from the mean increase of the control subjects (Fig. 7). The base of the BWS tongue was greater (increased symphysis-hyoid distance) when compared to the control, especially at the oldest age studied (Fig. 8). In addition, the hyoid bone had a more backward and downward position relative to the inferior border of the mandible in the BWS patient.

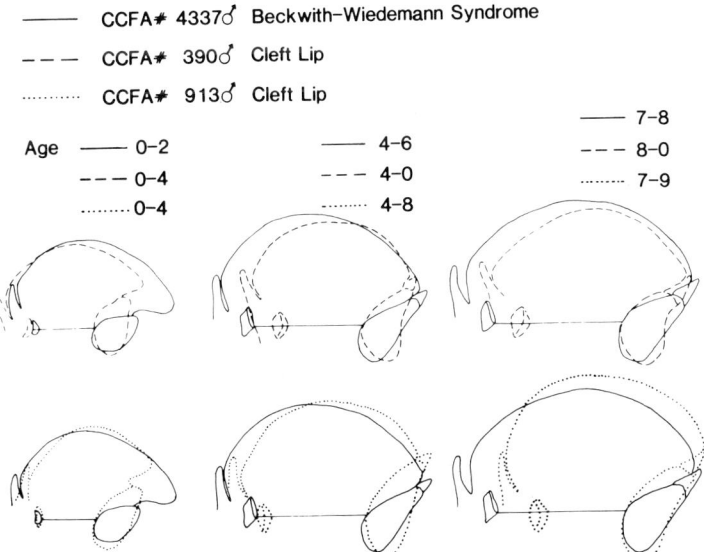

Fig. 8. Tongue tracings superimposed on symphysis-hyoid line comparing tongue shape of CCFA #4337 with two control patients at three different ages. Note the increase in length of the tongue base of the patient with BWS.

DISCUSSION

This paper presents *one* relatively mild case of BWS, and, therefore, some of the questions that triggered this study cannot be fully answered. Even though the macroglossia was judged to be clinically significant, it appeared much smaller than in some other cases reported in the literature [eg, Filippi and McKusick, 1970; Smith et al, 1982]. The accuracy in such comparisons would be enhanced if they were based on measurements from cephalometric radiographs rather than relying on clinical photographs. If available, cephalometric normative data for tongue size could be of great value for making a correct diagnosis of BWS. This would be especially true in cases with mild phenotypic traits of the syndrome and with a minor degree of macroglossia.

The limitations and difficulties in providing standard values for tongue size are acknowledged. In the lateral roentgencephalogram only the sagittal view of the tongue can be studied and the dorsal outline may occasionally be difficult to define. Alterations in head posture may make linear measurement appear inconsistent but this can be overcome by studying longitudinal records. With regard to tongue size, we agree with Vig and Cohen [1974] that minor changes in mandibular posture, such as from rest position to occlusion, do not significantly influence the measurements.

Tongue size in our BWS patient was above the normal but growth with age paralleled the norm. Therefore, this case does not support the suggestion that shrinkage of the tongue is the mechanism for clinical regression of the macroglossia. Instead, we would suggest that a change in the position of the base of the tongue, as reflected in the change to a more downward and backward position of the hyoid bone, makes the anterior part less protrusive. Moreover, the reposturing is sufficient to compensate for the growth of the tongue. Similar tongue shape and hyoid position could be seen in other case reports on BWS when lateral radiographs of the head were used to illustrate the condition [Arons et al, 1970; Lee, 1972]. Whether the elongated tongue base with a long genohyoid muscle would help to explain our patient's unusual ability to extrude his tongue remains an interesting speculation.

It is a well-known fact that the tongue influences the development of dentofacial structures. Therefore, it is reasonable to believe that the increased effective length of the mandible and the abnormally obtuse gonial angle of our BWS patient were related to his macroglossia. In spite of this mandibular morphology, the chin was in a normal "nonprognathic" position relative to the cranial base, which supports previous findings [Baer, 1975]. In addition, we did not find any real midfacial deficiency, again as previously reported by Baer [1975]. We suspect that this characteristic, mentioned in earlier investigations [Irving, 1971], was a clinical illusion due to the frontal bossing.

To account for the early anterior cross-bite in our patient and in the cases illustrated by Arons et al [1970] and Lee [1972] it is necessary to examine the effect the macroglossia has on the dental arch. It is accepted that incisor position and the shape of the dental arch are in part the result of muscle forces from the lips and the tongue. The protrusive, macroglossic tongue, present in the early years of life, results in excessive labial tipping of the lower incisors and the consequent anterior crossbite. If the dentoalveolar compensations do not regress spontaneously after the tongue is accommodated into the oral cavity, orthodontic treatment can be instituted. For the moderate cases of macroglossia, such conservative measures seem preferable to partial glossectomy in infancy [Schafer, 1968]. However, we realize that tongue surgery might be indicated in *extreme* cases for both morphological and functional reasons.

The cephalometric standards on tongue size that have been presented in this report can be used for objective evaluation of the macroglossia in patients where tongue reduction is under consideration. There is a need for further longitudinal roentgencephalometric investigations, either as case reports or group studies of patients with BWS. Knowledge of the natural history of this syndrome is an essential part of its diagnosis and treatment planning.

ACKNOWLEDGMENTS

Howard Aduss, D.D.S. reviewed the manuscript and made helpful suggestions. Julie Jordan provided artistic assistance; Steven Schnieder did the photography, and Joann Darrow typed the manuscript.

This investigation was supported in part by grants from the National Institutes of Health (DE 02872) and Maternal and Child Health Services, Department of Health and Human Services.

REFERENCES

Abelson SM, Brodie AG, Bronstein IP, Schreiber SL: Muscular macroglossia. Am J Dis Child 62:624–628, 1941.
Arons MS, Solitare GB, Grunt JA: The macroglossia of Beckwith's syndrome. Plast Reconstr Surg 45:341–345, 1970.
Baer LD: A cephalometric study of patients with the Wiedemann-Beckwith syndrome and subjects with class III malocclusion. Master Thesis, University of Washington, Seattle, Washington, 1975.
Broadbent BH, Sr, Broadbent BH, Jr, Golden WH: "Bolton Standards of Dentofacial Developmental Growth." St. Louis: C.V. Mosby Co., 1975.
Cohen MM, Jr: Comments on the macroglossia-omphalocele syndrome. Birth Defects V(2):197, 1969.
Cohen MM, Jr: The Beckwith-Wiedemann syndrome. Am J Dis Child 122:515–520, 1971.
Filippi G, McKusick VA: The Beckwith-Wiedemann syndrome. Medicine 49:279–298, 1970.
Hunter SW: The Michigan cleft twin study. J Craniofac Genet Dev Biol 1:235–242, 1981.
Irving I: The "E.M.G." syndrome (exomphalos, macroglossia, gigantism). Progr Pediatr Surg 1:1–61, 1971.
Lee FA: Radiology of Beckwith-Wiedemann syndrome. Radiol Clin North Am 10(2):261–275, 1972.
Pruzansky S: Editorial. Cleft Palate J 13:85–87, 1976.
Schafer AD: Primary macroglossia. Clin Pediatr 7:357–363, 1968.
Smith DF, Mihm FG, Flynn M: Chronic alveolar hypoventilation secondary to macroglossia in the Beckwith-Wiedemann syndrome. Pediatrics 70:695–697, 1982.
Sotelo-Avila C, Gonzalez-Crussi F, Fowler JW: Complete and incomplete forms of Beckwith-Wiedemann syndrome: Their oncogenic potential. J Pediatr 96:47–50, 1980.
Vig PS, Cohen AM: The size of the human tongue shadow in different mandibular postures. Br J Orthod 1(2):41–43, 1974.
Wiedemann H-R: E.M.G. syndrome and carbohydrate metabolism. Lancet II:104–105, 1968.

Cardiorespiratory Disease Associated With Hallermann-Streiff Syndrome: Analysis of Craniofacial Morphology by Cephalometric Roentgenograms

Hans Friede, Melvin Lopata, Elizabeth Fisher, and Ira M. Rosenthal

Center for Craniofacial Anomalies, (H.F.) Departments of Pediatrics (E.F., I.M.R.) and Medicine (M.L.), University of Illinois College of Medicine, Chicago

This paper analyzes the craniofacial morphology in a patient with typical Hallermann-Streiff syndrome (HSS) who developed symptomatic cardiorespiratory deficiency at the age of 48 years. The patient had obstructive sleep apnea (OSA), hypoxia, hypercarbia, pulmonary hypertension, tricuspid insufficiency, and right ventricular failure. Analysis of cephalometric roentgenograms, done 15 years earlier, revealed severe mandibular hypoplasia with marked underdevelopment of the ramus and body. The gonial angle was abnormally obtuse. The condylar and coronoid processes were reduced in size. The anteroposterior dimension of the upper airway was markedly narrowed. Cephalometric roentgenograms of six other HSS patients from our clinic were compared to those of the reference patient. Considerable variation in the features of the syndrome were noted. None of the other patients showed definitive airway obstruction. Comparison was also made with cephalometric roentgenograms of a patient with Treacher Collins syndrome and of a patient with progeria. The former showed airway obstruction associated with a deformed hypoplastic mandible; the latter had an unobstructed airway despite a small mandible because of associated hypoplasia of the maxilla and tongue.

The HSS reference patient improved after oxygen therapy, diuretics, antibiotics, and relief of OSA. Patients with HSS, as well as those with Treacher Collins syndrome, appear to be at risk for the development of cardiopulmonary disease if they have obstructed airways. OSA has been shown to have developed in two patients with HSS. The resultant cardiopulmonary insufficiency of such patients may be preventable if airway obstruction can be relieved relatively early in life.

Key words: cardiorespiratory insufficiency, cephalometry, Hallermann-Streiff syndrome, hypoplastic mandible, micrognathia, obstructive sleep apnea

INTRODUCTION

The Hallermann-Streiff syndrome (HSS) is characterized by typical craniofacial abnormalities, ophthalmologic defects, proportionate short stature, hypotrichosis, and skin atrophy, especially over the nose and the sutural areas of the scalp. Although case reports appeared as early as 1893, the syndrome, also known as oculomandibu-

---

Address reprint requests to Dr. Ira M. Rosenthal, Department of Pediatrics, University of Illinois College of Medicine, 840 South Wood Street, Chicago, IL 60612.

© 1985 Alan R. Liss, Inc.

lodyscephaly with hypotrichosis, was delineated as a distinct entity some 40 years later [Gorlin et al, 1976]. It has been noted that in HSS, serious respiratory problems may be present during infancy and childhood and may contribute to an early demise [Hoefnagel and Benirschke, 1965]. Cardiac problems have not been previously associated with this syndrome.

We are reporting a patient with HSS who developed cardiac and respiratory problems in her fifth decade. We believe these problems are related to chronic upper airway obstruction. Analysis of cephalometric roentgenograms indicates that the respiratory obstruction is associated with the malformations of HSS. The cephalometric roentogenograms have been compared with other patients with HSS from our center. Mandibular shape and airway have also been compared with those of Treacher Collins syndrome and progeria, two conditions also characterized by micrognathia.

CASE REPORT

The reference patient is a white female who was referred to the University of Illinois Hospital and the Center for Craniofacial Anomalies at the age of 20 years. Her birth weight was 2,820 gm after an apparently normal pregnancy, labor, and delivery. Facial abnormalities typical of HSS were recognized. Because of feeding difficulties, weight gain was slow; at 6 months she weighed 2.5 kg., at 1 year, 2.75 kg, at 2 years, 4.5 kg, and at 3 years, 7 kg. Cataracts were removed from her eyes at the age of 5 months, but vision remained severely impaired. The patient remained small as a child and as an adult. Sexual maturation was normal. She attended classes for the vision impaired and graduated from high school. She has been employed as a Braille proof reader.

Her parents were both 24 years old at the time of her birth. She has a younger brother and sister who are normal. There was no history of other family members affected with HSS.

On physical examination at the age of 20 years, the patient was 141 cm in height with a span of 125 cm. She weighed 32.4 kg. She appeared older than her chronologic age, with sparse scalp hair present mostly over the posterior portion of the head. There were no eyebrows and few lashes. Axillary and pubic hair, however, were normal in quantity and distribution. Breast development was normal.

The skull was mildly brachycephalic with a tendency to frontal bossing (Fig. 1). The nose was narrow and beaked. The small lower jaw together with the prominence of the upper anterior neck resulted in the appearance of a cutaneous "double" chin. The skin of the face appeared to be thin and stretched. Prominent nasolabial folds were present. A number of ophthalmologic abnormalities were noted. The lenses had been removed. The pupils were small, and the left pupil showed a sluggish response to light. Irregular nystagmus and convergent strabismus were noted.

Blood pressure was 150/70; pulse was 80 and regular. There were no heart murmurs, and heart sounds were normal.

Urinalysis and blood count were normal. Serum electrolytes, cholesterol, protein electrophoresis, and blood glucose were normal. Electrocardiogram was normal. The karyotype, prepared from peripheral blood lymphocytes, was 46, XX, normal. Psychologic tests revealed an IQ of 129 on the Stanford Binet L.

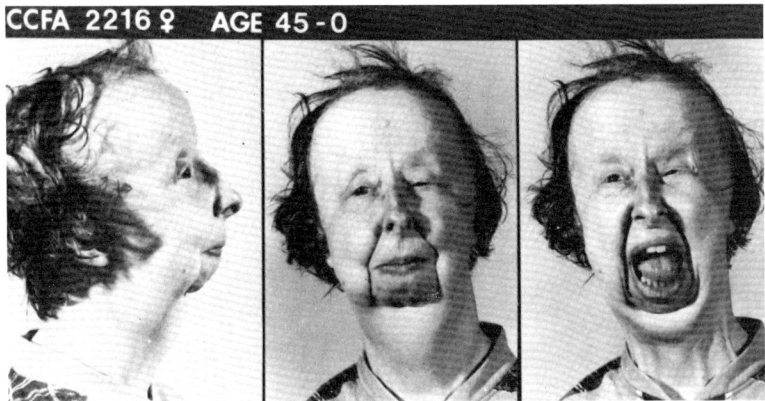

Fig. 1. Facial appearance of patient CCFA #2216 at rest and with maximal opening of the mouth. See text for description of featured characteristics of Hallermann-Streiff syndrome.

Roentgenograms revealed a diminished transverse diameter of the chest with gracile ribs and small clavicles. Bilateral coxa valga was present. Spina bifida of the upper sacral segment was noted.

Dental evaluation, done some years later at the age of 33 years, revealed retention of upper first primary molars and absence of 16 permanent teeth. It could not be established which of the teeth were congenitally missing and which had been extracted. The upper incisors displayed areas of hypoplastic enamel, and the overall quality of the teeth was further impaired by dental neglect. All of the lower incisors and canines were replaced by a prosthesis. There was severe class II malocclusion with anterior open bite. Cephalometric roentgenograms were done and are discussed below.

In October, 1983, at the age of 48 years, the patient complained of weakness and shortness of breath after exertion. A grade II apical systolic murmur was heard for the first time. An echocardiogram revealed left and right atrial enlargement; a Doppler study showed tricuspid regurgitation. A multigated cardiac scan revealed a left ventricular fraction of 57% and a right ejection fraction of 16%. A nuclear log scan revealed decreased perfusion of the right midlung consistent with parenchymal disease. Pulmonary function tests revealed a forced vital capacity 36% of predicted, a forced respiratory volume in 1 second 34% of predicted, total lung capacity 23% of predicted, and functional residual capacity 33% of predicted.

The patient gradually developed pedal edema. Because of progressive dyspnea of 3 days duration, she was admitted to the hospital on February 13, 1984. The systolic ejection murmur with radiation to the left sternal border was again noted. The liver was palpable 8 cm below the costal margin. There was severe edema of both legs extending to the thighs. Arterial blood gas analysis revealed a Po_2 of 41 mm Hg, Pco_2 of 47 mm Hg, and pH of 7.36. A right pleural effusion was noted on chest roentgenogram. There was no change in the echocardiogram. Lung ventilatory perfusion scan showed multiple nonsegmental perfusion deficits bilaterally, changes consistent with chronic obstructive pulmonary disease.

On the third day after admission, the patient developed lethargy and wheezing. Arterial blood gas analysis revealed increased Pco_2. It was noted that respiratory function appeared to deteriorate at night, suggesting the presence of obstructive sleep apnea (OSA). A nocturnal sleep study with polysomnographic monitoring revealed apnea plus hypopnea with 74 episodes per hour of sleep. These episodes were all obstructive in character, each resulting in significant oxygen desaturation. The minimum oxygen saturation documented was only 42%; the mean level of saturation was 69%. These results were consistent with severe OSA.

Treatment with nasal oxygen, diuretic agents, and antibiotics resulted in rapid improvement. The patient was discharged with oxygen per nasal catheter at night, theophyllin, furosemide, and an albuterol inhaler (two puffs every 6 hours). Since discharge she has improved further and can now walk without developing dyspnea. In addition to HSS and OSA, a diagnosis of pulmonary hypertension and secondary cor pulmonale was made.

ROENTGENCEPHALOMETRIC EVALUATION

The craniofacial morphology was analyzed by cephalometric radiographs at age 33 years 8 months and was compared to various normative data [Haas, 1952; Broadbent, et al, 1975; Costaras et al, 1982]. The cephalograms were also compared to those of a normal white female of similar age.

The analysis confirmed the clinical impression of slight microbrachycephaly and a flat forehead (Figs. 2, 3). The posterior bony contour of the head was uneven, displaying a step in the region above the lambdoid suture. The parietal bones appeared somewhat thin, and large areas of radiolucency indicated deficient calvarial ossification, particularly adjacent to the lambdoid suture. The cranial base showed platybasia (151°) caused by depression of the sella region in addition to some elevation of the anterior cranial fossa.

The midfacial skeleton was characterized by reduced bony interorbital distance, small orbits, and hypoplasia of the malar bones. The maxillary development was adequate (Figs. 2, 3).

The most striking morphologic feature revealed in the cephalogram of the reference patient was mandibular hypoplasia. This finding is in agreement with a detailed anthropometric description of another HSS patient [Haberman and Clement, 1979]. The ramus and the body of the mandible of the reference patient were markedly underdeveloped. The gonial angle between the mandibular ramus and body was 158° which is abnormally obtuse. In comparison to normal, the coronoid and condylar processes were very much reduced in size, the latter being more severely affected. The glenoid fossa and articular eminence of the temporal bone were poorly developed. The temporomandibular joints (TMJ) were displaced forward (porion-condyle distance, 27 mm) but appeared to function with both hinge and translatory movements (Fig. 4).

The anteroposterior dimension of the upper airway was markedly reduced as seen in the lateral cephalogram (Fig. 2). The hyoid bone was positioned at the normal level of the fourth cervical vertebra.

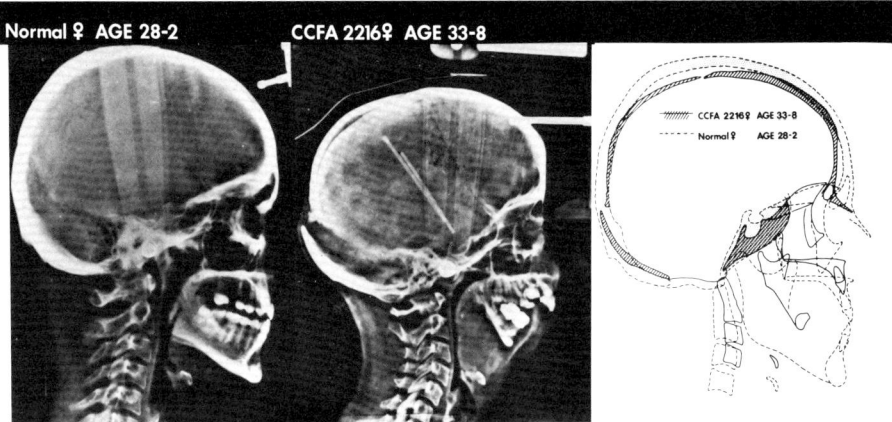

Fig. 2. Lateral cephalogram of patient CCFA #2216 compared to a normal case. Note particularly the small mandible, the narrow airway, and the displaced temporomandibular joint. See text for further discussion.

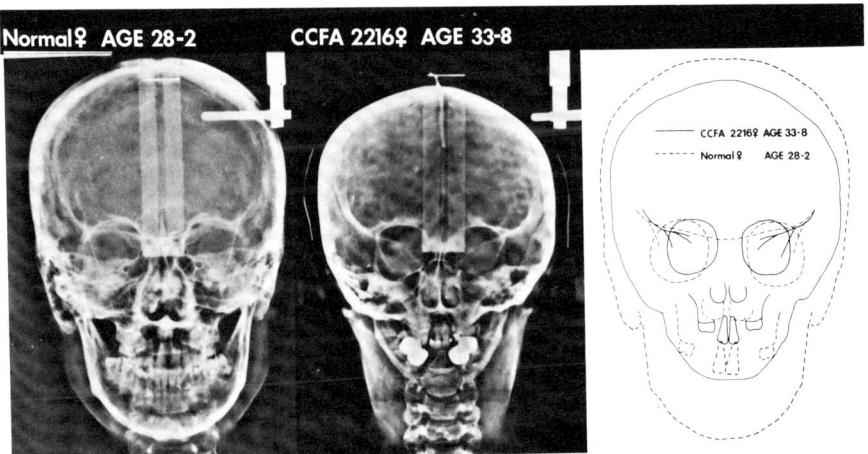

Fig. 3. Posteroanterior cephalogram of patient CCFA #2216 compared to a normal case. Note the hypoplastic mandible and small orbits. See text for additional description.

The craniofacial morphology of the reference patient was compared to that of six other HSS patients from our clinic (Table I). There was a wide range in the phenotypic characteristics of the syndrome. The reference patient was clearly the most severely affected, especially with respect to the mandible. The platybasia of the cranial base of the reference patient was also extreme in comparison to other cases, as were the extensive areas of ossification adjacent to the lambdoid suture. None of the other HSS subjects, including a 59-year-old male with sleep apnea, had an airway as restricted as the reference patient. The hyoid bone in all of our HSS patients followed the growth pattern of the cervical spine and was therefore at the normal vertebral level in spite of the variable mandibular abnormality.

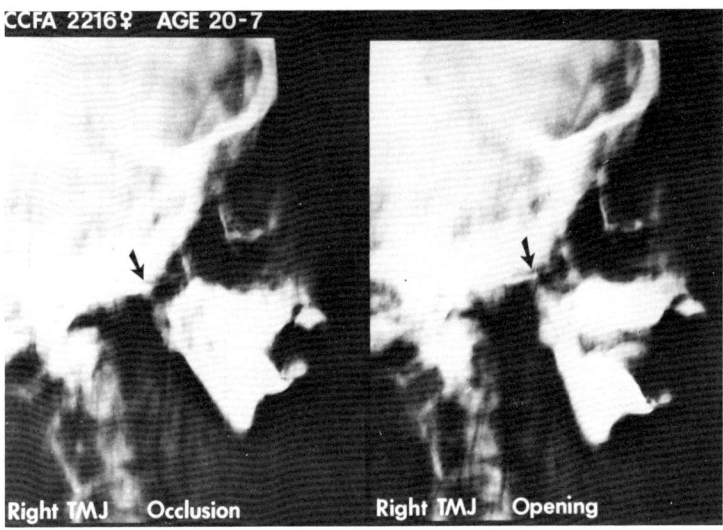

Fig. 4. Tomograms of right temporomandibular joint with the mandible in occlusion and in maximal opening position. The body and especially the ramus and condylar process (arrow) of the mandible are reduced in size. Note the forward movement of the condyle on opening.

Mandibular shape and the upper airway in HSS were compared to these structures in two other syndromes characterized by a small mandible: Treacher Collins syndrome and progeria. Patients with Treacher Collins syndrome can manifest restricted airway as do patients with HSS. OSA has been reported as well [Schafer, 1975]. However, the shape of the mandible in Treacher Collins syndrome differs from that of HSS by syndrome-specific features such as typical curvature of the lower border of the mandibular body [Roberts et al, 1975]. Moreover, the forward position of the TMJ, seen in most HSS patients, is not found in Treacher Collins syndrome.

The small mandible in progeria has a less abnormal shape than that of HSS. The TMJ is essentially normally positioned. It should be noted that not only the mandible but the whole facial skeleton is small in progeria [Gorlin et al, 1976]. Since in progeria the tongue is also reduced in size in proportion to the rest of the face, and the hyoid bone is in the proper position relative to the small cervical spine, no airway restriction would be expected, and none has been reported.

DISCUSSION

More than 80 cases of HSS have been reported. An excellent summary of the syndrome and relevant literature has been published [Gorlin et al, 1976].

The prinicipal abnormalities of HSS, including micrognathia, hypoplasia of the rami, anterior displacement of the TMJ, microphthalmia, cataracts, small pointed nose, and proportionate short stature were found in the reference patient. In addition she had other typical findings, including brachycephaly, delayed ossification of the sutures, hypoplasia of teeth, persistent primary teeth, atrophy of the skin of the nose and scalp, and hypotrichosis of scalp hair, eyebrows, and lashes.

TABLE I. Roentgencephalometric Characteristics of Patients With Hallermann-Streiff Syndrome (University of Illinois Center for Craniofacial Anomalies)

	#2216[1] (female, 33 yr 8 mo)	#4243 (male, 18 yr 6 mo)	#4752 (female, 17 yr 9 mo)	#5289 (female, 22 yr 11 mo)	#5512 (male, 12 yr 10 mo)	#5719 (male, 59 yr 11 mo)	#6263 (female, 2 yr 8 mo)
Calvaria							
Microbrachycephaly	+	0	0	+	0	0	+
Thin parietal bones	+	0	0	0	0	0	0
Radiolucent areas	++	+	0	0	0	0	0
Cranial base							
Platybasia	++	0	+	+	+	+	+
Depressed sella	+	+	+	+	0	+	+
Elevated ant. fossa	+	0	0	+	+	+	0
Midface orbits							
Malar hypoplasia	+	0	+	+	+	0	0
Beaked nose	+	+	0	+	0	+	+
Hypotelorism	+	0	+	+	0	0	0
Small orbits	+	+	0	+	+	0	0
Maxilla							
Adequate horizontal	+	0	+	+	+	+	+
Adequate vertical	+	+	+	+	+	+	+
Mandible							
Small ramus	++	+	++	+	+	+	+
Small body	++	+	+	++	+	+	+
Obtuse gonial angle	++	+	+	++	+	+	++
TMJ forward	++	0	++	+	+	+	0
Occlusion							
Class II:1	+	0	+	+	+	+	0
Open bite	+	+	0	+	+	0	+
Missing perm. teeth	+	+	+	+	+	+	+
Retained prim. teeth	+	0	+	+	+	+	+
Airway							
Reduced	++	0	0	0	0	+	0

++, Marked; +, present; 0, absent.
[1]Reference case. All cases are from the University of Illinois Center for Craniofacial Anomalies.

As with the reference patient, most cases are sporadic. There is no sex predilection. Both concordance and discordance have been reported in apparently monozygotic twins. Karyotypes, as in the reference case, have been normal. Although most cases appear to be the result of fresh mutations, autosomal recessive transmission cannot be excluded on the basis of available data.

In several reported cases there have been respiratory and feeding problems in infancy and childhood. Respiratory problems, as noted, apparently contributed to the early demise of some patients [Hoefnagel and Bernirschke, 1965]. We have, however, been unable to find reports of documented pulmonary hypertension, right ventricular hypertrophy, acquired tricuspid insufficency, or OSA.

The reference patient had severe OSA. Such sleep-induced apnea results from passive collapse and occlusion of the oropharynx caused by hypotonicity of dilatory upper airway muscles which are unable to maintain pharyngeal patency against negative inspiratory airway pressures [Hill et al, 1983]. This loss of pharyngeal and genioglossal muscle tone occurs in association with the development of sleep-induced periodic breathing, during which neural drive to both the respiratory and upper airway muscles waxes and wanes. The loss of upper airway muscle tonicity and resultant occlusive apnea occur during the waning phase of this process [Onal et al., 1982]. Although the cause of this periodic breathing is unknown, it appears to reflect a critical central neural component in the pathogenesis of OSA. However, in addition to this central mechanism, it is clear that a peripheral pathogenic component, represented by some degree of upper airway compromise, is necessary for the occlusive process to occur. Whether resulting from enlarged tonsils, micrognathia, macroglossia, hypertrophied and redundant pharyngeal musoca, or nasal obstruction, obstructive apnea develops by the generation of greater than normal negative inspiratory pressure caused by increased upper airway resistance, or the presence of a smaller than normal and thus more easily collapsible oropharynx, or a combination of both factors [Sukerman and Healy, 1979].

It is precisely this peripheral component that puts all HSS patients at risk for the development of OSA. In the reference patient, an exceedingly small upper airway appears to be a major factor in the development of this disease process. However, two caveats must be made concerning the role of upper airway obstruction in the pathogenesis of OSA. In the first place, although most, if not all, patients with OSA have some degree of anatomic upper airway obstruction, and the extent of such obstruction has been positively correlated with the severity of OSA, the degree of upper airway compromise is quite variable. The presence of airway compromise is frequently subtle and, even if diagnostic studies are made, may not be recognized [Guilleminault et al, 1976]. Moreover, not all patients with established upper airway obstruction develop OSA. This indicates that a central component must also be present. Thus, not all patients with HSS will necessarily develop OSA. If OSA does develop, the greater the upper airway compromise, the more severe the disease will tend to be. The risk of developing sleep apena apparently increases with age and obesity. Patients with HSS should be periodically monitored for the signs, symptoms, and sequelae of OSA. Daytime somnolence, excessive fatigue, loud snoring, recognized apnea during sleep, clinical evidence of cor pulmonale, or documented hypercarbia indicate the need for a nocturnal sleep study.

The reference patient had severe disease as reflected by two ominous complications of OSA, hypercapnic respiratory failure and cor pulmonale. The development of hypercarbia is felt to be secondary to the long-term detrimental effects of apnea, induced hypoxemia, and sleep disruption on the respiratory control system, such that at some point the patient lacks sufficent ventilatory drive to maintain adequate alveolar ventilation [Lopata and Onal, 1982]. This hypoventilation is especially likely to occur under conditions of extreme respiratory load or demand, such as marked obesity or, as in the reference patient, in the presence of peripheral airway obstruction, ie, asthma.

In patients with OSA, repetitive and often severe elevation of pulmonary artery pressure in conjuction with the apneic episodes has been documented and is in large part secondary to hypoxia-induced pulmonary vasoconstriction [Tilkian et al, 1976]. Sustained pulmonary hypertension and cor pulmonale probably occur after years of such stimuli, especially when daytime hypoxemia and hypercapnea intervene. Thus, although the reference patient was symptomatic only a few months, the presence of such severe sequelae of OSA indicates that she had OSA for many years, probably dating from childhood.

The optimal treatment for severe obstructive apnea with life-threatening complications is tracheostomy [Guilleminault et al, 1981]. However, because of the reference patient's blindness and other disabling effects of HSS and the difficulties these would present in terms of tracheostomy care as well as patient acceptance, a trial of continuous oxygen therapy was considered. The rationale for the use of oxygen was that it would not only correct the daytime hypoxemias, but also prevent apnea-related worsening of the Po_2 at night, and thus prevent hypoxia-induced pulmonary vasoconstriction. This treatment, found to be effective in some patients with sleep apnea, can be detrimental, since oxygen supplementation at night can lead to significant prolongation of the obstructive apnea [Martin et al, 1982]. However, it did prove effective in the reference patient, and she is presently only requiring supplemental oxygen during sleep.

Surgical correction of the facial abnormalities of HSS using the techniques of mandibular advancement has been attempted [Patterson et al, 1982]. There has been cosmetic as well as occlusal improvement, and the result appears to have been essentially stable. It is not clear, however, if there has been any effect on the airway. It is possible that reconstructive surgery in HSS can result in improvement in airway function. It should be noted that Tessier has not only improved the cosmetic appearance but also the obstructed airway of patients with Treacher Collins syndrome. In at least one case, however, improvement of airway obstruction has not been sustained [Pruzansky, 1982].

The signs and symptoms of cor pulmonale seen in the reference patient apparently developed as a result of pulmonary hypertension secondary to hypoxia and hypercarbia. In patients with upper airway obstruction, OSA and chronic obstructive pulmonary disease, pulmonary hypertension initially develops as a result of a direct vasoconstrictor effect of hypoxia or through the action of circulating vasoactive mediators such as angiotensin II or bradykinin [Rounds and McMurty, 1981]. With continued hypoxia, structural changes such as medial hypertrophy and extension of muscle peripherally into normally nonmuscular arteries occur [Rabinovitch et al, 1979]. In response to increased pulmonary artery pressure, the right heart chambers dilate and hypertrophy and systemic venous congestion develop. Tricuspid insufficiency, which the reference patient developed, was most likely due to tricuspid annular dilation which prevented complete coaptation of the tricuspid valve leaflet during systole. The etiology of the pulmonary edema, seen in some patients, is thought to be left ventricular dysfunction and increased capillary permeability, both secondary to hypoxia [Luke et al, 1966]. In addition, vigorous inspiratory effort against an obstructed airway may result in an increased transcapillary pressure gradient contributing to the development of pulmonary edema [Ainger, 1968].

Treatment of the cardiac problem is directed at relief of the airway obstruction. Prompt improvement in the signs and symptoms of heart failure, as in the reference patient, is usually seen [Cox et al, 1965]. In some patients, however, slow or incomplete recovery may be due to slow regression of structural changes in the pulmonary arteries or to presence of a central factor [Levin et al, 1975].

ACKNOWLEDGMENTS

This investigation was supported in part by grants from the National Institutes of Health (DEO2872) and Maternal and Child Health Services, Department of Health and Human Services.

REFERENCES

Ainger LE: Large tonsils and adenoids in small children with cor pulmonale. Br Heart J 30:356–362, 1968.
Broadbent BH, Sr, Broadbent BH, Jr, Golden WH: "Bolton Standards of Dentofacial Development Growth," St. Louis: C.V. Mosby Co., 1975.
Costaras M, Pruzansky S, Broadbent BH, Jr: Bony interorbital distance (BIOD), head size, and level of the cribiform plate relative to orbital height: 1. Normal standards for age and sex. J Craniofac Genet Dev Biol 2:5–18, 1982.
Cox MA, Schiebler GI, Taylor WJ, Wheat MW, Krovetz LJ: Reversible pulmonary hypertension in a child with respiratory obstruction and cor pulmonale. J Pediatr 67:192–197, 1965.
Gorlin RJ, Pindborg JJ, Cohen MM, Jr: "Syndromes of the Head and Neck," 2nd ed New York: McGraw-Hill Book Co., 1976, pp 557–561, 622–625.
Guilleminault C, Simmons FB, Motta J, Cummiskey J, Rosekind M, Schroeder JS, Dement, WC: Obstructive sleep apnea and tracheostomy. Ann Intern Med 141:985–988, 1981.
Guilleminault C, Tilkian AG, Dement WC: The sleep apnea syndromes. Ann Rev Med 27:465–484, 1976.
Haas LL: Roentgenological skull measurements and their diagnostic applications. Am J Roentgenol 67:197–209, 1952.
Haberman H, Clement PAR: The value of anthropometrical measurements in a case of Hallermann-Streiff syndrome. Rhinology 17:179–194, 1979.
Hill MW, Guilleminault C, Simmons, FB: Fiber-optic and EMG studies in hypersomnia-sleep apnea syndrome. In: Guilleminault C, Dement WC (eds): "Sleep Apnea Syndromes," New York: Alan R. Liss, 1983, pp 249–258.
Hoefnagel D, Benirschke K: Dyscephalia mandibulo-oculo-facialis (Hallermann-Streiff syndrome). Arch Dis Child 40:57–61, 1965.
Levin DL, Muster AJ, Pachman LM, Wessel WU, Paul MH, Koshaba J: Cor pulmonale secondary to upper airway obstruction. Cardiac catheterization, immunologic and psychometric evaluation in nine patients. Chest 68:166–171, 1975.
Lopata M, Onal E: Mass loading, sleep apnea and the pathogenesis of obesity hypoventilation. Am Rev Respir Dis 126:640–645, 1965.
Luke MJ, Mehrizi A, Folger GM, Jr, Rowe RD: Chronic nasopharyngeal obstruction as a cause of cardiomegaly, cor pulmonale and pulmonary edema. Pediatrics 37:762–768, 1966.
Martin RJ, Sanders MH, Gray RA, Pennock BE: Acute and longterm ventilatory effects of hyperoxia in the adult sleep apnea syndrome. Am Rev Respir Dis 125:175–180, 1982.
Onal E, Lopata M, O'Connor TD: Pathogenesis of apneas in hypersomnia-sleep apnea syndrome. Am Rev Respir Dis 125:167–174, 1982.
Patterson GT, Braun TW, Sotereanos GC: Surgical correction of the dentofacial abnormality in Hallermann-Streiff syndrome. J Oral Maxillofac Surg 40:380–384, 1982.
Pruzansky S: Craniofacial surgery, the experiment on nature's experiment: Review of three patients operated by Paul Tessier. Eur J Orthod 4:151–171, 1982.
Rabinovitch M, Gamble W, Nadas AS, Miettinen OS, Reid L: Rat pulmonary circulation after chronic hypoxia: Hemodynamic and structural features. Am J Physiol 236:H818, 1979.
Roberts FG, Pruzansky S, Aduss H: An x-radiocephalometric study of mandibulofacial dysostosis in man. Arch Oral Biol 20:265–281, 1975.
Rounds S, McMurty IF: Inhibitors of oxidative ATP production cause transient vasoconstriction and block subsequent pressor responses in rat lungs. Circ Res 48:393–400, 1981.
Schafer ME: Upper airway obstruction and sleep disorders in children with craniofacial anomalies. Clin Plast Surg 9:555–567, 1975.
Sukerman S, Healy GB: Sleep apnea syndrome associated with upper airway obstruction. Laryngoscope 89:878–884, 1979.
Tilkian AG, Guilleminault C, Schroeder JS, Lehrman KL, Simmons FB, Dement WC: Hemodynamics in sleep-induced apneas. Ann Intern Med 85:714–719, 1976.

Skeletal and Functional Craniofacial Adaptations in Plagiocephaly

Sven Kreiborg, Eigild Møller, and Arne Björk
Departments of Orthodontics (S.K., A.B.) and Oral Physiology (E.M.), The Royal Dental College, Copenhagen, Denmark

The present report aims to contribute to our understanding of craniofacial development in plagiocephaly. A previously unreported dry skull with plagiocephaly and two clinical cases with unoperated plagiocephaly are presented. The clinical cases were followed longitudinally with roentgencephalometry in lateral, frontal, and axial projections. In addition, in one of the cases, electromyographic analysis of the temporal, masseter, sternomastoid, and trapezius muscles was carried out. The dry skull revealed premature closure of the sphenofrontal suture in addition to the coronal suture. Furthermore, severe asymmetry of the cranial base and mandible was observed. The clinical cases revealed a similar marked asymmetry of the cranial base. Mandibular asymmetry was observed to develop in early infancy secondary and compensatory to the primary asymmetry of the cranial base. The electromyographic examination revealed that the muscles of mastication were less developed on the affected side. Furthermore, the analysis of the muscles of the neck would seem to indicate that the patient compensated for her cranial base asymmetry and lateral deviation of the orbital axis on the affected side by rotating the head to the opposite side to secure binocular vision. Based on these findings, it would seem pertinent to consider early surgical release of the sutures of the calvaria and cranial base in plagiocephaly to prevent asymmetric facial development.

Key words: plagiocephaly, craniofacial asymmetry, coronal synostosis, unilateral coronal synostosis, unilateral sphenofrontal synostosis, cephalometric study, electromyographic study

INTRODUCTION

Patients with plagiocephaly exhibit premature synostosis of the coronal suture unilaterally. A few reports have indicated that the sphenofrontal suture in the cranial base may also be involved [Seeger and Gabrielsen, 1971; Kreiborg, 1981; Kreiborg and Björk, 1981].

In a previous publication we reported on a dry skull with plagiocephaly and described marked asymmetry of the cranial base as a result of premature synostosis of sutures [Kreiborg and Björk, 1981]. The asymmetry of the cranial base, including the position of the glenoid fossae, was compensated for by asymmetric maxillary and

Address reprint requests to Dr. S. Kreiborg, Department of Orthodontics, The Royal Dental College, Jagtvej 160, DK-2100 Copenhagen, Denmark.

mandibular development, and the occlusion was close to normal. Another plagiocephalic skull, exhibiting very similar deviations, is illustrated in Figures 1 and 2. Mandibular asymmetry in plagiocephalic patients was reported by Fauré et al [1967], Kreiborg [1981], and Tulasne and Tessier [1981].

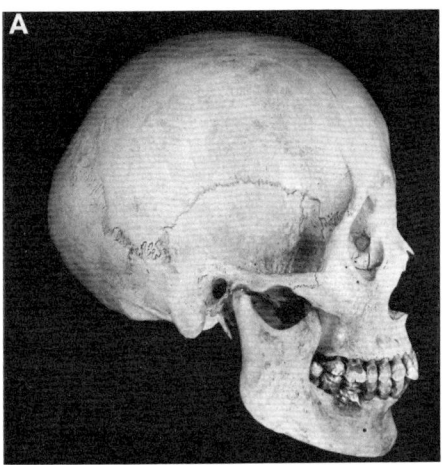 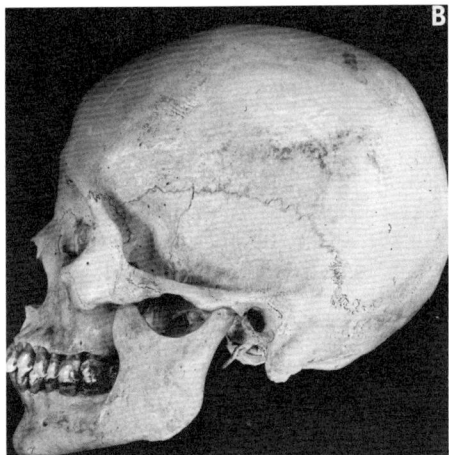

Fig. 1. A. Plagiocephalic skull from Professor Björk's collection. Right lateral view. Note the synostosis of the coronal suture and the short temporal fossa. B. Left lateral view. Note the greater width of the ramus on this side compared to the affected side.

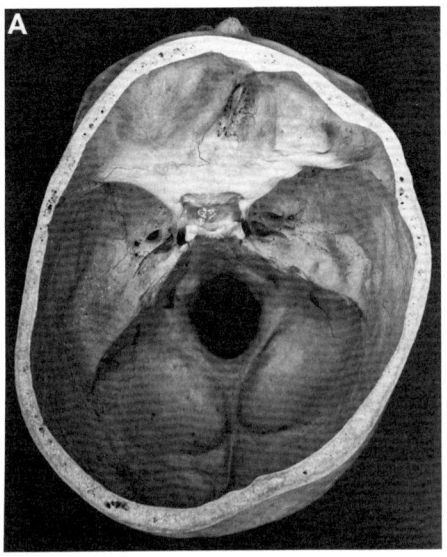 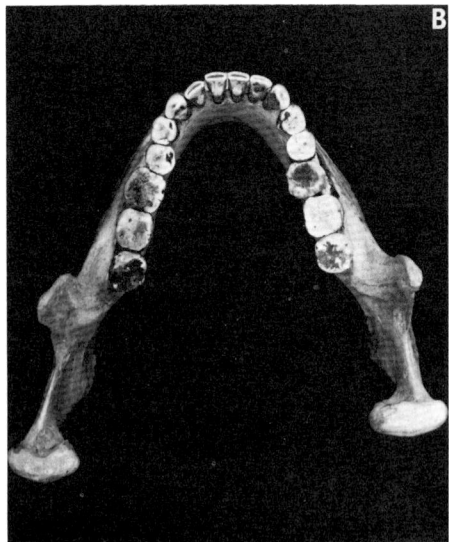

Fig. 2. A. The internal cranial base of the same skull as shown in Figure 1. Note the premature synostosis of the sphenofrontal suture on the right side, the short anterior and middle cranial fossae on the right, and the deviation of the midline of the anterior cranial fossa to the right side. B. The mandible from the same skull shown in Figure 1. Note the marked asymmetry.

Longitudinal roentgencephalometric studies of craniofacial growth in patients with plagiocephaly are rare [Kreiborg, 1981; Kreiborg and Pruzansky, 1981; Lilja et al, 1983] probably because of the methodological problems involved [Kreiborg, 1981]. The few unoperated cases previously studied by roentgencephalometry have indicated that the degree of asymmetry of the cranial base and the jaws remains relatively unaltered during the adolescent period. It was hypothesized that the most marked asymmetric adaptive development of the jaws occurs in early infancy in connection with the rapid growth of the cranial base [Kreiborg, 1981]. The present report aims to further our understanding of the skeletal and functional craniofacial adaptations in plagiocephalic patients.

MATERIALS AND METHODS

Two female patients, both with premature synostosis of the coronal suture on the right side, are reported. The ages of the patients and the duration of the observation periods are given in Table I.

Both patients were followed longitudinally with roentgencephalometric x-rays in the lateral, frontal, and axial projections. The roentgencephalometric methodologies employed herein are based on the principles and standards described by Björk [1968] and modified for infants by Kreiborg et al [1977]. The specific roentgencephalometric analyses employed in plagiocephalic patients have previously been described in detail [Kreiborg, 1981]. If the patient is positioned in the cephalometer according to the ear-rods (ear-rod position), the vertical beam of the light-cross, indicating the midsagittal plane in the cephalometer, will be projected on the unaffected side of the face (Fig. 3). In other words, the affected side of the face will be positioned more dorsally than the unaffected side. If, on the other hand, the patient is positioned so that the facial midline corresponds to the vertical light beam (light-cross position), the ears will be at different sagittal levels, and this is most often the position the patient will find natural. Provided the cephalograms are taken in the same position at every examination it is possible to make a fairly accurate estimate of the growth changes in the sagittal, vertical, and transverse planes from the lateral and frontal projections. The images of asymmetric structures are more susceptible to error than normal, and the evaluation is therefore rather rough. However, since the plagiocephalic deformity is primarily a sagittal asymmetry, additional information concerning the location and degree of asymmetry can be obtained from the basal projection [Cook, 1980; Kreiborg, 1981]. In the present study the ear-rod position was used for all exposures in the longitudinal series.

An electromyographic examination of the action of the temporal, masseter, sternomastoid, and trapezius muscles was carried out at adult age in one of the patients. The electromyograms were picked up bilaterally with bipolar surface elec-

TABLE I. The Ages of the Patients and the Duration of the Observation Periods

Case No.	Sex	Age at first examination	Age at last examination
1	F	4 months	3 years 11 months
2	F	10 years 4 months	32 years

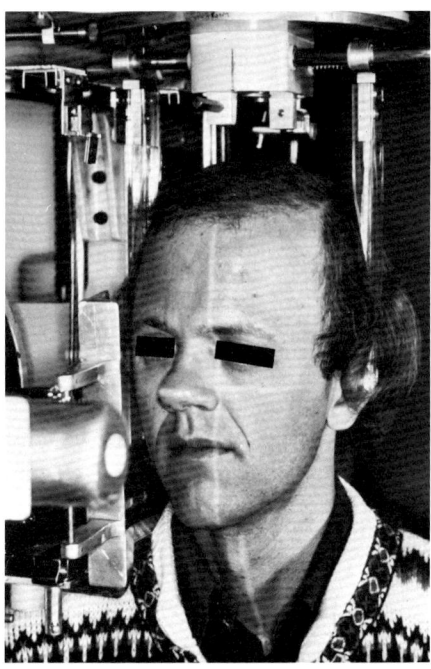

Fig. 3. A plagiocephalic patient with premature synostosis of the coronal suture on the right side positioned in the cephalometer according to the ear-rods. The vertical beam of the light-cross, indicating the midsagittal plane of the cephalometer, is projected on the unaffected side of the face [from Kreiborg, 1981].

trodes and were recorded simultaneously with their numeric mean voltages. The analysis of the temporal and masseter muscles included rest, maximal activity, and chewing. The sternomastoid and trapezius muscles were recorded during rest, maximal activity, and head movement.

CASE REPORTS
Case 1 (Fig. 4)

The patient was a white female referred at 4 months of age for evaluation. The facial appearance of the infant was characteristic of plagiocephaly (Fig. 4A). There was a depression of the supra-orbital region on the affected side, whereas the frontal bone protruded on the contralateral side. The eyes were at slightly different levels. The sagittal diameter of the skull was somewhat short and the cephalic index was increased. The head circumference was in the lower part of the normal range for age. The roentgencephalometric films revealed premature closure of the coronal suture on the right side. The lesser wing of the sphenoid exhibited a steep upward and lateral slope on the affected side (Fig. 5). The cranial base was asymmetric, being much shorter on the affected side than on the unaffected side. The lateral orbital wall deviated laterally on the affected side. The mandible was, however, fairly symmetric (Fig. 6A). The patient exhibited no sign of increased intracranial pressure and the neurological examination was normal.

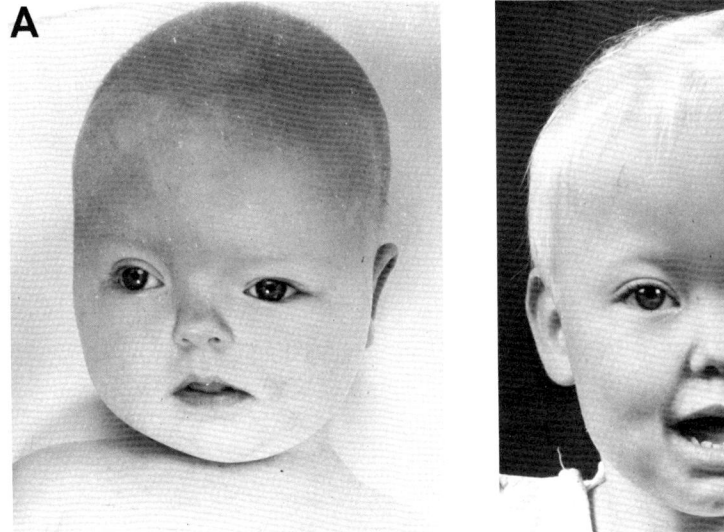

Fig. 4. A. Case 1. Facial appearance at 4 months of age. B. Facial appearance at 1 year 3 months of age. Note the progressive facial asymmetry.

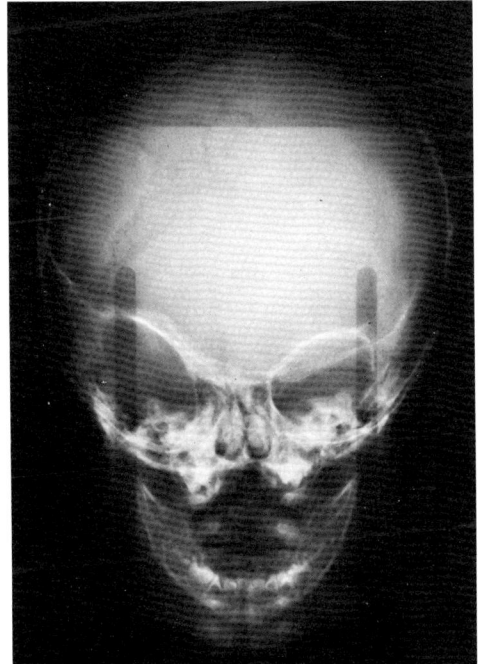

Fig. 5. Case 1. Frontal roentgencephalometric film at 4 months of age. Note the steep upward and lateral slope of the lesser wing of the sphenoid on the affected side.

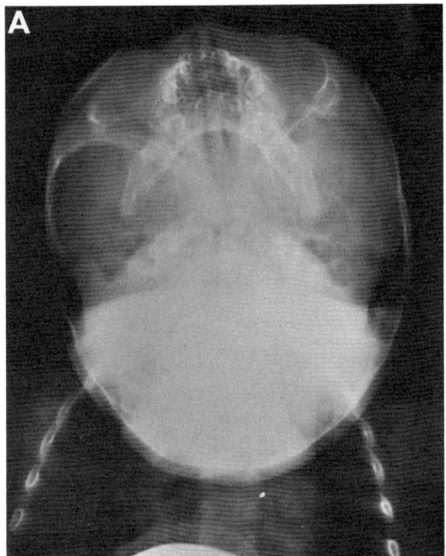 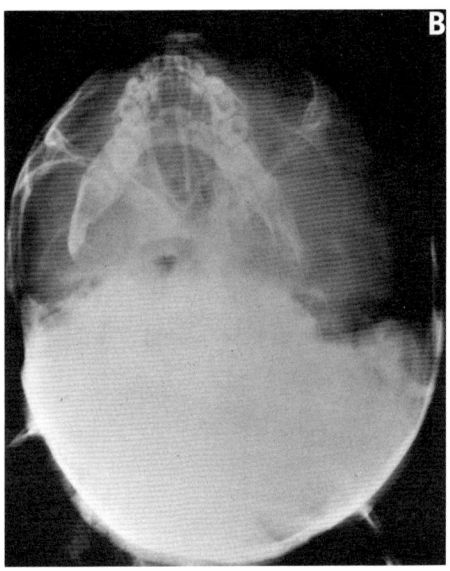

Fig. 6. A. Case 1. Axial roentgencephalometric film at 4 months of age. Note the marked asymmetry of the cranial base and the symmetric mandible. B. Axial projection at 1 year 3 months of age. Note the progressive asymmetry of the cranial base and the asymmetric development of the mandible.

A neurosurgical release of the synostotic suture with advancement of the frontal bone on the right side was recommended in order to treat the calvarial and orbital deformity and to prevent secondary asymmetric facial development. The parents were not interested in such treatment for their child but agreed to have the child's facial growth followed by roentgencephalometry.

The patient was examined again at the ages of 1 year 3 months (Fig. 4B), 2 years 1 month, and 3 years 11 months. During the observation period the asymmetry of the cranial base and the jaws, especially the mandible, progressed, as is clearly illustrated by the axial cephalometric film (Fig. 6B). Although these results were explained to the parents, who were told that the asymmetry could be expected to progress somewhat, they continued to refuse treatment for their child, who has otherwise developed quite normally without any medical or psychosocial problems. The facial appearance of the patient at age 3 years 11 months is illustrated in Figure 7.

Case 2 (Fig. 8)

This patient was a white female who at the age of 10 years 4 months was referred to the Department of Orthodontics for evaluation. Her facial appearance was characterized by marked asymmetry. She had a depression in the supra-orbital region on the right side and the eyes were at different levels (Fig. 8A). She had never received any neurosurgical treatment, nor had she had any neurologic problems.

Roentgencephalometric examination revealed premature closure of the coronal suture on the right side. The lesser wing of the sphenoid exhibited a steep upward and lateral slope on the affected side. The cranial base was markedly asymmetric. The anterior and middle cranial fossae were shorter on the affected side than on the unaffected side, whereas the posterior cranial fossa was fairly symmetric. The orbital

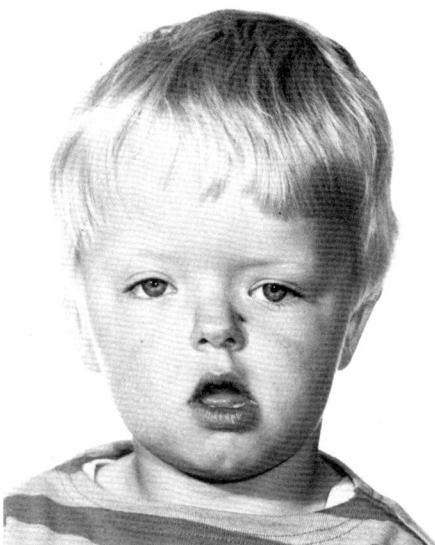

Fig. 7. Case 1. Facial appearance at the age of 3 years 11 months.

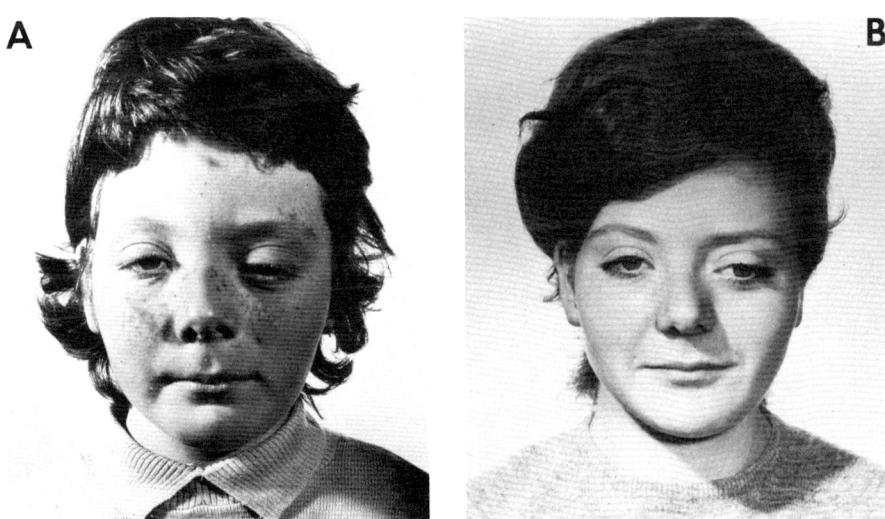

Fig. 8. A. Case 2. Facial appearance at the age of 10 years 4 months. B. Facial appearance at the age of 17 years 8 months.

axis on the affected side deviated laterally. The midline of the anterior cranial fossa deviated markedly toward the affected side. The deviation of the facial midline became less pronounced down through the nasal bones, the maxillae, and the mandible. The maxilla and especially the mandible were asymmetric, being shorter on the affected side than on the unaffected side. The mandibular asymmetry was localized to the region of the ramus and condyle (Fig. 9).

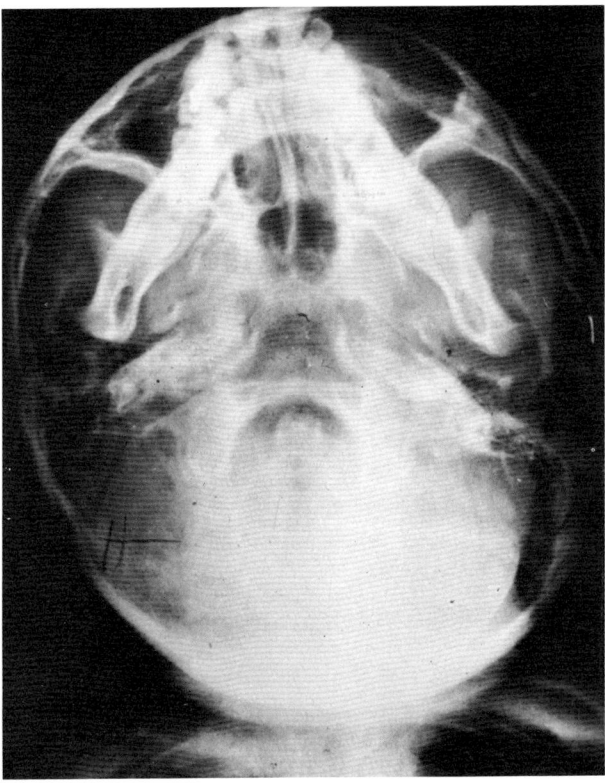

Fig. 9. Case 2. Axial roentgencephalometric film at 10 years 4 months of age. Note the marked asymmetry of the cranial base and the mandible.

The patient was followed longitudinally at approximately 2-year intervals until she was 17 years 8 months old (Fig. 8B). She was called back for a final examination at the age of 32.

The growth analysis based on the lateral, frontal, and axial roentgencephalometric projections obtained in the ear-rod position showed no marked change in the degree of asymmetry from the age of 10 years to adulthood. However, the frontal projection revealed that the mastoid process on the affected side increased more in size than on the unaffected side. The axial cephalograms showed no change of the angular relationships in the cranial base during the observation period. It was not possible to analyze accurately mandibular growth from the axial projection. This could have been carried out successfully using an oblique frontal projection [Björk, 1971], but this projection was not employed at our department in the early series of this patient.

An electromyographic (EMG) examination of the muscles of mastication and of the neck was carried out at the age of 32 years.

The electromyographic recordings for the temporal and masseter muscles during maximal bite in the intercuspal position are illustrated in Figure 10. It was noted that the activity in the left temporal muscle was about 30% higher than in the right, and

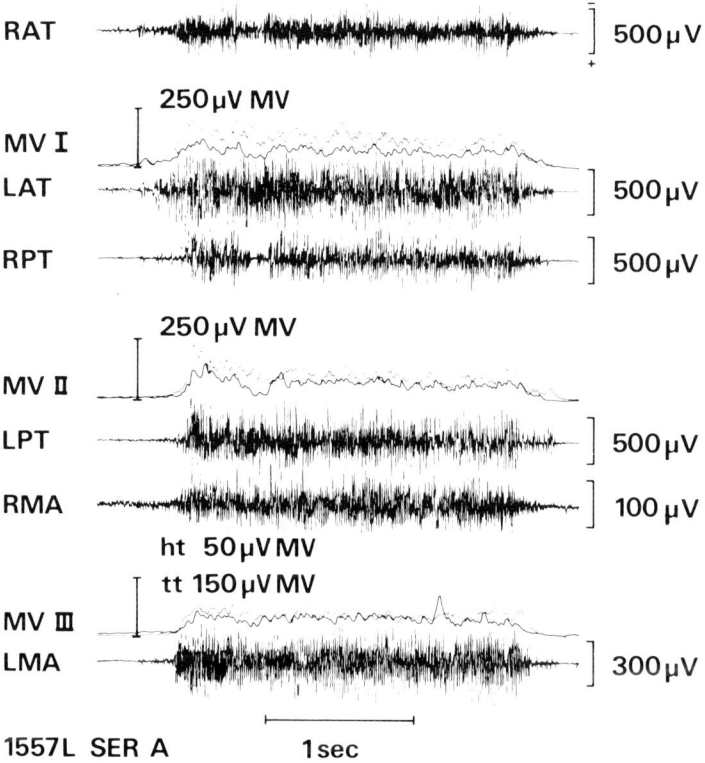

Fig. 10. Case 2. Action of the mandibular elevators during maximal bite. Electrical activity in the right and left anterior temporal muscles (RAT/LAT), right and left posterior temporal muscles (RPT/LPT), and right and left masseter muscles (RMA/LMA), and the corresponding mean voltages (MVI, MVII, and MVIII; heavy trace, right muscle; thin trace, left muscle). Note the weaker activity in the temporal and masseter muscles on the right side than on the left side. Recordings obtained at the age of 32 years; bipolar surface electrodes. Copy in india ink from ultraviolet recording.

the activity in the left masseter muscle was three times higher than the activity in the right.

Weaker activity in the temporal and masseter muscles on the affected side than on the unaffected side was also found at rest and during natural chewing. In an attempt to achieve symmetry in the muscular activity, the patient was fitted with an occlusal splint. However, the asymmetric pattern of activity in the musculature remained unaltered, suggesting that the temporal and masseter muscles were less developed on the affected side than on the unaffected side. Figure 11A illustrates the EMG-recordings at rest from the anterior temporal, sternomastoid, and trapezius muscles with the patient looking straight ahead. It was noted that in this position the activity in the right sternomastoid muscle was about twice the activity in the left. The trapezius muscles showed symmetric activity.

The recordings shown in Figure 11B indicate the activity in the same muscles as in Figure 11A, but now the patient had turned the head about 15 degrees to the right so that the ears were at the same sagittal level (ear-rod position). Note that the activity thereby became symmetric in the sternomastoid muscles.

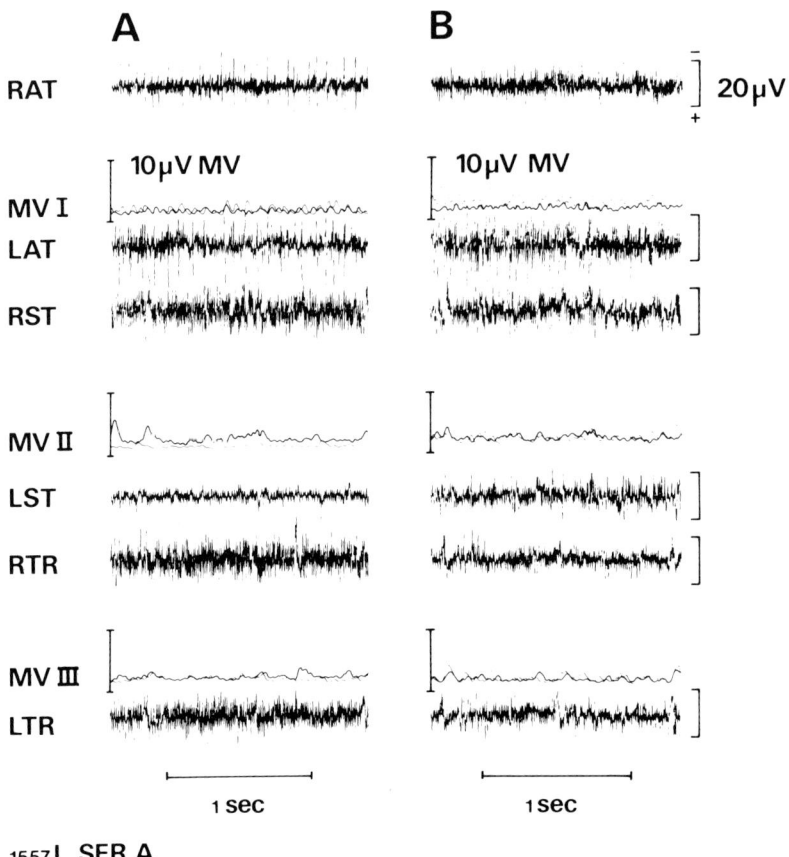

Fig. 11. A. Case 2. Action of the muscles of the neck with the patient looking straight ahead (light-cross position). Electrical activity in the right and left anterior temporal muscles as reference, and the right and left sternomastoid muscles (RST/LST), right and left trapezius muscles (RTR/LTR), and the corresponding mean voltages (MVI, MVII, and MVIII; heavy trace, right muscle; thin trace, left muscle). Note the asymmetry in activity of the sternomastoid muscles on the two sides, the right muscle exhibiting about twice the activity of the left. B. Action of the same muscles when the patient had turned the head about 15° to the right, so that the ears were at the same sagittal level (ear-rod position). Note that the electrical activity in the sternomastoid muscles became symmetric in this situation. Recordings obtained at the age of 32 years; bipolar surface electrodes. Copy in india ink from ultraviolet recording.

DISCUSSION

The results of the growth study performed in case 1 would seem to support the hypothesis that asymmetric development of the jaws in patients with plagiocephaly occurs secondarily to the primary asymmetry of the cranial base in early infancy in conjunction with the rapid growth of the cranial base. This asymmetric adaptive development of the jaws serves to compensate for the asymmetry of the cranial base and thereby maintain a normal occlusal relationship. However, as a result the face becomes progressively more asymmetric in early childhood, and it would seem pertinent to consider early surgery of the calvaria and cranial base to prevent asymmetric facial development, as previously suggested by Whitaker et al [1977].

The craniofacial growth pattern observed in case 2 revealed no marked progression in the asymmetry during the observation period. This finding is in close agreement with a previously published growth analysis of a plagiocephalic patient followed during adolescence [Kreiborg, 1981]. These findings would seem to support the hypothesis that the major part of the compensatory asymmetric jaw development in plagiocephaly occurs early ie, during the first 6–7 years of life.

The electromyographic examination performed in case 2 suggested that the temporal and masseter muscles were less developed on the affected side than on the unaffected side. This finding was probably related to the diminished development of the temporal fossa and the mandible on the affected side.

The stronger activity in the right sternomastoid muscle than in the left when the patient was looking straight ahead, combined with the symmetric activity that could be recorded when the patient turned the head to the right until the ears were at the same sagittal level, suggests that when looking straight ahead, in fact, the patient had turned the head slightly to the left in relation to the cervical column. The altered head posture could serve to compensate for the lateral deviation of the orbital axis on the affected side, and thereby secure binocular vision with fusion, which the patient had. A similar mechanism is known to the ophthalmologist as visual torticollis, often found in patients with strabismus. In other words, the plagiocephalic patient seemed to function with the head in the "light-cross position," whereas the natural position of the cranial base to the cervical column and the musculature of the neck would correspond to the "ear-rod position."

The presence of a dento-alveolar compensatory mechanism has been documented in several investigations [Björk and Skieller, 1972; Solow, 1980]. Björk and Björk [1964] and Kreiborg and Björk [1981] have suggested the possibility of compensatory asymmetric development of the maxilla and mandible in studies of dry skulls with asymmetry of the cranial base. The findings in the present study would seem to suggest the presence of a more general compensatory or adaptive mechanism, including the skeletal system as well as muscle function. The marked asymmetry of the cranial base in the plagiocephalic patients was compensated for by asymmetric maxillary and mandibular growth. Furthermore, the marked lateral deviation of the orbital axis on the affected side, in the case examined was compensated for by stronger activity in the sternomastoid muscle on that side, producing an altered head position to secure binocular vision.

CONCLUSIONS

Based on the literature and the findings in the present study it would seem justified to draw the following conclusions:

1) Both the coronal and the sphenofrontal sutures are prematurely fused in most cases of plagiocephaly.

2) In unoperated cases of plagiocephaly, the cranial base is asymmetric, the anterior and middle cranial fossae being much shorter on the affected side than on the unaffected side. The orbital axis deviates laterally on the affected side and the glenoid fossae are at different sagittal levels.

3) In unoperated cases of plagiocephaly, the maxilla and especially the mandible exhibit secondary asymmetric development during early childhood, becoming shorter on the affected side than on the unaffected side.

4) In unoperated cases of plagiocephaly, adaptive changes can be observed in the masticatory musculature and in the muscles of the neck controlling head posture.

It is suggested that the described skeletal and functional craniofacial adaptations should be taken into account in various clinical contexts.

ACKNOWLEDGMENTS

This study was supported by a grant from the Danish Dental Association (F.U.T.).

REFERENCES

Björk A: The use of metallic implants in the study of facial growth in children: Method and application. Am J Phys Anthropol 29:243–254, 1968.
Björk A: Kaebernes relationer til det øvrige kranium. In: Lundström A (ed): "Nordisk Lärobok i Ortodonti Uppl 3." Stockholm: Sveriges Tandläkarforbunds Förlagsförening, 1971, p 163.
Björk A, Björk L: Artificial deformation and craniofacial asymmetry in ancient Peruvians. J Dent Res 43:353–362, 1964.
Björk A, Skieller V: Facial development and tooth eruption. An implant study at the age of puberty. Am J Orthod 62:339–383, 1972.
Cook JT: Asymmetry of the craniofacial skeleton. Br J Orthod 7:33–38, 1980.
Fauré C, Bonamy P, Rambert-Misset C: Les craniosténoses par fusion prématurée unilatérale de la suture coronale. Ann Radiol (Paris) 10:32–42, 1967.
Kreiborg S: Craniofacial growth in plagiocephaly and Crouzon syndrome. Scand J Plast Reconstr Surg 15:187–197, 1981.
Kreiborg S, Björk A: Craniofacial asymmetry of a dry skull with plagiocephaly. Eur J Orthod 3:195–203, 1981.
Kreiborg S, Dahl E, Prydsoe U: A unit for infant cephalometry. Dentomaxillofac Radiol 6:107–111, 1977.
Kreiborg S, Pruzansky S: Craniofacial growth in patients with premature craniosynostosis. Scand J Plast Reconstr Surg 15:171–186, 1981.
Lilja J, Friede H, Svendsen P, Aggeryd J, Lauritzan C, Möller M, Andersson H, Johanson B: Cephalometric radiography and computed tomography in infants undergoing major craniofacial surgery—A comparison. Scand J Plast Reconstr Surg 17:63–72, 1983.
Seeger JF, Gabrielsen TO: Premature closure of the frontosphenoidal suture in synostosis of the coronal suture. Radiology 101:631–635, 1971.
Solow B: The dentoalveolar compensatory mechanism: Background and clinical implications. Br J Orthod 7:145–161, 1980.
Tulasne JF, Tessier P: Analysis and late treatment of plagiocephaly. Unilateral coronal synostosis. Scand J Plast Reconstr Surg 15:257–263, 1981.
Whitaker LA, Schut L, Kerr PL: Early surgery for isolated craniofacial dysostosis. Improvement and possible prevention of increasing deformity. Plast Reconstr Surg 60:575–581, 1977.

Craniofacial Dysmorphology in Syndromes Associated With Abnormal Physical Growth

Nobuyoshi Motohashi
Department of Orthodontics II, School of Dentistry, Tokyo Medical and Dental University, Tokyo, Japan

> Nine syndromes associated with varying patterns of abnormal physical growth were selected to study quantitative craniofacial dysmorphology with cephalometric analysis. A schematic diagram was developed in which a hexagon measures the neurocranium and facial skeletal size and form. This hexagon offers the possibility of quantitative dysmorphic roentgencephalometry to study the effects of various growth disorders on the craniofacial complex.

Key words: craniofacial dysmorphology, craniofacial anomalies, abnormal somatic growth, cephalometric pattern analysis

INTRODUCTION

Abnormalities of the craniofacial complex have been described in a number of syndromes characterized by dysmorphic physical growth. However, quantitative descriptions of craniofacial dysmorphology are rarely reported. Furthermore, the literature in roentgencephalometry is so complex and replete with tables of measurements and multivariate analysis that it is of value only to the expert in the field. In this paper, I have attempted to develop a discriminant set of measurements that may be useful in showing significant differences readily apparent to the dysmorphologist untutored in roentgencephalometry. Accordingly, nine syndromes have been selected for study, each of which seems to affect somatic and craniofacial growth in a different way.

MATERIALS AND METHODS
Materials

Cephalometric data on 30 patients (11 males and 19 females) with nine syndromes formed the basis of this study. Serial sets of lateral and postero-anterior radiographic material were available for one group of 15 patients (5 males and 10 females) and one set of films for the other 15 patients. Data are summarized in Table I. The nine

EDITORS' NOTE: Dr. Pruzansky contributed to the research reported in this paper and was listed as a co-author prior to his death.

Address reprint requests to Nobuyoshi Motohashi, Department of Orthodontics II, School of Dentistry, Tokyo Medical and Dental University, 5-45, Yushima, 1-chome, Bunkyo-ku, Tokyo, 113 Japan.

TABLE I. Description of Patients Analyzed by Roentgencephalometry

Syndrome	CCFA No.	Sex	1	2	3	4	5	6	7	8	9	10	11	12	13	14	15	16	17	18
Progeria	2102	Female	X	X																
	1867	Female										X								
Progeroid	1996	Female	X																	
Johanson-Blizzard	4447	Male			X		X													
	5699	Male	X				X													
Russell-Silver	3571	Male			X		X	X	X	X										
	4035	Male				X						X								
	4911	Female				X	X													
	4827	Female							X		X									
Turner																				
(45,X)	569	Female		X	X	X		X												
(45,X)	1428	Female					X													
(mosaic)	2283	Female								X	X			X	X					
(mosaic)	2275	Female						X	X	X		X	X		X					
Down																				
(mosaic)	955	Female	X							X	X	X	X		X		X			
(21 trisomy)	1687	Female								X	X		X							
(21 trisomy)	4204	Male						X												
(21 trisomy)	4218	Male			X															
(21 trisomy)	5477	Female														X			X	
(21 trisomy)	5639	Male														X				
Cornelia de Lange	1006	Female	X																	
	5294	Male		X			X													
Cerebral gigantism	4932	Male	X		X			X												
	5451	Female											X							
Marfan	3124	Male																		
	4921	Female														X			X	
	4922	Female																		
	4923	Male																		
	4924	Female									X									
	4925	Female																		X
	2919	Female			X	X														

Age at cephalometry (years)

syndromes examined in this study were diagnosed by professional staff of the Center for Craniofacial Anomalies, University of Illinois-College of Medicine.

Methods

Principles and standards for roentgencephalometry have been detailed elsewhere [Broadbent, 1931, Pruzansky and Lis, 1958]. In this study, Bolton standards were used for normative data of the craniofacial complex. To estimate neurocranial size, Haas's data [1952] were used for the younger age group and Costaras's data (personal communication) for older patients.

The hexagon, utilized to illustrate deviations from the norm, includes six discriminant measurements, three of which relate to the neurocranium and three to the face. Of those related to the face, one measures the maxilla and two measure the mandible. The limitations of this format are obvious; measures of interorbital distance, head shape, craniovertebral dysplasia and so forth are not included. However, in this initial effort, the main interest focused on an estimate of the impact of a generalized growth disorder on the neurocranium, where rate and growth differ from that of the face. Within the face, the focus was to separate maxilla from mandible, since the rate and pattern of growth of one vary from those of the other.

The six measures include the following (Fig. 1):

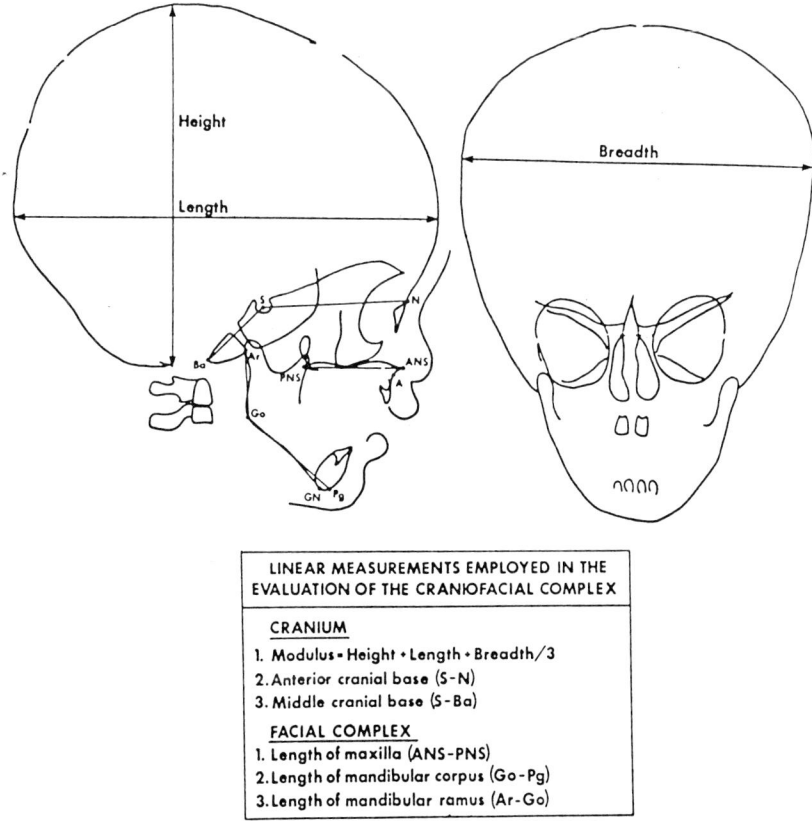

Fig. 1. Tracing of lateral and postero-anterior cephalometric radiographs to illustrate landmarks and constructed planes utilized in study.

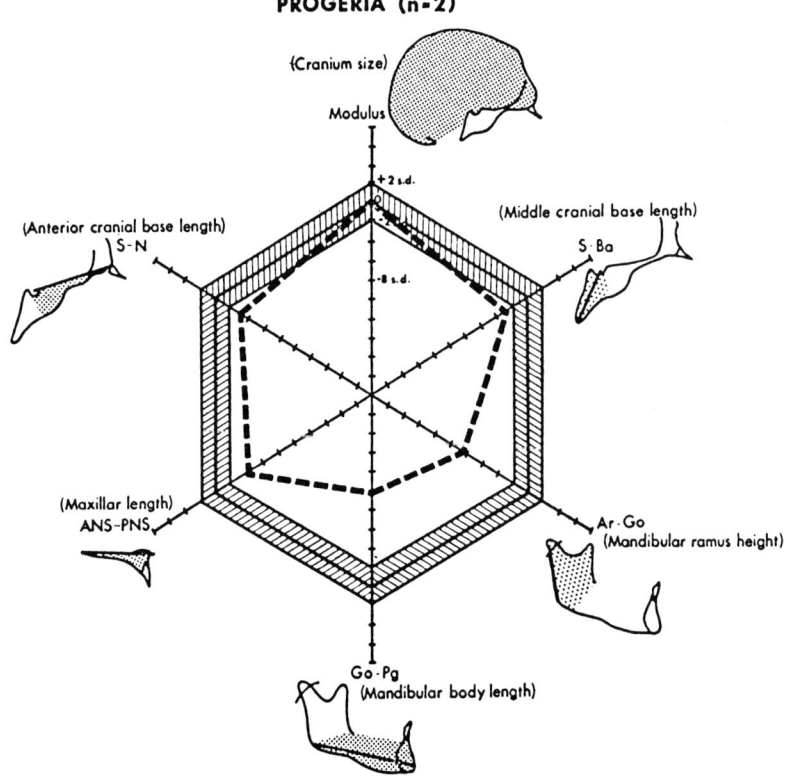

Fig. 2. Schematic diagram to illustrate the effect of growth disorders on the development of the craniofacial skeleton utilizing three parameters to define neurocranial growth and three parameters for facial bone growth. The hexagon encompasses the mean and ±2 standard deviations of the norm matched for age and sex. The standard score for each parameter is plotted on the radiating axes in accord with their deviation from the norm. For progeria, the neurocranial volume, as measured by the modulus, is within the norm. The facial skeleton seems to be most retarded in its development.

A. *Neurocranium.* It is assumed that all of the measures under this heading follow a neural growth curve [Scammon et al, 1930].

1. Modulus: This is an indirect measure of intracranial volume as defined by Haas [1952]. Altogether, this measure reflects the combined contribution of sutural growth of the calvarium and of the cartilaginous cranial base.

2. Anterior cranial base length (Na–S).

3. Length of the middle cranial fossa (S–Ba). Measurements 2 and 3 attempt to fractionate the contributions of components of the cartilaginous cranial base.

B. *Splanchnocranium.* Since facial growth follows a somatic growth curve, it is expected that growth increments in this area will continue long after neurocranial growth has plateaued. Thus, a differential long-term deceleration or acceleration of generalized somatic growth will occur. It is also recognized that there are sexual dichotomies in rates and duration of mandibular growth and that maxillary growth differs in several ways from growth of the mandible.

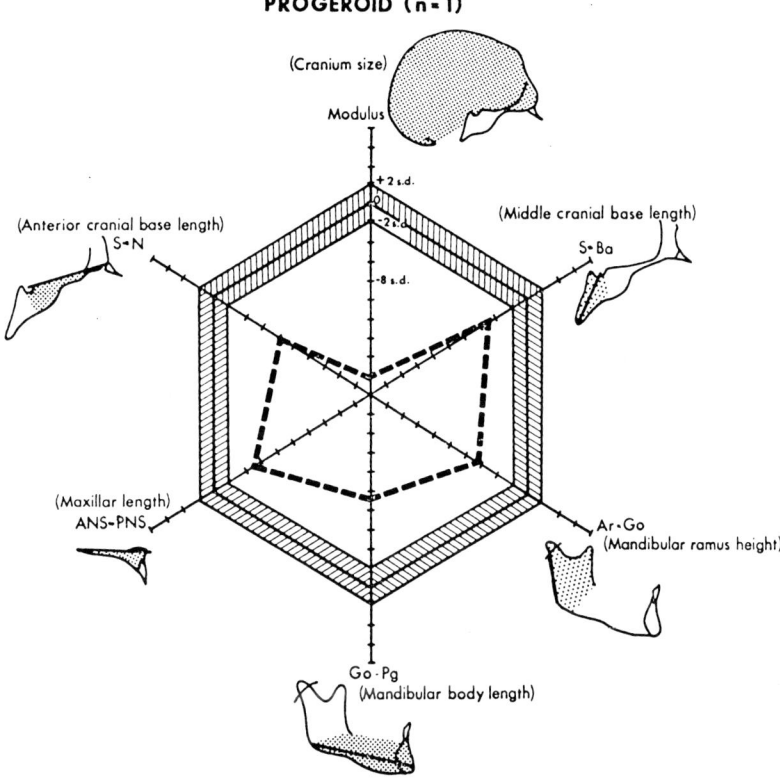

Fig. 3. The craniofacial skeletal pattern of progeroid is marked by microcephaly and an extremely small facial component. The comparison of two hexagon charts of progeria and progeroid clearly demonstrates the different craniofacial dysmorphology of both conditions, characterized by the neurocranial size.

1. Anterior nasal spine to posterior nasal spine (ANS–PNS): measures the length of the maxilla.

2. Gonion to pogonion (Go–Pog): measures the length of the corpus of the mandible.

3. Articulare to pogonion (Ar–Go): measures the height of the ramus. The decision to employ two separate measures for the mandible reflects previous experiences in finding disproportions in these dimensions among various syndromes.

Statistical Methods

In this study, the pattern of craniofacial dysmorphology and the growth pattern of each syndrome are examined by cross-sectional analysis based on standard scores and by longitudinal analysis of the growth increment ratios.

Cross-Sectional Analysis. With small numbers and each subject in a given diagnostic category which varies in age and sex, it is difficult to summarize the findings in terms of actual values. Through standard scores, each patient can be compared with normal values matched for age and sex. Since the mean of any

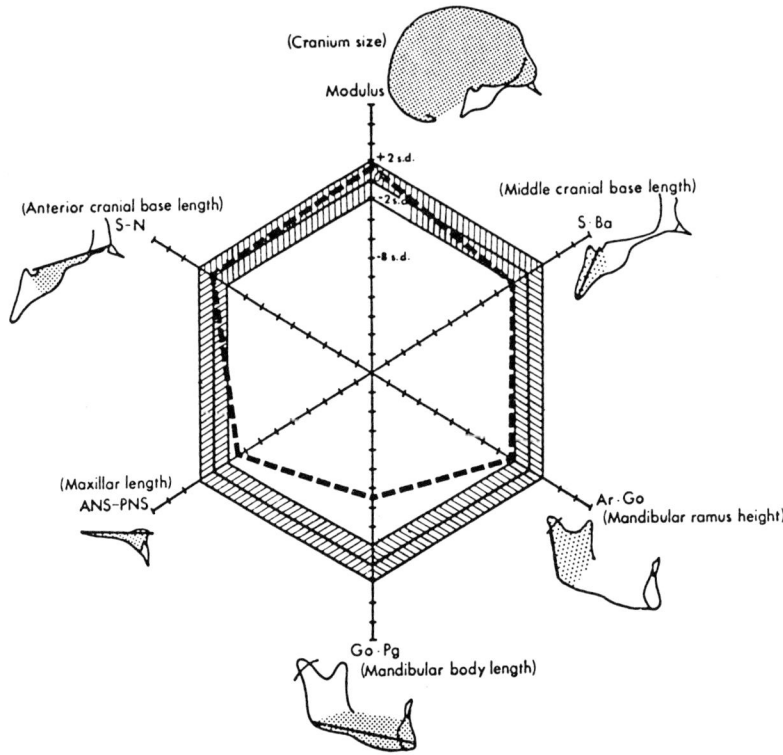

Fig. 4. The craniofacial dysmorphology of Johanson-Blizzard syndrome is distinguished by normocephaly and small face.

distribution of standard scores is always equal to zero and the variance is always equal to 1.00, standard scores from one distribution can be compared with standard scores of another distribution of comparable form.

In this study, all data of the six parameters obtained from x-ray films were converted to standard scores. The standard score of each set of measurements was calculated by matching each patient's measurement with that of the norm paired for age and sex, according to the following formula:

$$Z = \frac{X - \bar{X}}{s}$$

where Z = standard score; X = original measurement; $\bar{X}$ = the mean of the distribution in normal controls paired for age and sex; and s = the standard deviation of the distribution. The average standard score for each syndrome was computed from the combined data for the subjects in the group.

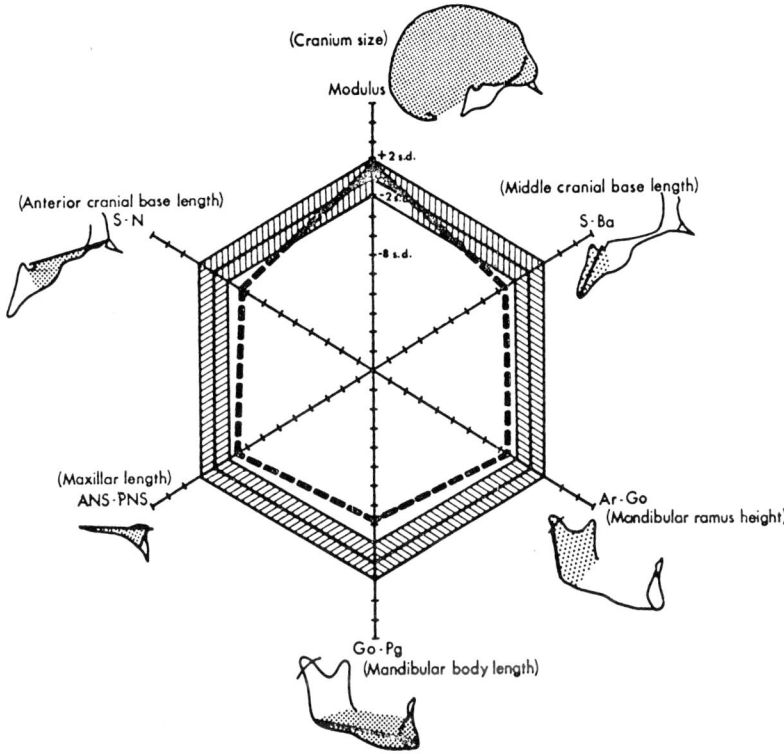

Fig. 5. Russell-Silver syndrome is characterized by pseudohydrocephaly owing to normocephaly and marked small facial components including anterior and middle cranial base.

For the purpose of a simple schematic presentation of standard scores, a hexagon was developed. Accordingly, the average of the six parameters in each syndrome was plotted along six radiating axes. The shaded perimeter of the hexagon represents ±2 standard deviations about the mean applicable to all age levels of the normal for each of the six parameters.

Longitudinal analysis. The sex and age of each patient at the time of cephalometry are shown in Table I.

When serial data were available, it was possible to calculate a growth increment ratio (GIR) for a given age and sex from the original measurement, as follows:

$$\text{GIR}\% = \frac{\text{growth increment ratio of affected}}{\text{growth increment ratio of normal}} \times 100$$

When several subjects were available, the average of the subjects was utilized to illustrate the growth pattern for the syndrome. An exception was made for Cornelia

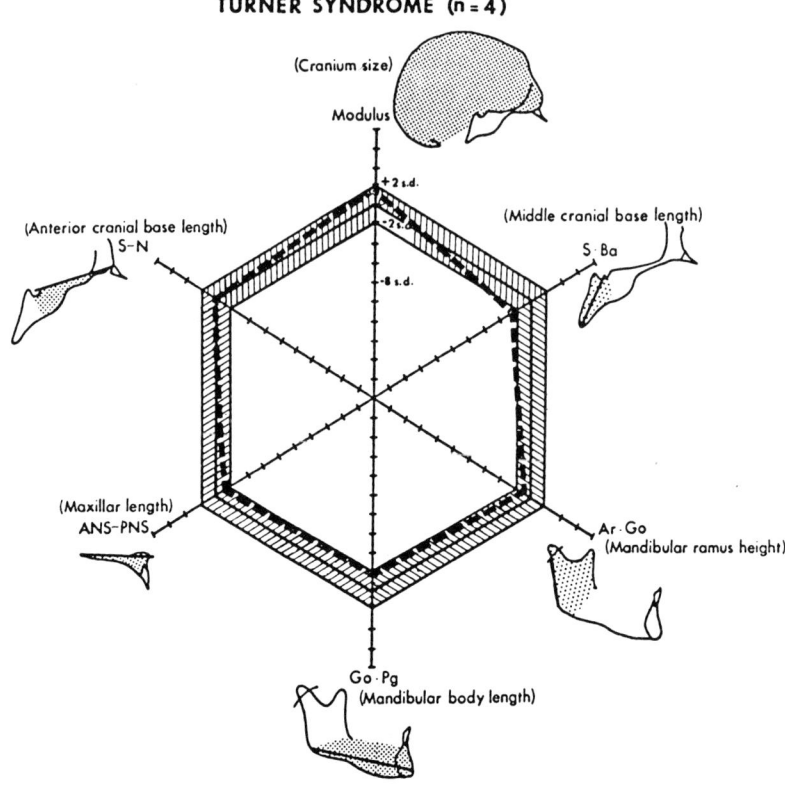

Fig. 6. Four patients with Turner syndrome showing normocephaly and somewhat smaller face as their common cranifacial characteristics, irrespective of karyotype.

de Lange syndrome, where considerable variance in severity was encountered. Under such circumstances, it was deemed best to illustrate each individual.

RESULTS

Average standard scores for each syndrome are shown in Figures 2–11. Growth increment ratios are presented in Figure 12.

Progeria (Figs. 2, 12)

The discriminant effect of growth retardation was strikingly apparent in the hexagon. The neurocranium was relatively normal in contrast to the marked retardation of facial growth, especially the mandible. On the basis of clinical reports, it is emphasized that the disorder is not apparent at birth but is manifested as the child grows older. In an earlier report [Rosenthal et al, 1969], Pruzansky suggested that a constant growth deceleration operating postnatally is most likely to exert the greatest braking effect on those organs having to travel further distances over time, such as the lower face. The fact that patients with progeria have normal mentation further testifies to the relatively sparing effect of this growth-decelerating process on the brain and the bony capsule that houses it.

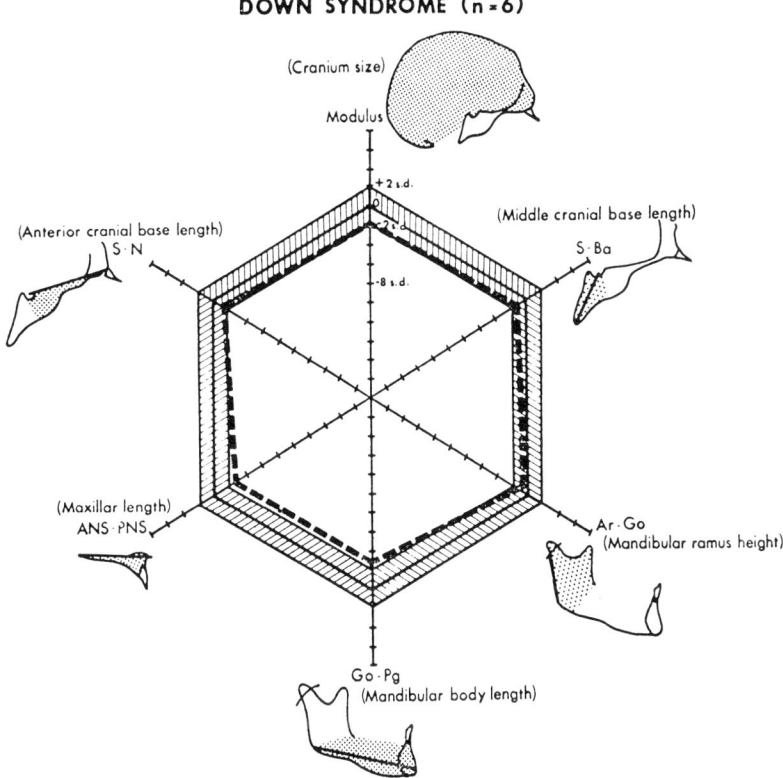

Fig. 7. Note the microcephaly and the smaller than normal face characterizing Down syndrome.

Progeroid (Figs. 3, 12)

The progeroid phenotype is not a clearly defined entity.* It is not implied that this patient is representative of any given group. However, the patient does serve as a special example in terms of time of onset and severity of growth arrest.

In contrast to Progeria, the progeroid phenotype demonstrates not only a smaller head size but one in which the neurocranium is particularly affected. Onset of growth retardation is prenatal, extending into postnatal life, and it is evident that the cumulative impact will be on the neurocranium, which manifests the greatest incremental growth during this period. The face will not be spared but will be less affected than the neurocranium.

Johanson-Blizzard Syndrome (Figs. 4, 12)

According to the hexagonal grid, neurocranial growth is similar to the norm but facial growth is retarded. The length of the mandible appears more severely affected

---

Editors' note. This phenotype is based on a paper written in 1955. By today's standards, it might represent cockayne syndrome or a cockayne syndrome variant.

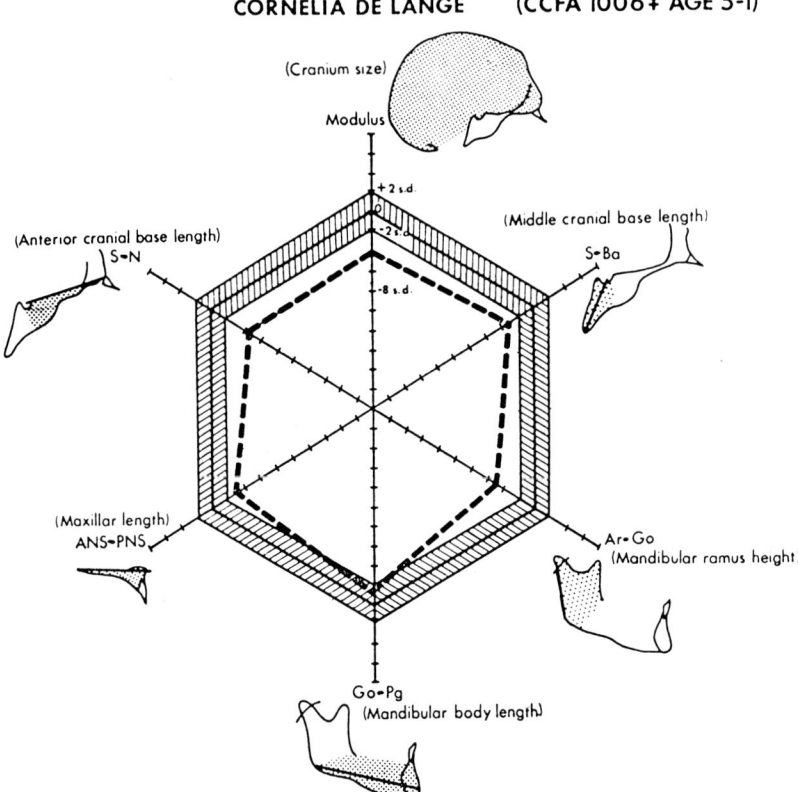

Fig. 8. CCFA 1006 with Cornelia de Lange syndrome, characterized by a severely affected neurocranial and facial component.

than the length of the maxilla. Calculation of the growth increment ratio over time shows a rate of change that suggests that if the process were to continue, the maxilla would become more severely affected than the mandible.

Russell-Silver Syndrome (Figs. 5, 12)

Inspection of each patient in this study demonstrates within-group variation. Two subjects show standard scores for the modulus well in excess of the norm, while two fall below the norm. Cranial base measurements fall beneath the norm, as do all facial measurements.

Turner Syndrome (Figs. 6, 12)

Of the four patients studied, two were 45,X and two were (45,X/46,XX) mosaics. All four, irrespective of karyotype, showed essentially normal neurocranial development. The middle cranial base was shortened in all cases. Facial components were somewhat smaller than the norm.

Down Syndrome (Figs. 7, 12)

The karyotypes of five of the six patients were trisomy 21 and one was mosaic. No differences in phenotype could be attributed to the karyotypic variability. Micro-

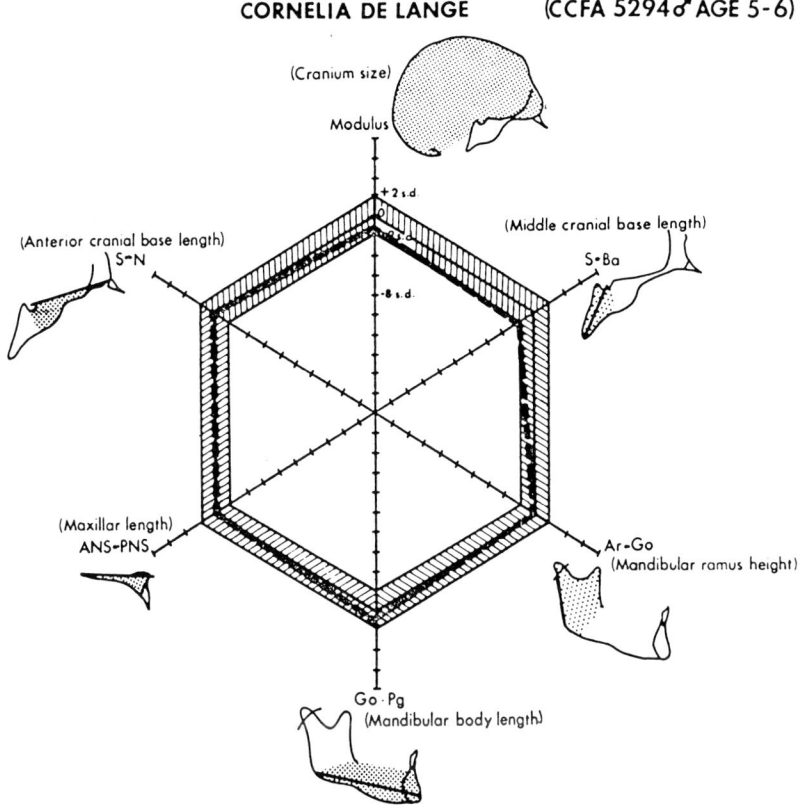

Fig. 9. CCFA 5294 with Cornelia de Lange syndrome. Note the different pattern of craniofacial dysmorphology in the two cases (CCFA 1006 and 5294) with this syndrome. The common feature in both cases is the abnormal disproportion of mandibular corpus length and ramus height.

cephaly and smaller facies characterized the sample. Comprehensive roentgencephalometric studies of this syndrome have appeared in papers by Gosman [1951] and Roche et al [1972].

Cornelia de Lange Syndrome (Figs. 8,9,12)

Clinical experiences suggest a wide spectrum of variable expression in this syndrome [Pashayan et al, 1969,1975] and this variability was also observed in our population. An earlier report from the Center for Craniofacial Anomalies based on a series of severely affected institutionalized patients showed greater homogeneity in craniofacial dysmorphology. However, with ascertainment of less severely affected cases from other sources, the concept of a syndrome-specific craniofacial skeletal profile was not supported. For this reason, two different patterns in patients judged by experienced syndromologists to qualify as examples of Cornelia de Lange syndrome were demonstrated in this study.

Figure 8 shows a severely retarded patient. Neurocranial size is clearly below the norm in all three measures. The mandible is unusual; body length is normal and ramus height is shortened. Moreover, the growth increment ratio shows that ramus height was 25% of normal, while mandibular body length was 153.1% of normal.

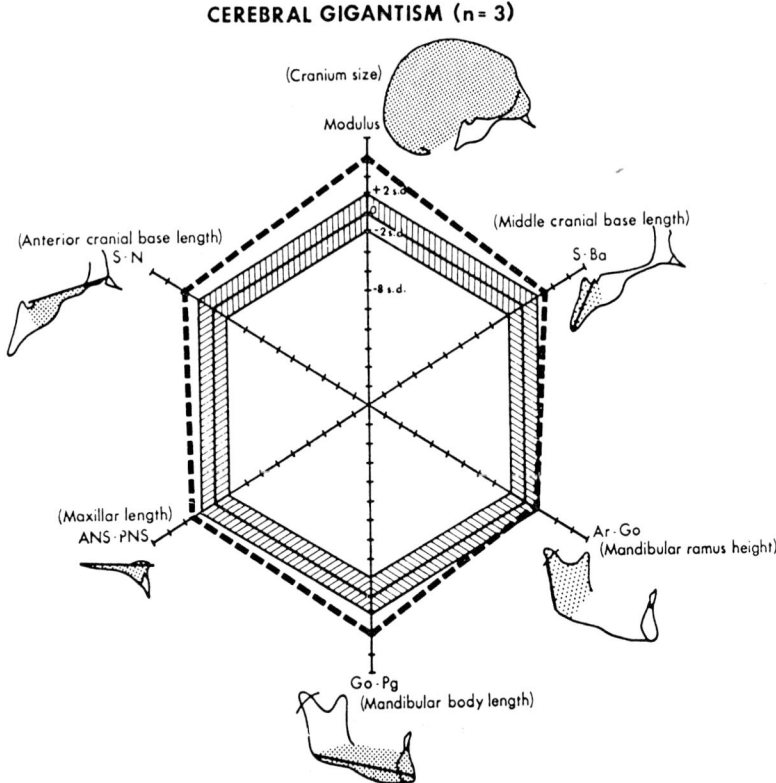

Fig. 10. Cerebral gigantism is distinguished by macrocephaly and facial size larger than the norm.

The patient in Figure 9 is currently observed on an outpatient basis and is not severely retarded. The neurocranium is within normal limits for two parameters but reduced for anterior cranial base length. In this instance, as in the previous case, mandibular body length is greater than ramus height.

Despite the different hexagonal displays of these two patients, a common denominator is evident in the growth increment ratio of the mandible (Figure 12). Both patients show greater than normal increments in mandibular body length and less than normal increments in ramus length, thereby contributing to what may be a syndrome-specific imbalance in the ratio of mandibular ramus to mandibular body length.

Cerebral Gigantism (Figs. 10, 12)

The effect of accelerated growth was manifest in both the neurocranium and the facial skeleton. In two of the three patients, mandibular growth showed increased mandibular body length in the presence of normal ramus height, producing a disproportion in mandibular shape.

Marfan Syndrome (Figs. 11, 12)

Five of the six patients studied showed neurocranial measurements greater than normal (macrocephaly). All six patients had facial measurements within normal limits.

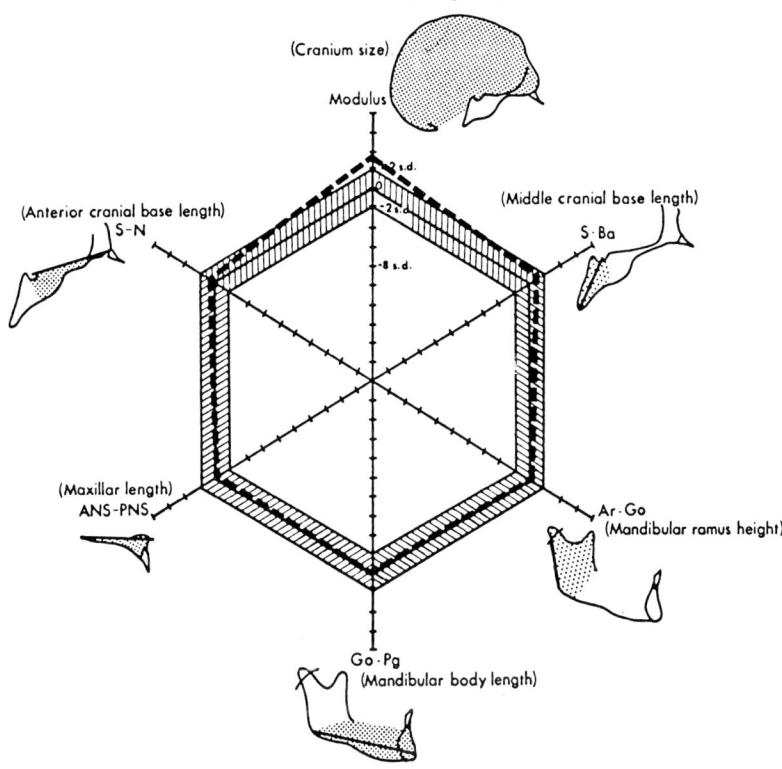

Fig. 11. In contrast to cerebral gigantism, Marfan syndrome demonstrates macrocephaly with normal-sized face.

DISCUSSION

Disorders of growth vary in many ways. Some accelerate growth; others decelerate growth. Time of onset varies in each from intrauterine development to late in postnatal growth. The duration of effect may be relatively short with subsequent recovery, as in transient malnutrition, or may involve a continuing process of variable intensity.

Certain growth disorders exhibit a generalized somatic effect; others are tissue specific, as in achondroplasia with affected cartilage of the long bones and cranial base. In still other instances, imbalance in remodeling processes may produce distortions in the growth of the skull as well as the limbs.

In considering the impact of such variable growth disorders on the craniofacial skeleton, it is useful to reconsider its biology. The skull is a community of bones of different phylogenetic origin and variable ontogeny. The neurocranium is derived in part from a desmocranium influenced by sutural growth and in part from a cartilaginous cranial base. Each component of the skull relates to a different functional matrix, such as those concerned with neural function and neural growth curves, respiratory functions, and masticatory and speech functions.

On the basis of the foregoing, it is not unexpected that the impact of growth arrest on any given individual will vary in kind and severity. Serial studies by

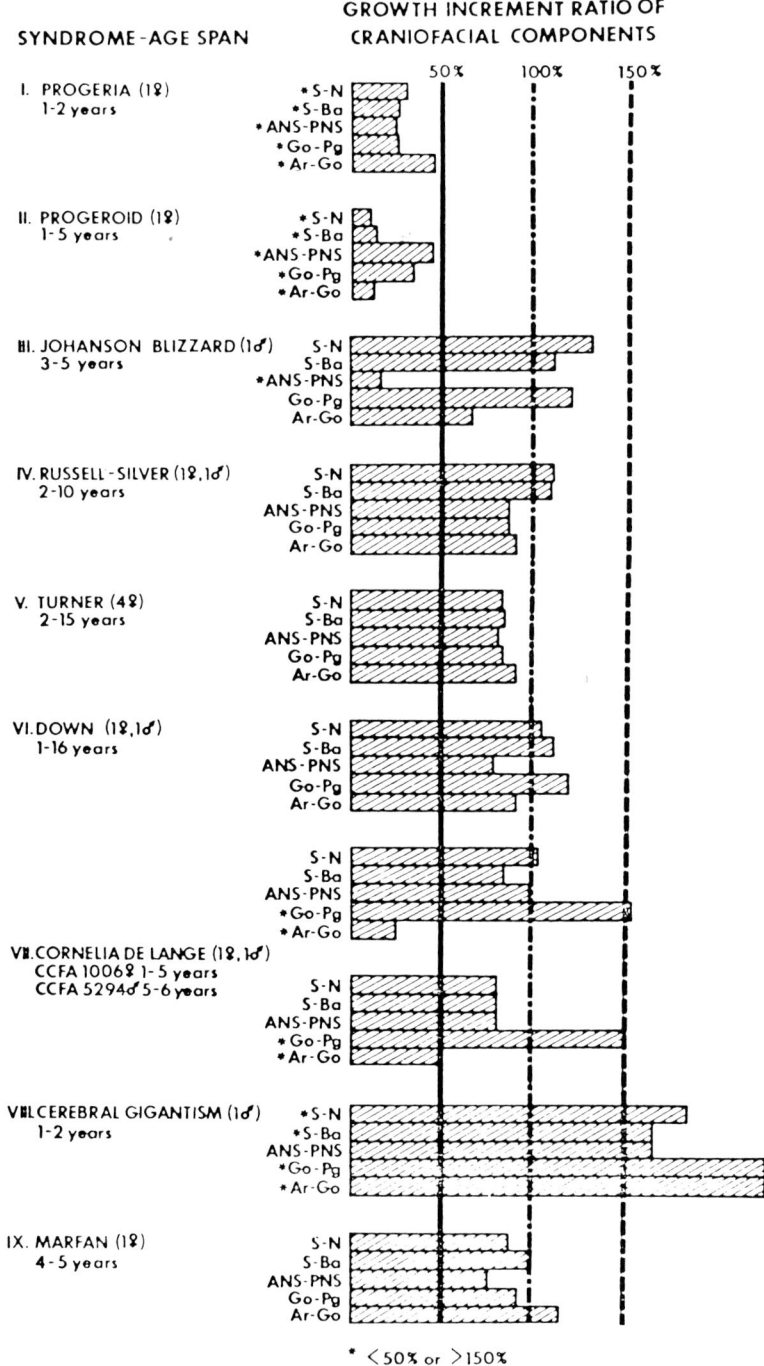

Fig. 12. Growth increment ratio of each craniofacial component in nine syndromes associated with various physical growth disorders.

quantitative measures provide a means for documenting and analyzing the process, at least at the macroscopic level.

CONCLUSIONS

A schematic diagram in the form of a hexagon that measures neurocranial and facial skeletal size and form as determined by six variables serves to summarize the effect of various growth disorders on the craniofacial complex. It offers the possibility of a quantitative dysmorphology based on roentgencephalometry.

ACKNOWLEDGMENTS

When I was a research associate at the Center for Craniofacial Anomalies in Chicago from 1978 to 1980, I was particularly interested in craniofacial dysmorphology in various syndromes associated with abnormal physical growth. This study was my final work with Dr. Pruzansky at the Center. In his last letter to me dated December 26, 1983, he recommended that I submit this paper for this volume. I sincerely appreciated his kindness, supervision, and the opportunities he gave me to study birth defects.

REFERENCES

Broadbent BH: A new X-ray technique and its application to orthodontics. Angle Orthod 1:45–66, 1931.
Broadbent BH Sr, Broadbent BH Jr, Golden WH: "Bolton Standards of Dentofacial Developmental Growth." St. Louis: C.V. Mosby Company, 1975.
Gosman SD: Facial development in mongolism. Am J Orthod 37:332–349, 1951.
Haas LL: Roentgenological skull measurements and their diagnostic applications. Am J Roentgenol 67:197–209, 1952.
Pashayan H, Whelan D, Guttman S, Fraser FC: Variability of the de Lange syndrome: Report of 3 cases and genetic analysis of 54 families. J Pediatr 75:853–858, 1969.
Pashayan HM, Fraser FC, Pruzansky S: Variable limb malformations in the Brachmann-Cornelia de Lange syndrome. Birth Defects Original Article Series XI (5):147–156, 1975.
Pruzansky S, Lis EF: Cephalometric roentgenography of infants: Sedation, instrumentation, and research. Am J Orthod 44:159–186, 1958.
Roche AF, Roche PJ, Lewis AB: The cranial base in trisomy 21. J Ment Defic Res 16:7–20, 1972.
Rosenthal IM, Bronstein IP, Dallenbach FD, Pruzansky S. Rosenwald AK: Progeria: Report of a case with cephalometric roentgenograms and abnormally high concentrations of lipoportines in the serum. J Pediatr 18:565–577, 1969.
Scammon RE, Harris JA, Jackson CM, Patterson DG: "The Measurement of Man." Minneapolis: University of Minnesota Press, 1930.

The Degenerative, Regenerative Mandibular Condyle: Facial Asymmetry

J. Daniel Subtelny
Department of Orthodontics, Eastman Dental Center, Rochester, New York

Studies of longitudinal cephalometric radiographs are presented for several patients with condylar fracture or hemifacial microsomia to illustrate condylar regeneration, presumably under functional influences. Implications of new condylar development and growth to facial and mandibular symmetry are presented. Clinical implications are introduced and the hypothesis of necessity of function for maintenance of relative facial symmetry is considered.

Key words: condylar regeneration, condylar degeneration, condylar fracture, facial asymmetry, mandibular asymmetry, mandibular condyle, hemifacial microsomia

INTRODUCTION

Controversy exists as to whether the mandibular condyle is a primary growth site in the growth of the mandible [Robinson and Sarnat, 1955; Sarnat, 1983] or whether condylar growth is adaptive in nature to functional demands associated with mandibular jaw activity. If one subscribes to the functional matrix concept of growth, it might be said that growth in the condylar region is regulated by the growth and function of the oral cavity itself [Moss and Saletijn, 1969]. One way or the other, the direction and the extent of growth in the condylar region is known to have an effect on facial appearance and facial asymmetry. Any defect leading to asymmetric condylar growth on one or both sides of the mandible has been shown to cause facial asymmetry.

This paper evaluates damage to one of the condylar regions and the consequences of the ensuing alteration in its positional and functional relationships to contiguous structures. Three cases are analyzed longitudinally. It is hoped that some insight may be gained into the importance of the condyle for the developing mandible and the maintenance of mandibular symmetry.

With a congenitally absent condyle or trauma to the condyle, deficient growth on one side and continued full expression of mandibular growth on the unaffected side causes the chin to deviate progressively further toward the affected side (Fig. 1). This

---

Address reprint requests to Dr. J. Daniel Subtelny, Department of Orthodontics, Eastman Dental Center, 625 Elmwood Avenue, Rochester, NY 14620.

© 1985 Alan R. Liss, Inc.

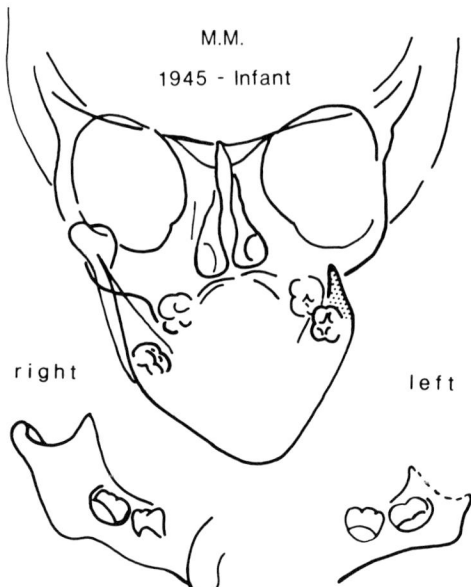

Fig. 1. Tracings of hospital radiographs of infant (M.M.) born with microtia. Congenital agenesis of the left condyle and minimal development of the left ramus with a diminutive coronoid process is noted.

observation can best be demonstrated through the three case presentations of patients with unilateral mandibular growth problems illustrating, with longitudinal records, the eventual effects of restriction or reduction of mandibular growth on one side or the other.

CASE REPORTS

Case 1

The first case represents agenesis of the condyle and ramus on the left side. The patient also had microtia, absent external auditory meatus, left cleft lip, and a left supernumerary thumb. The craniofacial radiographs taken during infancy clearly revealed skeletal discrepancies. Frontal radiographs indicated the presence of a foreshortened coronoid process and no ramus on the left side with definite agenesis of the left mandibular condyle. This was corroborated by the oblique radiographs, which demonstrated a normal ramus, coronoid process, and condyle on the right side and no condylar process, a diminutive coronoid process, and a deficient ramus on the left side (Fig. 1). In infancy, facial asymmetry was already noted on the frontal radiograph with the chin deviated toward the affected side.

Orthodontic treatment was instituted at 12 years of age with the realization that facial asymmetry would probably become more pronounced with continued facial growth. At this time considerable facial asymmetry was noted; the lower face, mouth, and jaw were displaced to the left with considerable depression in the left cheekbone area. Upon opening the chin deviated severely to the left and full opening could not be achieved. However, function was evident. When the teeth were brought into occlusion, the lower dental midline deviated to the left. Both the upper and lower

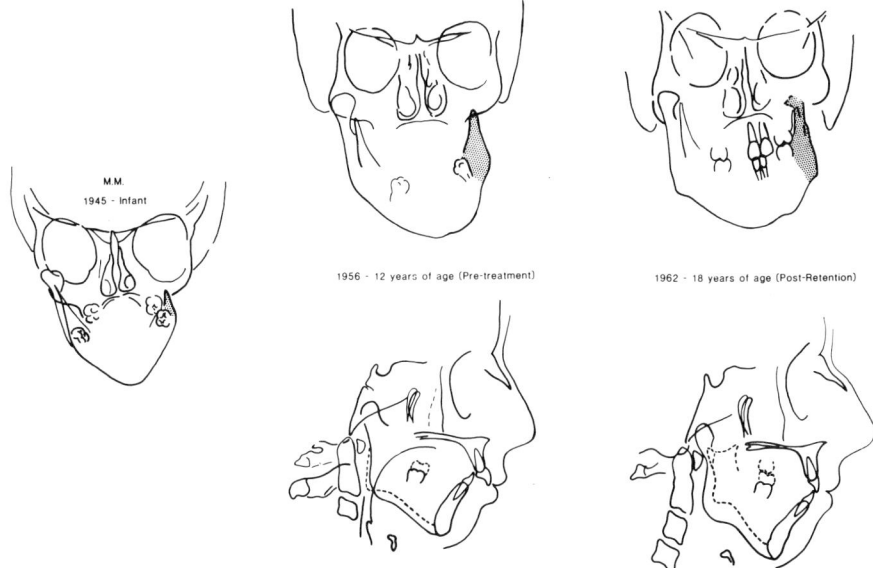

Fig. 2. Tracings of lateral and frontal cephalometric radiographs (M.M., Fig. 1) taken prior to orthodontic treatment at 12 years of age and several years after completion of orthodontic treatment at 18 years of age. Note facial asymmetry; also note initiation of development of the congenitally missing left ramus as denoted by the stippled area on the frontal radiographs and broken lines on the lateral radiographs.

posterior teeth on the left side were infra-erupted, so there was a strongly discernible upward cant of the occlusal plane. The frontal radiograph showed the left side of the skeletal face to be underdeveloped, both in the zygomatic bone area and in the left aspect of the ramus. The left ramus was considerably shorter in height than the right ramus, although it seemed to have grown to some extent when compared to the original hospital radiograph (Fig. 2). The left occlusal level of the molar teeth was discernibly higher—that is, closer to the cranium or the floor of the nasal cavity when compared to the unaffected side. Antegonial notching was becoming evident on the affected side.

With orthodontic treatment, reasonable occlusion was achieved and maintained for many years after retention removal. Appliance therapy was instituted to retract the protruding maxillary dental arch (cervical appliance); elastic force was also used to retract the upper arch. The elastic force had a forward pull on the mandibular arch as well as a distally directed force on the upper arch; in addition, there was forward pull on the movable mandible while there was distal traction on the maxilla. A maxillary acrylic bite plate was placed in the palatal region to disarticulate the upper and lower dentition. The bite plate had an additional occlusal splint on the left side. Vertical elastics were used first on the right side and then on the left side in an attempt to level the two sides of the occlusal plane as much as possible.

Cephalometric radiographs following orthodontic treatment showed that the mandible did not grow on the affected side comparable to the unaffected side. A ramus was observed to be developing on the congenitally affected side—an unexpected

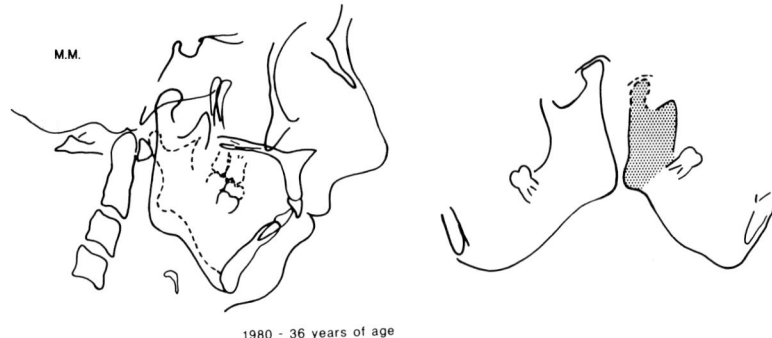

1980 - 36 years of age

Fig. 3. Tracings of lateral and oblique cephalometric radiographs of M.M. taken at 36 years of age. Note apparent development of left ramus and condyle (broken line and stippled area). Note also what appears to be a flattening of the head of the right condyle.

finding (Fig. 2). The new left ramus was considerably smaller than the right ramus, antegonial notching was marked, and a condylar process was observed (Fig. 3). No surgical reconstruction of a new ramus was attempted, and it can only be surmised that muscular function and the influence of muscle activity on bone and periosteum was instrumental in the new bony development. In addition to achieving some degree of functional movement of the mandible, the patient also had additional functional stimulation from the use of elastic forces on the affected side. This served to reposition the mandible, to perhaps stretch the soft tissues associated with the affected ramus, and to maintain functional activity on that side.

Although function was probably instrumental in new development on the affected side, less than ideal functional movements may have resulted in condylar problems on the normal side. Cephalometric oblique radiographs showed some flattening of the head of the condyle (Fig. 3). Clinically, a snapping or clicking noise was noted on functional opening. Compensatory functional movements on the normal side resulting from aberrant functional movements on the affected side may have altered the configuration of the condyle.

Case 2

Case 2 deals with fracture and dislocation of one condyle in a 6-year-old boy. It is known that a fractured and displaced condyle will atrophy and can regenerate at early ages [Walker, 1960; Blevins and Gores, 1961]. It is also known that mandibular function and functional control of mandibular posture can be helpful to continued mandibular growth [Harvold, 1975; Hotz, 1978]. Cephalometric radiographs taken at the time of the fracture indicate that the fractured condylar process was displaced medially, anteriorly, and inferiorly (Fig. 4). With displacement of the mandibular condyle, immediate shortening of the vertical height of the ramus was noted. By 19 years of age, the patient was approaching the time of completed mandibular growth. During this time span, the patient had undergone continued orthodontic treatment and continued stimulation of mandibular development on the side of the condylar fracture. Throughout treatment there was periodic use of functional stimulation by elastic therapy, class II mechanics when indicated, bite plate therapy when indicated, bite

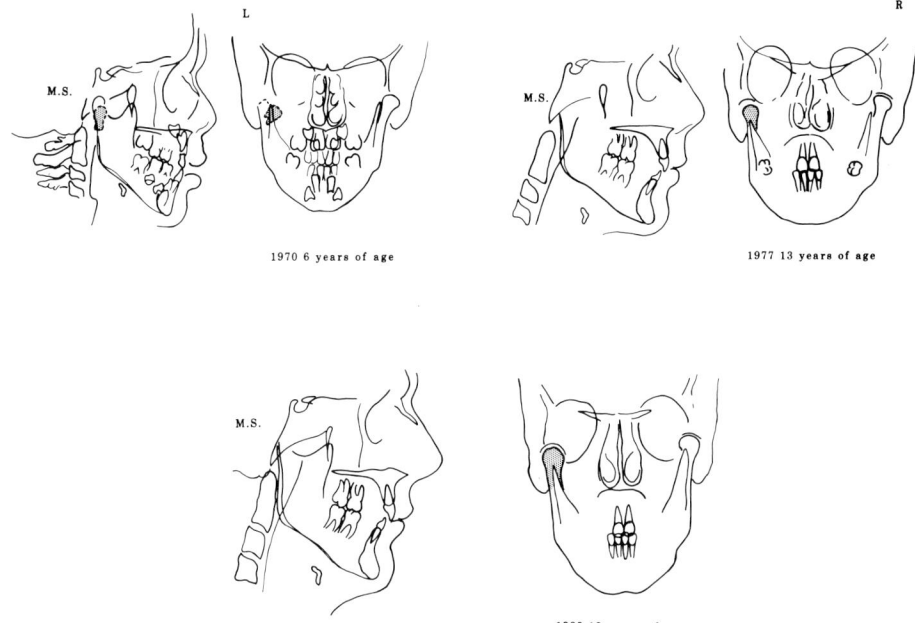

Fig. 4. Tracings of longitudinal lateral and frontal cephalometric radiographs of a growing youngster (M.S.) with an early-age fracture of the left mandibular condyle (stippled area). Note size, shape, and position of the regenerated left condyle and reasonable skeletal facial symmetry.

block therapy when indicated, and orthodontic tooth movement to maintain reasonable occlusion and to maintain acceptable facial symmetry. As can be seen from the oblique radiographs, regeneration of the fractured condyle occurred (Fig. 5) with gradual developmenmt of a condylar process and then a condylar head. The new condyle was larger and more bulbous than the normal condyle (Figs. 3–5).

The vertical height of the affected ramus never achieved the same vertical ramal height noted on the non-fractured side. The posterior border of the ramus on the affected side seemed to become progressively more posterior in its location than the other mandibular ramus. Mobility in both condylar regions was clearly evident on cephalometric laminagraphs taken with the mandible in a wide open position. Considerable alteration in bony architecture was noted anterior to the gonial region on the non-fractured side. This may be related to compensatory function on the non-fractured side. With time, a snap or click was noted on the non-fractured side during temporomandibular joint function. Without therapy, it is possible that deficient growth on the affected side would have been more severe, with the eventual development of considerable facial asymmetry.

Case 3

The patient was an 8-year-old girl with a left condylar fracture. Clinical radiographic findings revealed a fracture dislocation of the left condyle with a deviation of the mandible to the left side. Under general anesthesia, intermaxillary fixation was established. Three years following the fracture, the patient was referred for orthodontic consultation and care. Facial asymmetry was evident, the chin deviating to the

232 Subtelny

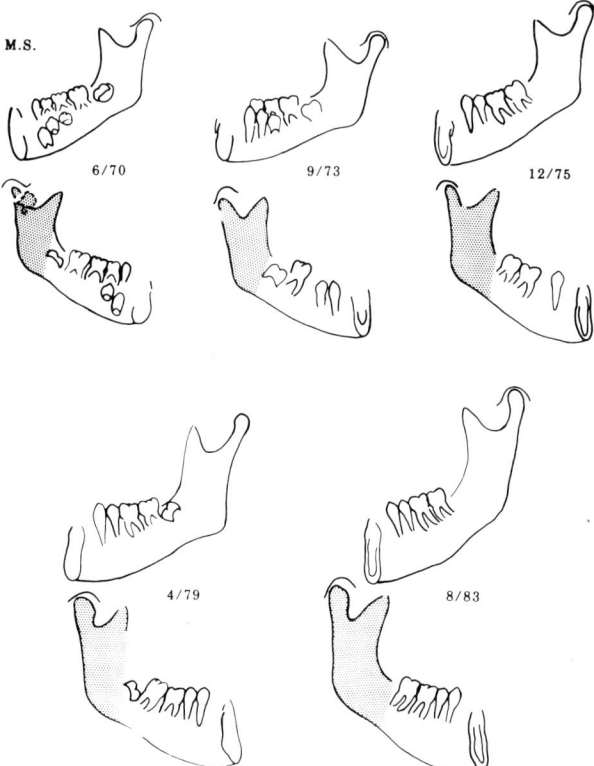

Fig. 5. Tracings of longitudinal cephalometric oblique radiographs of the right and left mandibles of the subject depicted in Figure 4. The displacement of the fractured condyle and the regeneration of a new condyle is illustrated (stippled ramus). The shape and size of the new condyle can be compared with the non-fractured side.

left. She had restricted movement of the left temporomandibular joint on mandibular excursion to the right, and there was pronounced deviation to the left upon opening. Frontal, lateral, and oblique cephalometric radiographs showed some lack of development of the left side of the mandible (Fig. 6); there was deficient vertical and horizontal growth on the left side of the mandible. Jaw orthopedic therapy was initiated. A functional appliance followed by a unilateral bite block were constructed to counteract progressive asymmetry with continued growth, to stretch muscle fibers and soft tissue components, and to attempt to improve functional movements on the side of the fracture. In addition to the facial and functional problems, the maxillary and mandibular alveolar processes on the left side were underdeveloped with tilting of the occlusal plane from right to left (Fig. 6). This possibly resulted from contraction of tissue as well as muscle on the left side. The vertical height of the alveolar processes on the fractured side was also corrected. After three years of functional therapy, mandibular movements improved. Radiographically, a small new malformed condyle appeared (Fig. 7). Facial asymmetry seemed to be increasing with growth, but with soft tissue masking the patient appeared more symmetrical with the chin closer to the midline.

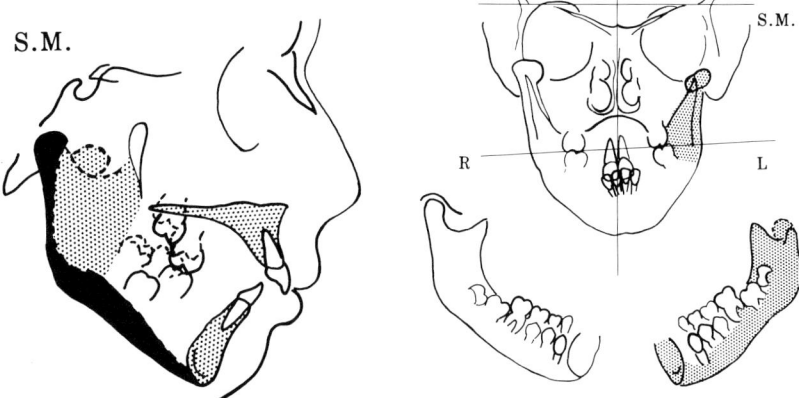

Fig. 6. Tracings of cepholometric lateral, frontal and oblique radiographs of a young girl (S.M.) taken 3 years after fracture of the left condyle; stippled area represents the left side as well as the hard palate and symphysis. Note the skeletal facial and mandibular asymmetry and the two different levels of the occlusal surfaces of the molar teeth (occlusal line on the frontal tracing); solid line and the broken line (fracture side) represent molar teeth on the lateral tracing.

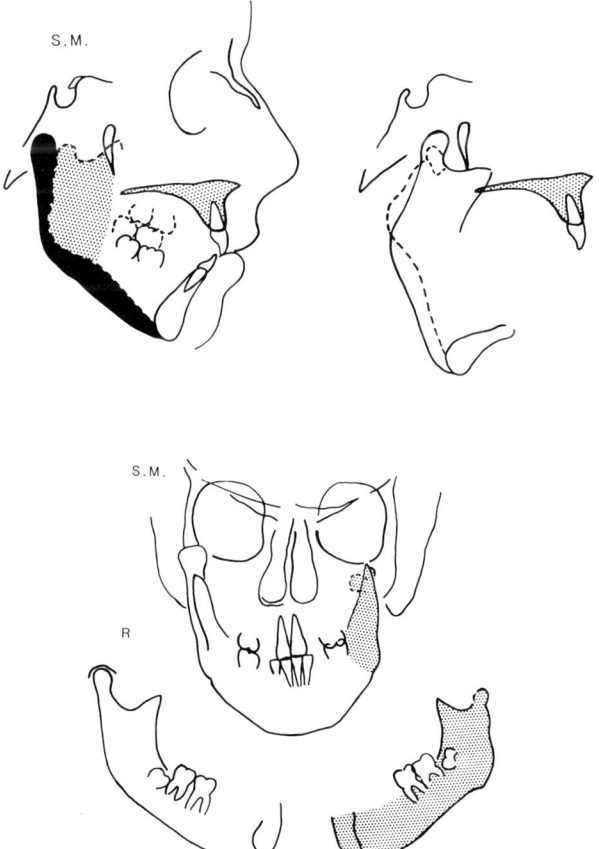

Fig. 7. Tracings of cephalometric radiographs of individual depicted in Figure 6. It can be noted that a new condyle, diminutive in size, seems to be forming on the fractured side (stippled area and broken line).

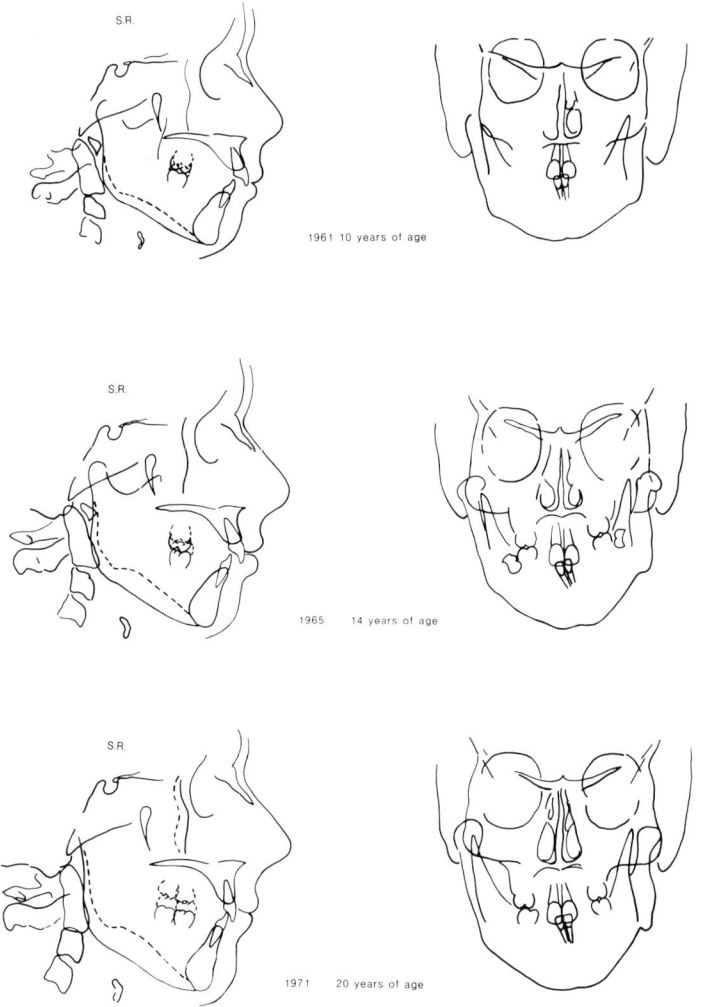

Fig. 8. Tracings of lateral and frontal cephalometric radiographs taken on the same individual (S.R.) at 10, 14, and 20 years of age. Progressive development of mandibular and skeletal facial asymmetry is depicted. On the lateral radiograph tracings, the side of reduced development is depicted by the broken line. Deviation of the chin, reduced ramal height, and considerable antegonial notching is evident on the side of reduced development.

Case 4

In this case, the developing mandibular asymmetry was not recognized at the initiation of orthodontic therapy, but was noted when the patient was completing orthodontic treatment. During retention, it was recognized that there was deficient growth on one side of the mandible. The patient was treated to a fine occlusion, which maintained itself many years after retention. However, with continued growth, the mandibular asymmetry became more prominent. Skeletal chin deviation and reduction in the size of the left ramus and left body of the mandible became visible

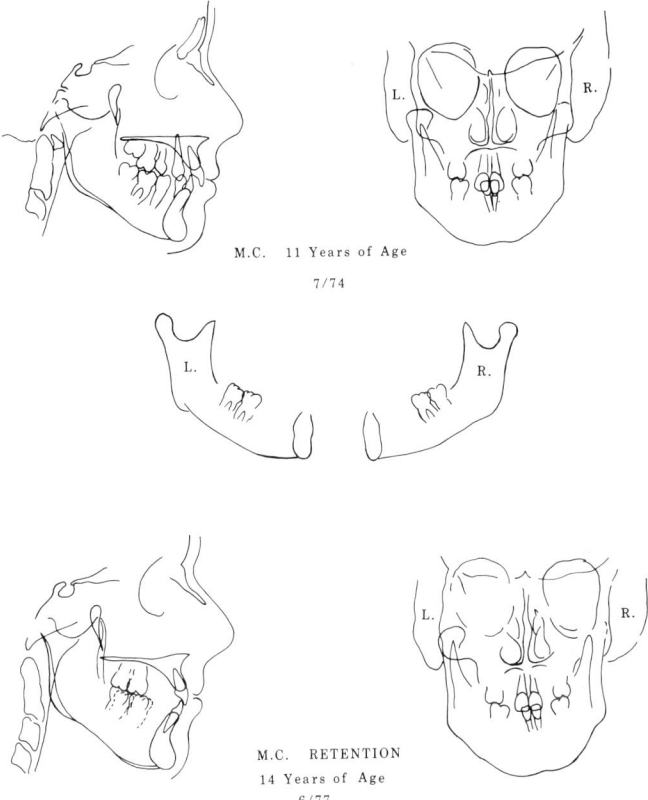

Fig. 9. Cephalometric tracings of radiographs taken on the same individual (M.C.) at 11 and 14 years of age. An indication of developing skeletal facial asymmetry can be noted. A disparity in the images of the posterior borders of the two rami is depicted. Deviation in the position of the chin and the mandibular dental midline has become more evident.

on cephalometric radiographs (Fig. 8). A similar case, although less dramatic, is noted in Figure 9. In this instance, mandibular and facial asymmetry became more noticeable on completion of orthodontic treatment. Follow-up cephalometric radiographs taken at 20 years of age, after the asymmetry was visually obvious, revealed partial degeneration or reduction in the size of the condyle on one side (Fig. 10). The cause was unknown.

DISCUSSION

It should be emphasized that asymmetrical growth of the mandible should be recognized as early in life as possible, so that procedures can be instituted to control mandibular development. If permitted to develop to late teenage years, greater mandibular asymmetry will be evident. At present, more mandibular asymmetry is being noted in young children, either because of improved diagnosis or because the condition may be more common now. One of the major problems associated with mandibular asymmetry is concomitant malrelationship in vertical development of the

236   Subtelny

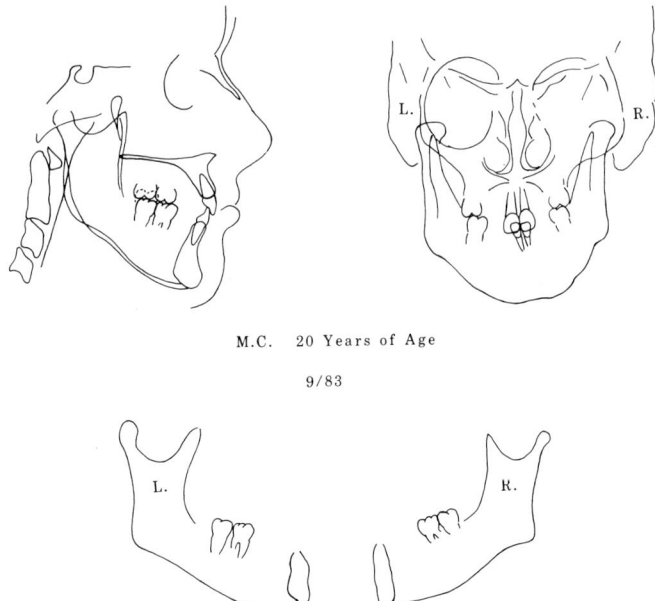

Fig. 10. Tracings of cephalometric radiographs taken at 20 years of age of the individual illustrated in Figure 9. Mandibular asymmetry and skeletal and chin deviation are more clearly evident. Differences in the left and right (affected side) condylar regions are observable; the right condylar region appears reduced in dimension.

maxillary and mandibular posterior dento-alveolar process on the affected side. In these instances, it can be noted that the ramus on the affected side has been growing inadequately in vertical dimension when compared to the unaffected side (Fig. 6). This results in reduction of the vertical height of the maxillary and mandibular posterior dento-alveolar processes on the affected side. When the teeth are in occlusion on the affected side, the posterior occlusal plane will be more closely situated to the cranial base than on the unaffected side (Fig. 6). This will be recognized on frontal and lateral cephalograms (Figs. 6,8).

It is our premise that developing mandibular asymmetry should be functionally treated as soon as it is recognized and that the two occlusal levels should be orthodontically treated at as young an age as possible to improve vertical symmetry and to level—as much as possible—the two posterior occlusal planes relative to the cranial base. At present, a unilateral occlusal bite block or a pronounced occlusal wedge is being placed on the unaffected side. This serves to stretch the postural muscles on both the affected and unaffected side, while opening a sizable interocclusal dimension on the affected side. This will permit vertical dento-alveolar growth on the affected side and prevent such occurrence on the unaffected side since, in growing children, the bite block prevents eruption of the buccal teeth [Buck, 1979]. Furthermore, it facilitates vertical development of the dento-alveolar processes via orthodontic influences on the side with an open inter-occlusal space. Subsequent to vertical repositioning of the mandible and vertical development of the two alveolar processes on the affected side, teeth are permitted to erupt into occlusion on the unaffected side by removal of the unilateral bite block.

It should also be noted that what may appear to be mandibular asymmetry may in reality be the result of an asymmetric vertical repositioning of the mandible to achieve full occlusal contact. Overtly, facial appearance may be the same, but the causative mechanism may differ. It may be the result of developing maxillary skeletal asymmetry rather than developing mandibular asymmetry. In these instances, definite asymmetry is noted in the vertical levels of the right and left nasal floor, while right and left oblique radiographs of the mandible may indicate symmetry. Here, treatment is similar; unilateral bite block therapy is instituted in the lower arch and an attempt is made to increase maxillary posterior dento-alveolar height on the affected side with vertical elastic and/or arch wire therapy in an effort to obviate the necessity for the mandible to shift unilaterally into vertical malposition to achieve full occlusal contact. This should be treated orthodontically as early as possible to avoid more severe facial asymmetry and dental malrelations. It should also be recognized that treatment may have to be instituted—off and on—over prolonged periods of time to achieve desirable and acceptable end results in facial symmetry and occlusal relationships.

REFERENCES

Blevins C, Gores RJ: Fractures of the mandibular condyloid process: Results of conservative treatment in 140 patients. J Oral Surg 19:392–407, 1961.

Buck R: A study of the treatment effects of the posterior occlusal bite block. Unpublished Senior Certificate Research Presentation, Department of Orthodontics, Eastman Dental Center, Rochester, New York, 1979.

Harvold EP: Experiments in mandibular morphogenesis. In McNamara JA (ed): "Determinants of Mandibular Form and Growth," Monograph 4. Ann Arbor: University of Michigan Center for Human Growth and Development, 1975, pp 155–178.

Hotz RP: Functional jaw orthopedics in the treatment of condylar fractures. Am J Orthod 73:365–377, 1978.

Moss ML, Saletijn L: The primary role of functional matrices in facial growth. Am J Orthod 56:474–490, 1969.

Robinson IB, Sarnat BG: Growth pattern of the pig mandible. Am J Anat 96:37–64, 1955.

Sarnat BG: Normal and abnormal craniofacial growth; some experimental and clinical considerations. Angle Orthod 53:263–289, 1983.

Walker RV: Traumatic mandibular condylar fracture dislocations: Effect on growth in the Macaca rhesus monkey. Am J Surg 100:850–863, 1960.

V. OTHER CONTRIBUTIONS

Agnathia-Holoprosencephaly: A Developmental Field Complex Involving Face and Brain. Report of 3 Cases

David Bixler, Richard Ward, and David D. Gale

Departments of Oral Facial (D.B., R.W.) and Medical Genetics (D.B., R.W.), Indiana University Schools of Dentistry and Medicine, Indianapolis, and College of Allied Health and Nursing (D.D.G.), Eastern Kentucky University, Richmond, Kentucky

> Agnathia-holoprosencephaly (A-H) is a developmental field complex involving a graded series of defects in the jaws, mouth, tongue, ears, eyes, and brain. Two general groups can be recognized: agnathia with holoprosencephaly (more severe) and agnathia without holoprosencephaly (less severe). This report describes three new cases of agnathia without holoprosencephaly and reviews the recent literature. By combining published cases with those ascertained through a survey of genetic centers in the United States, it appears that there have been at least 24 occurrences of A-H in the past 25 years. An inductive defect of the prechordal mesoderm that also affects neural crest cells is presented as the cause for this developmental field complex. Because of the etiologic heterogeneity associated with developmental field defects, the genetic counselor must provide a wide range of recurrence risks when dealing with the A-H complex.

Key words: Agnathia-holoprosencephaly, developmental field, neural crest, prechordal mesoderm

INTRODUCTION

The rare lethal syndrome of agnathia with microstomia, aglossia, synotia, and brain malformations has been designated by Pauli et al [1983] agnathia-holoprosencephaly (A-H), being a developmental field defect. To date, over 80 cases of agnathia-holoprosencephaly have been reported in the literature dating back into the 1800s [Pauli et al, 1983]. At least two groups of agnathia can be recognized, those which have varying degrees of cyclopia with a holoprosencephalic brain and those which do not. Those cases with holoprosencephaly more often appear to have accompanying developmental abnormalities of other organ systems. However, the data of Wright and Wagner [1934] on the inbred guinea pig shows this to be a continuum of face-brain defects, and Opitz [1980] has reviewed the findings that support A-H's being a developmental field defect.

The purpose of this paper is threefold: to present and discuss three new cases of agnathia in which the brain is either normal or at least there are no cyclopia-like facial malformations; to present the results of a survey of clinical geneticists in the United States regarding recent incidence of this malformation complex; and finally, to

---

Address reprint requests to David Bixler, Department of Oral Facial Genetics, Ball Residence, Rm. 026, 1226 W. Michigan Street, Indianapolis, IN 46223.

© 1985 Alan R. Liss, Inc.

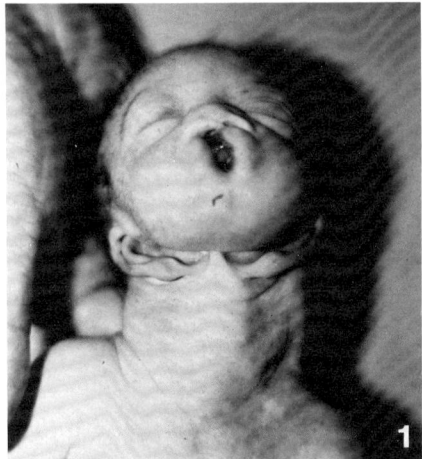 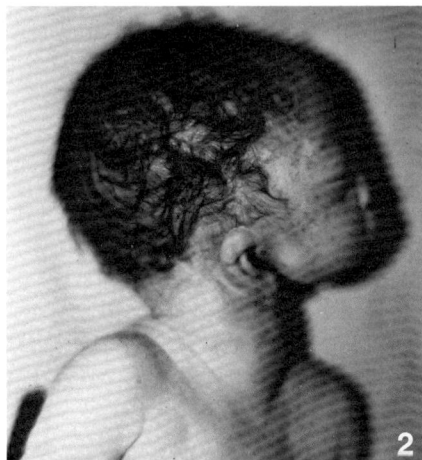

Fig. 1. Front face and neck of case 1, showing absence of mandible, right cleft lip and palate, and synotia.

Fig. 2. Lateral face of case 1.

comment on the developmental embryology and genetics of this unique developmental field defect relating it to the very similar if not identical trait reported in the guinea pig and mouse [Wright and Wagner, 1934; Juriloff et al, 1980].

Case 1

Case 1 was a black female born to a 28-year-old gravida 4, para 3-4 (G4P3-4) mother whose estimated gestational age by sonar was 30 weeks. This mother had previously had three children by the same father. All three were alive, well and without any birth defects. This pregnancy was complicated by alcohol abuse (1 pint of vodka/day early in the pregnancy but reduced to three beers/day near delivery). There was no other history of drug abuse. Labor was spontaneous and delivery was vaginal without problems. Polyhydramnios was diagnosed by ultrasound just prior to delivery. Severe congenital anomalies of the ears, nose, mouth, and throat were noted immediately, and attempts to establish an airway by oronasal intubation were unsuccessful. Repiratory efforts were vigorous for a few seconds but quickly ceased. A bag and mask were used over the face but no air movement was heard in the lungs. The infant was pronounced dead after 30 minutes and permission for postmortem examination was denied.

This was an essentially normal-appearing, deceased newborn with the notable exception of major malformations of the face. Length was 42 cm (75th %tile for a 30-week gestation), occipital-frontal circumference (OFC) 25 cm (below 3rd %tile for 30-week gestation), and weight 1.25 kg (<25th %tile for a 30-week gestation). The anterior fontanel, skull bones, and scalp hair pattern were normal. The face showed down-slanting palpebral fissures with normal-sized eyes (Fig. 1). There was epicanthus inversus of both eyelids. The palpebral fissures measured 1.3 cm on both sides (normal for a 30-week gestation). The canthal index was .38 (borderline for primary telecanthus). There was a hypoplastic nose and a right cleft lip that distorted the nares. Severe microstomia was present and the lip cleft extended in a U-shaped fashion from the midline of the mouth up into the nose. There was no palpable

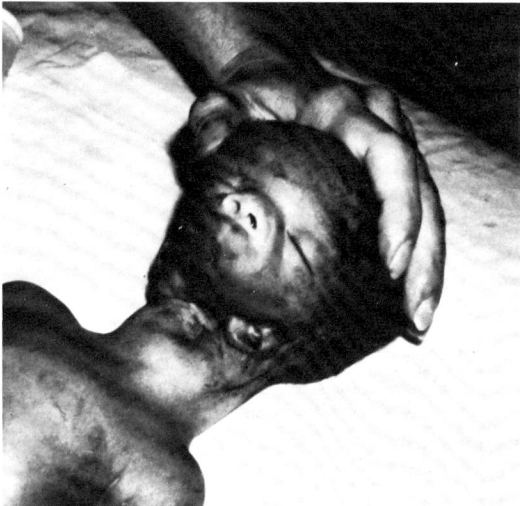

Fig. 3. Front face of case 2, showing synotia, microstomia, and down-slanting palpebral fissures.

mandible. Intraoral examination revealed a cleft palate and an absent tongue. The ears were so low-set on the face that they met in the midline beneath the maxilla. Two openings present in the midline of the neck probably represented the external auditory meati. The pinnae of both ears were well formed (Fig. 2) with the exception of the tragus. The right ear measured 3.5 cm, but the left ear measured 4.0 cm (at or above the 25th %tile for a 36-week gestation).

The neck was broad at the base and slightly webbed. Cervical vertebrae were palpably normal, and the joints of the extremities were lax but within normal limits. No abnormalities of the chest were noted, and prior to expiring the infant was reported to have a regular heart rate and rhythm. The abdomen was soft without masses, and the genitalia were those of a premature female infant. The extremities appeared somewhat long in proportion to the trunk, but no gross abnormalities were noted. Examination of the placenta showed three vessels in the cord. A banded karyotype gave a normal, 46,XX chromosome constitution.

Case 2

Case 2 was a premature black male infant whose gestational age was estimated at 28 weeks. This was the first pregnancy for this 19-year-old mother. The pregnancy was uncomplicated except for premature rupture of the membranes 48 hours prior to delivery. At delivery the baby was noted to have extensive malformations of the face. Apgar scores of 1 and 1 were recorded at 1 and 5 minutes and no access to an airway could be obtained. The baby lived approximately 1 hour before expiring. At the time of postmortem examination the weight was 1.2 kg, length 38 cm, and OFC 28 cm (all values at or above 50th %tile for a 28-week gestation). The head was normocephalic and covered with black curly hair. The eyes appeared to be normally formed but had cloudy corneas. The nose had nares that ended blindly consistent with a choanal atresia. The mouth had a very small opening (microstomia), which ended blindly against the maxillary bone (Fig. 3). The mandible was absent and the ears located below the maxilla. External auditory meati could not be probed in either ear. The neck had excessive skinfolds anteriorly. The chest and abdomen were grossly normal. The umbilical cord had three vessels. Extremities were thin but normal, although the nails were poorly developed. Genitalia were appropriate for a premature male and showed undescended testes. There was a small pigmented dimple on the lower sacrum.

At autopsy, dissection of the neck revealed a dilated pharynx leading into a normal-sized esophagus. The epiglottis, trachea, and esophagus were normal in relation to the pharynx. All internal organs appeared to have normal development and positioning. The brain weighed 180 g and had congested meninges, but the hemispheres were symmetrical, normally formed and had convolutions consistent with those of a premature infant. Serial sections through the cerebrum and cerebellum revealed congestion but no apparent congenital anomalies. Histologic sections of tissue from the pharynx failed to reveal remnants of tongue or tonsils. Banded chromosome studies showed a normal 46,XY karyotype.

Case 3

Case 3 was a 5-week-old white male infant, the product of a 29-week gestation, born to a 32-year-old G2P1-2 mother. Vaginal bleeding was present on and off during the last 6 weeks of the pregnancy, but there was no fever. Fetal monitoring at that time was normal. Delivery was vaginal and Apgar scores of 5 and 5 were recorded at 1 and 5 minutes, respectively. Because of marked microstomia, a nasotracheal tube was blindly inserted, and the baby was oxygenated through that tube. Respiratory distress continued and a tracheostomy was performed. Throughout these few weeks of life the medical course was stormy and a grade 2-3/6 cardiac murmur compatible with a patent ductus arteriosus was audible. The baby died of acute respiratory distress and compromised pulmonary function at 5 weeks of age, and an autopsy was performed.

At the postmortem examination, this infant had a weight of 2.95 kg, length of 44 cm, and OFC of 30 cm (all above the 25th %tile for a 35-week-old infant). The head was normocephalic and the hair thin and brown. The eyes were normal in size and position (Fig. 4). A very small mouth opening measuring .7 cm in diameter was present. Intraorally, a small tongue could be identified and the palate was intact. The mandible was extremely small but palpably present. The ears were slightly low-set, dysplastic, and markedly cupped with shortened anterior-posterior dimensions (Fig. 5). However, their length appeared normal. External meati were present bilaterally. The abdomen was soft, not distended, and without masses. The left testis was descended but the right was not palpable. No abnormalities of the back or spine were seen. Extremities were normal. The heart had a patent foramen ovale, ventricular septal defect, pulmonary stenosis, and a patent ductus arteriosus. Hypoplasia of the right ventricle was also noted. A small mucosal defect was present in the esophagus 1.5 cm from the proximal end of the trachea but no tracheo-esophageal (TE) fistula was demonstrated. All the internal organs were normal in their appearance and position. Bones of the middle ear were examined (malleus, incus, and stapes) and found to be well formed. The very small mandible and small tongue were confirmed at this time. The brain showed minimal myelination and was too soft to be examined without fixation. After fixing, brain sections revealed no abnormalities within the cerebral hemispheres, and the ventricles were normal but dilated. The cerebellum was also normal to examination.

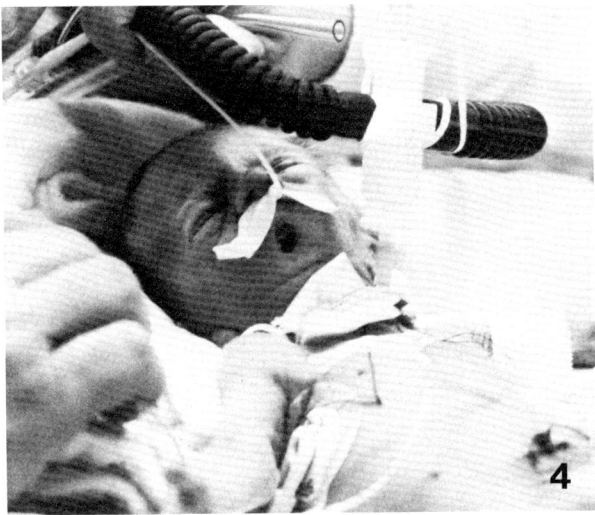

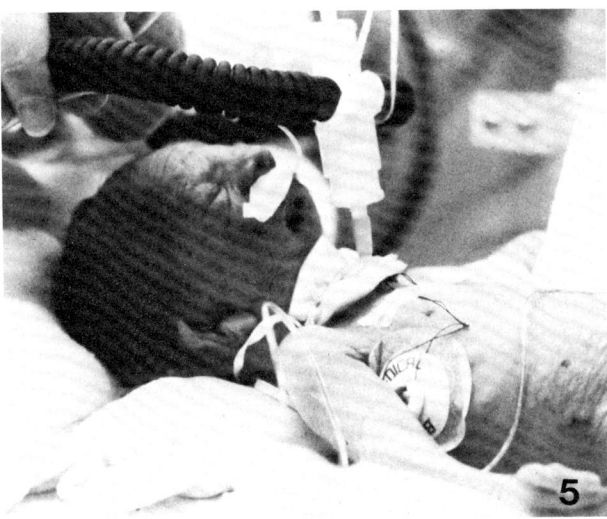

Fig. 4. Face of case 3, aged 2 weeks, showing tracheostomy tube in place, small mandible with microstomic mouth.

Fig. 5. Lateral face showing small mandible and dysmorphic ear.

DISCUSSION

Table I is a summary of the physical findings in published cases of agnathia without holoprosencephaly since 1961. Included in this table are the three cases reported here. Four of the 13 cases are known to be black and the male to female sex ratio was 1:1. All of these infants represented premature births with gestational ages under 36 weeks with one exception; birth weights were below the 10th %tile for gestational age in at least 7 of the 13 cases. Polyhydramnios was a common finding that is expected if there is persistence of the oropharyngeal membrane. Such an airway blockage would not permit circulation of amniotic fluid and lead to its

TABLE I. Published Cases of Agnathia Without Holoprosencephaly Since 1961

Traits	Case I	Case II	Case III	(1)	(2)	(3)	(4)	(5)	(6)	(7)	(8)	(9)	(10)
Race	B	B	W	B	B	?	W	W	?	?	W	W	?
Sex	F	M	M	F	?	M	F	F	F	F	F	M	M
Gestational age (weeks)	30	28	29	34	36	34	34	32	24	34	34	40	36
Birth weight[2]	−	−	−	+	+	?	+	+	?	+	−	+	+
Polyhydramnios	+	?	−	+	+	?	+	+	+	+	+	+	+
Agnathia	+	+	−	+	+	+	+	+	+	+	+	+	+
Microstomia	+	+	+	+	+	+	+	+	+	+	+	+	+
Aglossia	+	+	−	+	+	+	+	+	+	?	?	?	+
Blind mouth	+	+	−	+	+	+	+	+	+	?	+	+	?
Ear position[3]	b	b	a	b	a	b	b	c	c	c	b	c	b
Middle ear anomalies	?	?	−	?	+	+	?	+	+	?	?	?	?
Cleft lip, cleft palate	CL	−	−	CP	CP	CP	−	−	CP	?	?	?	?
Down-slanting palpebral fissures	!	+	+	+	+	+	+	+	+	?	+	+	+

[1](1) Black et al, 1973; (2) Johnson and Cook, 1961; (3) Lawrence and Bersu, 1982, (4) Leckie, 1975; (5) Le Marec et al, 1976; (6) Libersa and Heritier, 1974; (7) Scholl, 1977; (8) Ursell, 1972; (9) Van de Sande, 1966; (10) Woon and Tan, 1979.
[2]⩽ 10th %tile for gestational age [standards from Freeman et al, 1970].
[3]a, Low-set but not fused; b, approach midline but are not fused; c, fused.

accumulation with time. The clinical diagnosis of a blind-ending mouth also supports the persistence of an oropharyngeal membrane. Thus, the often described inability to pass an oral-pharyngeal tube to establish an airway confirms the presence of this anatomic defect. Agnathia, microstomia, and aglossia, common features of this syndrome, were present in almost every case. Even though this developmental field complex has been termed otocephaly by many authors, ear position in these 13 cases was variable. In two instances the ears were low-set but not closely approximated. In the 11 remaining cases, there were 7 instances in which the ears were low-set and approached each other in the midline but were not fused. Only four cases reported the ears to be fused in the midline. The frequency of middle ear anomalies was impossible to determine since most reports did not include autopsy or x-ray data. However, in only one of the five cases with middle ear examination (our case 3) were no middle ear bone anomalies found. Finally, involvement of the maxilla in this developmental field complex is apparent from the last two listed categories of defects, cleft lip and palate and down-slanting palpebral fissures, the latter occasionally accompanied by an author's comment on hypoplasia of the zygoma.

These new cases stimulated our interest in the frequency of this condition in the United States. To obtain an estimate of this frequency we sent out a questionnaire to 32 of the major genetic centers in the United States. Essentially all replies were negative for cases of the agnathia-holoprosencephaly series in the memory of the respondent with the following exceptions. Dr. John Optiz recalled a probable case of agnathia without holoprosencephaly seen in 1981 in Madison, Wisconsin. He also recalled a case of agnathia with holoprosencephaly born in 1981 to a couple from Idaho that he counseled. Dr. Cynthia Currie of Fresno, California made known to us a case of agnathia in a Mexican infant. This case was unusual in that it also had a frontal encephalocele and hydranencephaly. Thus, there was insufficient brain to diagnose a holospheric state. Dr. John Graham commented on two cases known to him in Seattle. One of these was reported by Pauli et al [1981] and the other case was reported by Jones et al [1980]. Finally, case 3 of this report was ascertained by Dr.

Wayne Finley at the University of Alabama. In summary, this survey revealed six cases—one reported here, two already in the literature, and another (Opitz's case 1) that is probably one of the two stillborn sisters reported by Pauli et al [1983]. Thus, this survey found only two unreported cases in the United States in recent years. A rough estimate of the A-H cases occurring in world literature in the last 25 years then is 24: the 13 cases reviewed here plus the 2 sisters reported by Pauli et al [1981], which represent agnathia without holoprosencephaly, and 9 cases of agnathia with holoprosencephaly [Blanc, 1980; Gaba et al, 1982; Mollica et al, 1979; Pauli et al, 1983; Jones et al, 1980; Usandizasa, 1966]; in addition there are the 2 as yet apparently unreported cases of Winter and Opitz. Thus, with an average of less than one case reported per year, the rarity of this syndrome is confirmed.

In spite of its infrequent occurrence in humans, A-H is a well-recognized malformation complex that has been reported in the mouse [Juriloff et al, 1980], guinea pig [Wright and Wagner, 1934], rabbit [Faller and Rossier, 1969], sheep [Willson, 1966], and pig [Malynicz, 1982]. The experimental work of Wright and Wagner [1934] with an inbred strain of guinea pigs is noteworthy because the anatomic sequence they described resembles that reported in man. They defined 12 grades of severity based on anatomical structures involved. The first four grades (which they called otocephaly) encompass the new cases reported in this paper (Table I). Their series ranged from specimens with partial mandibles to complete agnathia, from hypoplastic to missing tongue, and with variable malformation of middle ear and palatine bones. In all of these cases (as in our own) the brain appeared to be normal, and middle face involvement was moderate. Grades 5–12 in this series were characterized by increasing severity of malformation of the middle face and brain. Human cases of agnathia with holoprosencephaly can also be placed in such a spectrum ranging from the minimally affected case reported by Pauli et al [1981] to the extreme, cyclopic form reported by Mollica et al [1979]. Interestingly, with the exception of the two affected sibs reported by Pauli et al [1983], all human cases of A-H have been sporadic. However, data from the guinea pig [Wright and Wagner, 1934] and mouse [Juriloff et al, 1980] support the existence of an inherited type.

Some authors have viewed agnathia (otocephaly) and agnathia with holoprosencephaly (cyclocephaly) as distinct entities. Justification for this dichotomy would seem to stem from their apparently different etiologies. Thus, the primary defect producing a holoprosencephalic brain is probably related to a failure of induction of neural tube by prechordal mesoderm [Johnston and Sulik, 1979; Cohen et al, 1971]. This implies that gastrulation movements leading to formation of anterior mesoderm are inadequate to induce anterior neural plate formation. Agnathia, on the other hand, is viewed as a defect in the ventral portion of the first branchial arch secondary to defective neural crest migration or proliferation [Wright and Wagner, 1934; Johnston and Sulik, 1979]. This would explain the mandibular defect (hypoplasia to agnathia) and also account for maxillary defects (zygomatic insufficiency, down-slanting palpebral fissures, and cleft lip and palate). Persistence of the oropharyngeal membrane often present is probably a secondary effect since experiments with amphibian neurula show that an intimate interaction between pharyngeal endoderm and future mouth ectoderm is necessary to initiate membrane rupture [Arey, 1965]. This essential future mouth endoderm is largely of first branchial arch origin; endoderm transplanted from a mid-trunk level does not have this inducing capacity.

Since A-H is a developmental field defect, an amalgamation of these two developmental mechanisms is called for. A neural crest cell problem can account for the features seen in agnathia without holoprosencephaly but does not account for the conjoint appearance of these two entities. Considering only the agnathia portion of this series, the mildest defect resides in the ventral mandibular arch and ranges all the way from mandibular hypoplasia to agnathia, which involves maxilla and even parts of the second branchial arch. Those structures affected in the mild cases come from neural crest cell migrations of the greatest distance [Johnston and Sulik, 1979] and are structures most likely to be affected by an anterior neural crest cell deficit. Thus, the A-H complex involves a graded series of defects ranging from a deficiency in neural crest cell formation, migration, or proliferation at one end of the spectrum to a failure in prosencephalon formation at the other end of the spectrum. The uniting concept seems to us to be a prechordal mesoderm inductive defect. There is evidence [Arey, 1965; Sperber, 1981] that the same neuralizing inductive influence of prechordal mesoderm on neural tube formation is also utilized in the formation of cranial neural crest cells. The gradient of severity in the A-H developmental field could be explained by variable loss of inductive effect by the prechordal mesoderm ranging from a loss sufficient to minimally reduce anterior neural crest cell formation to a loss severe enough to drastically reduce neural crest cell formation and also to produce the neural tube defect, holoprosencephaly with its associated facial defects. Such an induction defect may even be able to account for the failure to form normal midline structures as reported in the cases of agnathia with situs inversus by Pauli et al [1981].

In conclusion, the A-H complex is best viewed as a developmental field defect. Opitz [1982] defines developmental fields as those parts of the embryo in which the "process of development of complex structures appropriate to those parts are controlled and coordinated in a spatially ordered, temporally synchronized and epimorphically hierarchical manner." In other words, a developmental field consists of a group of embryonic structures that respond as a single developmental unit. In this situation one anticipates that different etiologic agents acting on the same developmental field will produce a highly similar complex of malformations. Opitz [1980] noted that, as expected in developmental field defects, A-H occurs in a variety of species and shows causal heterogeneity. Thus the clinician is faced with the reality that genetic counseling for such developmental field defects must be flexible in order to encompass the range of sporadic and genetic causation.

ACKNOWLEDGMENTS

The authors greatly appreciate the efforts of Dr. Wayne Finley, Laboratory of Medical Genetics, University of Alabama, in supplying the information about case 2. We are also indebted to all those individuals who took the time to reply to our questionnaire on cases of agnathia-holoprosencephaly. This work was supported in part by the Oral Facial Genetics Training Grant DE 7043.

REFERENCES

Arey LB: "Developmental Anatomy," 7th ed., Philadelphia: W.B. Saunders Co., 1965.
Black FO, Myers EN, Rorke LB: Aplasia of the first and second branchial arches. Arch Otolaryngol 98:124–128, 1973.
Blanc L: Sur l'otocephalie et la cyclotie. J Anat Physiol 31:187–309, 1980.
Cohen MM, Jirasek JE, Guzman RT, Gorlin RJ, Peterson MQ: Holoprosencephaly and facial dysmorphia: Nosology, etiology and pathogenesis. Birth Defects: OAS VII(7): 125–135, 1971.

Faller A, Rossier B: Reconstruction of brain and ventricle system in an anchyote prosophthalmic otocephalic newborn cephalothoracopagus rabbit. Acta Anat 73:2–31, 1969.

Freeman MG, Graves WL, Thompson RL: Indigent Negro and Caucasian birth-weight gestational age tables. Pediatrics 46:9–15, 1970.

Gaba AR, Andersen GJ, VanDyke DL, Chason JL: Alobar holoprosencephaly and otocephaly in a female infant with a normal karyotype and placental villitis. J Med Genet 19:78, 1982.

Johnson WW, Cook JB: Agnathia associated with pharyngeal isthmus atresia and hydramnios. Arch Pediatr 78:211–217, 1961.

Johnston MC, Sulik KK: Some abnormal patterns of development in the craniofacial region. Birth Defects:OAS XV(8) :23–42, 1979.

Jones KL, Higginbottom MC, Smith DW: Determining role of the optic vesicle in orbital and periocular development and placement. Pediatr Res 14:703–708, 1980.

Juriloff DM, Sulik KK, Roderick TH, Hogan BK: Morphogenesis of spontaneously occurring otocephaly in a newly developed mouse mutant. Teratology 21:47A–48A, 1980.

Lawrence DK, Bersu ET: An anatomical study of otocephalic malformation. Teratology 25:58A, 1982.

Leckie GB: Aplasia of the first and second branchial arches. J Laryngol Otol 89:1263–1269, 1975.

Le Marec B, Bourdiniere J, de Clech G, de Freche JN, de Villartays A: A case of otocephaly. J Genet Hum 24(Suppl): 253–260, 1976.

Libersa JC, Heritier M: Orofacial anomalies in an otocephalic fetus. Rev Stomatodontal Nord Fr 29:101–105, 1974.

Malynicz GL: Complete polydactylism in Papua New Guinea village pig with otocephalic homozygous monsters. Ann Genet Sel Anim 14:415–420, 1982.

Mollica F, Pavone L, Nuciforo G, Sorge G: A case of cyclopia: Role of environmental factors. Clin Genet 16:69–71, 1979.

Opitz JM: Letter to the editor. Clin Genet 17:238, 1980.

Opitz JM: The developmental field concept in clinical genetics. J Pediatr 101:805–809, 1982.

Pauli RM, Graham JR, Barr M Jr: Agnathia, situs inversus and associated malformations. Teratology 23:85–93, 1981.

Pauli RM, Pettersen JC, Arya S, Gilbert EF: Familial agnathia-holoprosencephaly. Am J Med Genet 14:677–698, 1983.

Scholl HW: In utero diagnosis of agnathia, microstomia and synotia. Obstet Gynecol 49(Suppl 1):815–835, 1977.

Sperber GH: "Craniofacial Embryology," 3rd ed. Boston: Wright PSG, 1981.

Ursell W: Hydramnios associated with congenital microstomia agnathia and synotia. J Obstet Gynaec Br Commw 79:185–186, 1972.

Usandizasa JA: An unusual case of otocephalic cyclopic fetus of 7 months. Acta Gynaecol Obstet Hisp Lusit 15:18–28, 1966.

Van de Sande PL: A case of otocephalus. Ned Tijdschr Verloskel Gynaecol 66:471–474, 1966.

Willson JE: Congenital otocephalus in a lamb. Vet Med Small Anim Clin 61:58–59, 1966.

Woon KY, Tan KL: Aplasia of the first and second branchial arches. Aust Paediatr J 15:275–277, 1979.

Wright S, Wagner K: Types of subnormal development of the head from inbred strains of guinea pigs and their bearing on the classification and interpretation of vertebrate monsters. Am J Anat 54:383–448, 1934.

A Computerized Multi-Use Craniofacial Patient Record

Carla A. Evans and Richard L. Christiansen
Craniofacial Program, Children's Hospital, Boston, (C.A.E.), and School of Dentistry, University of Michigan, Ann Arbor, (R.L.C.)

A computerized craniofacial patient record reinforces the link between clinical research and the treatment process. The availability of microcomputers and appropriate software has made it feasible for most craniofacial groups to organize patient data for easy retrieval and analysis. Selection of the computer system and programs follows careful planning and systematic delineation of the desired functions of the system. An example of a working computerized craniofacial patient record system is described.

Key words: craniofacial anomalies, computerized patient records, classification system

INTRODUCTION

The increasing pace of innovation in the craniofacial anomalies field and the corresponding evolution of highly specialized craniofacial anomalies treatment centers has accentuated the importance of useful and accessible patient records. How patient information is acquired, organized, and stored directly influences the quality and success of clinical research efforts, as well as the delivery of clinical treatment. The formal linking of clinical research with the treatment process via the patient record is critical to ensuring a strong research component in the treatment center. The research/treatment connection is especially important in the realm of craniofacial anomalies because of the many unresolved problems in elucidating etiology, naming and classifying anomalies, and developing effective treatment measures [Christiansen and Evans, 1975, 1979]. An example of a computerized, multi-use patient record system and a description of its evolution follows in this paper.

Key to the whole issue of organizing craniofacial patient records for clinical research purposes is the need to simplify and standardize "core" patient records for efficient information retrieval by various members of the craniofacial team. The "core" record parallels the concept of a multi-disciplinary craniofacial clinic and its many advantages. The burden of maintaining a computerized record base for general craniofacial clinic use would be too great for any one discipline to assume but instead should be integrated into the clinic structure. A suitable "core" record should be used

---

Address reprint requests to Dr. Carla A. Evans, Craniofacial Program, Children's Hospital, 300 Longwood Ave., Boston, MA 02115.

© 1985 Alan R. Liss, Inc.

both for clinic management and promotion of clinical research, thus reducing the duplication of energy and cost inherent in maintaining a variety of separate records.

Cost is a very important aspect of developing the multi-use patient record. Since most centers or clinics are highly dependent on patient-derived revenue, the multi-use record should be similarly supported. Existence of the multi-use record should not depend on the cyclical nature of external funding. The focus on cost will also limit data collection to those items truly necessary for achieving practical goals. Computerization is an essential step in using available resources to maximize the research potential of every craniofacial program and to maintaining the effort through all funding situations. The impact of productivity, low cost, and widespread availability of microcomputer systems makes the office-based computerized patient record achievable now for most craniofacial groups.

The craniofacial team at Children's Hospital in Boston, Massachusetts, follows approximately 800 patients designated as craniofacial patients, as distinguished from cleft lip/palate or orthognathic patients. The craniofacial deformities include congenital anomalies and defects resulting from trauma or disease. The number of patients has increased markedly over the last 10 years and the manila-folder approach to recordkeeping became inadequate for coordinating the large number of complex patients with the multitude of clinicians involved. To develop more effective communication and increase efficiency, the patient record has been reorganized and partially computerized within a computerized office framework.

The hardcopy craniofacial records are stored in the craniofacial office where the craniofacial coordinator organizes the clinics, schedules appointments and operations, handles correspondence, and maintains the records. Each individual record is kept in a looseleaf notebook with a clear pocket on the front cover for a computer-printout summary insert so the record need not be opened to check identifying information, diagnoses, or dates of operations. All those items are shown on the cover. The first inside page contains the mailing list of people who need to be informed about the patient's progress, eg, referring pediatrician, local orthodontist, etc. The record itself is organized into five sections. Section 1 contains the dictated notes from craniofacial clinics and patient reviews. Section 2 has all operative sketches and dictated operative summaries. Section 3 contains the result of tests and evaluations such as those done by the psychologist, hearing and speech specialists, radiologist, etc. Section 4 contains correspondence, and section 5 has financial information. Stored within a spun-bonded olefin envelope at the back of the hardcopy records are the photographs and cephalometric and panoramic radiographs. Dental casts are kept nearby and hospital radiographs are stored in the radiology department. While the hardcopy record format provides a good way to review the status of individual patients very quickly, it does not lend itself to efficient retrieval of information; hence the need for computerization.

Design of the computerized record takes considerable planning since it is difficult to change computer software once a protocol is established. Most first attempts at computerized records seek to record everything and are too global in scope. Any data collection process not oriented toward an immediate useful goal will soon be dropped. The effort must be limited because it is impossible to record everything or study all problems. Similarly, computerization of raw data such as radiographic information must be carefully considered. The Boston craniofacial team decided against trying to digitize radiographs routinely, not just because some landmarks are missing and others must be invented for these dysmorphic patients, but because one cannot determine prior to doing a study which measurements are needed. It is more important to control the quality and frequency of radiographs and analyze them later in relation to very specific guidelines developed to answer particular questions. Maximum gain relative to effort will be realized if the quality of raw data such as radiographs, photographs, and dental casts is monitored closely and if the data to be analyzed are selected objectively.

Several features were specified for the computer system. First, the system must be physically located for easy access to the users and must be sufficienty simple that the user does not need a technician or secretary to access the program. Second, costs must be controllable. In the initial trial of a computer system, a terminal was used to reach a mainframe computer on a time-sharing basis. Recurring expenses were too high, programming problems occurred continually, access was limited, and long-term use was not practical. The microcomputer has startup costs but minimal expenses afterward. Third, the software package(s) must have several capabilities.

The most important software capability is database management. In order to update the patient record summary sheet and retrieve lists of patients by complex searching and sorting criteria, it is necessary to select a maximum-flexibility database management program. Also, a full-performance word processing program that accesses record files in the database program is needed for correspondence and preparation of manuscripts. Other desirable programs for the efficient operation of a craniofacial program office are a spreadsheet program for scheduling and business management, communications software for accessing other computers, pedigree drawing programs, and digitizing programs. If possible, the software package should be available commercially to increase reliability and interchangeability and to lower costs by eliminating or reducing the need for a programmer. A commercial package that can be customized by a programmer for special applications is most useful, however. Programs are now available that have these features and are sufficiently powerful for fast retrieval of craniofacial patient information.

A classification scheme for use with treatment-oriented craniofacial records could be based on a variety of characteristics such as etiology, morphology, timing of initiation of defect, biochemical markers, or chromosomal aberrations. A morphological classification based on visually detected physical characteristics is the most useful for several reasons:

1. All patients in a craniofacial program will be included. None will fall outside the limits of the classification because they all have anatomic craniofacial defects.
2. The classification doesn't require special tests to include patients who are seen briefly.
3. Many of the patients have no specific diagnosis—that is, specific syndrome or disease identification—or the diagnosis may be provisional or inaccurate. Also, today's diagnosis may change as subgroups are found or as more is known about etiology.
4. The system has enough flexibility to retrieve patients with multiple diagnoses.
5. Many craniofacial problems are a spectrum of defects. For example, there is considerable overlap in morphology in the craniofaciosynostosis syndromes. Using specific syndrome labels, one will probably not be able to find all cases of acrocephalosyndactyly, and the labels actually used may place artificial barriers in undertaking many types of growth and treatment studies.
6. The system is simple and easy to use. Broad categories of clinical dysmorphology are understandable by support staff as well as professionals.

Too rigid a classification will not work because changing the classification and coding sytem is difficult. Moreover, many patients seen at a craniofacial treatment center are undiagnosed, that is, not given a syndrome or disease label. A system of diagnoses such as the March of Dimes Birth Defects Information System (BDIS) diagnoses is too specific to be the primary classification in a treatment center. If a patient is classified inappropriately, information about that patient cannot be retrieved. Using a classification based on dysmorphology, one could go to a broader category of abnormality.

Organizing the database and selecting the software package are interrelated activities. Decisions regarding the type and extent of data to be collected are made first, but modifications may be necessary if the computer software does not permit all of the desired database applications. It is also necessary to have a well-defined application in mind when judging whether commercially available computer programs or custom programming is more satisfactory for the tasks.

Elements of data to be entered in a database management program, such as the patient's name and telephone number, are called fields. A major limitation of many commercial database programs for microcomputers is that the number of fields and the characters per field are too low. Also, the number of permissible patient records may be smaller than the number of records to be stored. Consequently, when evaluating potential database management programs, one should know roughly the number of required fields, the number of patient records, and the types of desired sorting and searching applications. Speed and flexibility are also desirable attributes of a useful database management program.

A description of the Boston system may be helpful. Several types of data are collected and entered into the computer: (1) identifying and demographic information such as name, hospital identification number, addresses, sex, and date of birth; (2) classification categories by craniofacial dysmorphology (Table I); (3) referral source and people requiring patient progress notes; (4) dates and names of operations; and (5) BDIS diagnosis and BDIS defect codes. Thus, each individual patient record is quite large and requires many fields. The tasks demanded of the computer program are also complex. In addition to preparing custom reports such as the facesheet for the hardcopy patient record and mailing lists, one can also match; search; order; sort; and exclude records by fields, fragments of fields, combinations of fields, or numeric relationships. The reports obtained are easily transferred into the word-processing program for inclusion into letters or manuscripts.

Choice of the computer system depends primarily on the applications desired by the craniofacial center. For the requirements described above, the Boston craniofacial program utilizes the following setup very successfully. The Boston system is described as an example of a feasible method for those who are not aware of the potential of the most recent database programs written for microcomputers, but other groups may find different systems more suitable to their needs. The IBM-XT microcomputer with 256K and hard disk provides sufficient storage and accessible memory for the database. The software package chosen for the craniofacial applications, MMSForth, was developed by Miller Microcomputer Services, and consists of a word-processing program (Forthwrite), a database management program (Datahandler-Plus), a spreadsheet program (General Ledger), and communications capabilities (Forthcom).[1] All of the programs are written in Forth, a popular interactive structured

---

[1]The MMSForth software system (1984) was developed and is available from Miller Microcomputer Services, 61 Lake Shore Road, Natick, MA 01760.

TABLE I. Classification Categories—Craniofacial Patients[1]

Congenital—Developmental Deformities
  Cranial deformity
    Craniofacial dysostosis
      Craniosynostosos alone (skull)
        1. Scaphocephaly
        2. Oxycephaly or turricephaly
        3. Plagiocephaly
        4. Trigonocephaly
        5. Other craniosynostosis
      Craniofaciosynostosis (skull and face)
        1. Crouzon syndrome
        2. Other craniofaciosynostosis
      Craniofaciosynostosis + extremity anomalies
        1. Apert syndrome
        2. Other craniofaciosynostosis +
          Extremity anomalies (eg, Pfeiffer,
          Carpenter, Saethre-Chotzen, etc.)
    Other cranial deformity
  Orbital Deformity
    Abnormality of inter-orbital distance
      Hypertelorism
        1. Encephalocele
        2. Median facial dysraphia
        3. Other hypertelorism
      Pseudohypertelorism (Telecanthus)
      Hypotelorism
    Abnormality in size shape of orbit(s)
    Abnormality of eyelid(s)
    Abnormality of eye(s)
  Midface and lower face deformity
    Nasal deformity
    Midface hypoplasia (without cranial deformity)
      Midface hypoplasia secondary to cleft lip/palate
      Midface hypoplasia—idiopathic
      Midface hypoplasia—other (eg, with
        nasal deformity, choanal atresia or obstruction)
    Mandibulofacial dysostosis (Treacher Collins syndrome)
    Facial microsomia (1st–2nd branchial arch syndrome)
      Isolated microtia
      Jaw + ear deformity (hemifacial microsomia)
      Jaw + ear + eye (epibulbar dermoids) + vertebral
      anomaly (Goldenhar syndrome)
    Facial cleft
      Cleft lip/palate
      Rare facial cleft
    Maxillary deformity
      Sagittal
        1. Maxillary protrusion
        2. Maxillary retrusion

(Continued)

TABLE I. Classification Categories—Craniofacial Patients[1] (continued)

    Vertical
      1. Maxillary vertical excess
      2. Maxillary vertical deficiency
    Frontal
      1. Maxillary width abnormality
      2. Maxillary asymmetry
    Dento-alveolar malformation (maxilla)

Mandibular Deformity
  Sagittal
    1. Mandibular prognathism
    2. Mandibular retrognathism
  Vertical
  Frontal
    1. Mandibular width abnormality
    2. Mandibular asymmetry
  Dento-alveolar malformation (mandibular)
  Chin deformity
    1. Macrogenia
    2. Microgenia
  Temporomandibular joint
    1. Ankylosis
      Fibrous
      Bony
    2. Trismus
    3. Other TMJ[2]

Occlusal abnormality
  Class I malocclusion
  Class II malocclusion
  Class III malocclusion
  Anterior open bite
  Crossbite (buccoversion, linguoversion)
  Deep bite

Abnormality of teeth
  Hypodontia
  Anodontia
  Supernumerary teeth
  Abnormal eruption of teeth
  Abnormal quality of teeth

Facial atrophy
  Romberg disease
  Lipodystrophy
  Other

Vascular lesion
  A-V-L malformation
  Hemangioma

Miscellaneous
  Facial Palsy
  Neurofibromatosis
  Encephalocele without hypertelorism
  Macroglossia
  Uncategorized asymmetry (cranial and/or facial)
  Other facial deformity (eg, orofacial digital syndrome)

(Continued)

TABLE I. Classification Categories—Craniofacial Patients[1] (continued)

Acquired Deformities

  Trauma
    Postcranial (skull) trauma deformity
    Postorbital trauma
    Postnasal trauma
    Postmidface fracture deformity
      Lefort 1
      Lefort 2
      Lefort 3
    Post-zygomatic trauma
    Post-mandibular trauma

  Neoplasm
    Benign neoplasm
    <u>Malignant neoplasm</u>
    <u>Post-radiation defect</u>
    <u>Post-surgery defect</u>

  Facial palsy

  Miscellaneous
    <u>Fibrous Dysplasia</u>
    <u>Infection</u>
    <u>TMJ dysfunction</u>
    <u>TMJ—rheumatoid arthritis</u>
    TMJ—other

[1] The clinical classification of craniofacial anomalies shown was developed by the craniofacial team at Children's Hospital, Boston. While many categories are available as choices when classifying patients by dysmorphic craniofacial features, only those underlined have actually been used for the computerized patient record. This classification serves as a first sort for retrieving patients. If the most specific category does not yield the desired information, a broader category can be used.

[2] Abbreviations used: TMJ, temporomandibular joint; A-V-L, arterial-venous-lymphatic.

language similar in philosophy to PASCAL. It provides its own operating system without DOS and allows the user to change disk format, execution speed, and other parameters, but the files can be read by non-Forth programs. Source code is given so that a programmer can customize individual features. The program can be purchased on an institutional license so that multiple clinicians in multiple offices within the same institution can all use the software package.

The MMSForth database management program will accept 255 fields per file with variable field length up to 255 characters. This is more than sufficient for the craniofacial patient records. The string and value selection mechanisms are very sophisticated and include normal compares and values inside or outside a range. Because the program is memory-based, the speed is very rapid. For example, records in memory can be selected conditionally on any field or fragment thereof with delay time of less than a half-second. Another type of computer program that may be useful to a craniofacial team is a computer-aided design program (such as AUTOCAD).[2] A drafting program helps to prepare family pedigrees that can be revised easily. Such a

---

[2] AUTOCAD (1984) is a product of Autodesk, Inc., 150 Shoreline Highway, Building B, Mill Valley, CA 94941.

program is used with a plotter and accepts input from the computer keyboard, lightpen, or digitizer.

The classification categories shown in Table I are entered directly into the computer. No coding is necessary because the computer matches sequences of letters, numbers, or in this instance, word categories. Consequently, the classification choices must follow Table I exactly without alterations or substitutions. In the database program at Children's Hospital, up to five choices may be entered. For example, a Treacher Collins patient with cleft palate would be classified as (1) mandibulofacial dysostosis and (2) cleft lip/palate. This system works well for general sorting of patients. The database program has also been set up for BDIS diagnoses and defect codes. If a specific diagnosis has been determined by the genetics consultant, a BDIS diagnosis is entered. For many patients, the physical examination has also been coded according to the BDIS method. Thus, very detailed information can be retrieved for some patients. For example, a list can be generated of male Treacher Collins patients who have congenital heart disease and short stature, but not cleft palate. This list can be arranged by year of birth, zip code, or other desired traits. Because of the strong interest in craniofacial abnormalities at Children's Hospital, other defect codes have been introduced for more accurate description of oral, facial, cranial, and radiographic findings. These added codes are distinguishable from the BDIS codes because they all end with an "X." Another advantage of including BDIS defect codes is the added ability to communicate with other craniofacial centers and genetics groups using common terminology and codes.

Computerized patient records will aid in organizing the documentation and follow-up needed to answer recurring questions about timing, sequence, and efficacy of various treatment regimens; diagnosis, inheritance patterns, and risk factors; and opportunities for laboratory research. They will also benefit current treatment if clinicians are more aware of the patients' problems and progress.

ACKNOWLEDGMENTS

Portions of the recordkeeping system described in this paper result directly from the insights and efforts of Drs. Joseph E. Murray, Park S. Gerald, Leonard B. Kaban, and John B. Mulliken of the Children's Hospital, Boston, Massachusetts. Their patients will continue to benefit from their commitment to developing new and improved treatment methods.

REFERENCES

Christiansen RL, Evans CA: Habilitation of severe craniofacial anomalies—The challenge of new surgical procedures: An NIDR workshop. Cleft Palate J 12:167–176, 1975.

Christiansen RL, Evans CA: Nomenclature and classification of craniofacial anomalies. In Kopel H (ed): "Teaching of Human Genetics in Dental Education." Los Angeles: Dental Concepts, 1979, pp 77–82.

March of Dimes/Birth Defects Founation Center for Birth Defects Information Services: "The Computerized Birth Defects Information System." Center for Birth Defects Information Services, Box 403, 171 Harrison Avenue, Boston, MA 02111, Techical Guide, 1982.

Evaluation of Chromosomal Damage in Males Exposed to Agent Orange and Their Families

Celia I. Kaye, Sita Rao, Stacy J. Simpson, Flori S. Rosenthal, and Maimon M. Cohen

Lutheran General Hospital, Park Ridge, Illinois; (C.I.K.) Cook County Children's Hospital, Chicago, (S.R., F.S.R.) and Children's Memorial Hospital, (M.M.C., S.J.S.) Chicago

Agent Orange (AO), a phenoxyherbicide, and dioxin, an impurity found in AO, are considered clastogens, mutagens, and teratogens in plants and animals. AO has come under suspicion in humans following claims that it causes chromosome damage and birth defects in offspring of exposed individuals. No well-designed edipemiological studies are available to support this conclusion. Of ten exposed individuals studied for chromosome breaks and sister chromatid exchange frequencies, eight were ascertained because they had children with congenital defects. No consistent pattern of anomalies was observed. Five children had neurologic deficit, one child had a central nervous system anomaly, and one child was affected with glaucoma. Although all individuals studied had normal karyotypes, a statistically significant increase in chromosome breakage was observed in exposed males compared to their unexposed wives and children; sister chromatid exchange frequency was not increased.

Key words: dioxin, chromosome breakage, sister chromatid exchange, birth defects, Agent Orange

INTRODUCTION

Agent Orange (AO), an extensively used defoliant, consists of equal parts of the n-butyl esters of 2,4,5-trichlorophenoxyacetic acid (2,4,5-T) and 2,4-dichlorophenoxyacetic acid (2,4-D). 2,3,7,8-tetrachlorodibenzo-p-dioxin (TCDD), also called dioxin, is an impurity which is formed naturally during the manufacture of chlorinated benzene compounds, including 2,4,5-T and hexachlorophene [Wasson et al, 1978] and also by the combustion of 2,4,5-T [Epstein, 1973]. AO or its components has been implicated as a possible clastogen, mutagen, teratogen, and carcinogen in various experimental systems [Grant, 1979; Giavini et al, 1983]. Although data are sparse and contradictory, AO has also come under suspicion in humans owing to claims of chromosome damage in exposed individuals [Yoder et al, 1973] and abnormalities in their offspring. We report observations on chromosome breakage and sister chromatid exchanges in the peripheral lymphocytes of a group of individuals exposed to AO and their non-exposed family members.

The current address for Dr. Maimon M. Cohen is the Division of Human Genetics, Departments of OB/GYN and Pediatrics, University of Maryland Medical School, 655 West Baltimore Street, Baltimore MD 21201.

Address reprint requests to Celia I. Kaye, M.D., Ph.D., Director, Section of Genetics, Lutheran General Hospital, 1775 Dempster Street, Park Ridge, IL 60068.

© 1985 Alan R. Liss, Inc.

PATIENT POPULATION

The individuals studied included ten Vietnam veterans who reported exposure to AO from 10 to 16 years prior to laboratory investigation, nine of their spouses, and four children ranging in age from 9 months to 4 years. Six of the the ten developed a skin rash after exposure, and five of the ten had peripheral neuropathy, which is commonly noted in exposed persons. All had at least one of these symptoms. The families were ascertained because of a history of pregnancy wastage, children with birth defects, or anxiety concerning childbearing. None of these families had had children before AO exposure and all who attempted pregnancy were successful; thus sterility was not observed. Of 20 conceptions in the group, 5 resulted in spontaneous abortions (25%), which is probably not different from the normal population frequency. Table I describes the clinical findings of the abnormal offspring in this group of families and their respective pregnancy history.

CYTOGENETIC STUDIES

Chromosome analysis was performed, using phytohemagglutinin (PHA)-stimulated peripheral lymphocytes, on "G-banded" karyotypes constructed after trypsinization. Chromosome damage was assessed from "unbanded" preparations in a sample of 50 cells per individual by the method of Cohen et al [1967]. All slides were coded

TABLE I. Clinical History of Families Referred Because of Pregnancy Wastage, Birth Defects, or Anxiety

Family	Normal children[1]	Abnormal children[1]	Reason for referral	Miscarriages
A	None	1	Male, aged 9, with heart murmur, learning disability, behavior problem, "pigeon toes"	None
B	None	1	Child with large kidneys, hypoplastic lungs, normal chromosomes, died at birth	None
C	None	2	Female with acqueductal stenosis; male with nystagmus, developmental delay, hypotonia	None
D	None	1	Child with rare form of glaucoma	None
E	None	1	Male with multiple endocrine adenomatosis	2
F	2	None	No abnormal children	None
G	None	None	Spouse pregnant	None
H	1	1	Male with neurological disorder and seizures	None
I	1	2	Male with aortic stenosis; male with cerebral palsy, speech problem, club feet	2
J	2	1	Male with cerebral palsy, developmental delay	None

[1]After exposure to AO.

and studied microscopically with no observer-knowledge of the origin of the cells. Open breaks were scored as single events and were classified as either chromatid or isochromatid lesions. Rearrangements, including dicentric or ring chromosomes and multiradial configurations, were considered as two break events. Chromatid and isochromatid gaps were noted but not included in calculation of chromosome damage.

Sister chromatid exchanges (SCE) were produced by the method of Perry and Wolff [Perry and Wolff, 1974]. PHA-stimulated lymphocyte cultures were incubated with 10 μg/ml bromodeoxyuridine (Sigma) for the final 48 hours. Slides were stained in a solution of 0.5 mg/ml Hoechst 22358 (Aldrich) for 12 minutes, dried, and exposed to a mixture of long- and short-wave UV light (distance of 20 cm) for 1–2 hours in a 0.3 M phosphate buffer. The slides were then rinsed in distilled water, dried, and stained with 4% buffered Giemsa (pH 7) and the frequency of SCE's per individual was scored from photomicrographs of second division cells. In all but one individual at least 15 metaphases were scored, with a mean of 22.3 cells per person.

RESULTS

All individuals had numerically and structurally normal karyotypes. Table II presents the chromosome breakage data observed in the exposed males. The range of damage was 0.02–0.20 breaks/cell with a mean and S.D. of 0.12 ± 0.057 breaks/cell. Several of the individuals in this group clearly fall within the normal range observed in this laboratory (0.00–0.06 breaks/cell). The three rearrangements observed were all dicentric chromosomes. Table III describes the chromosome damage observed among the unexposed wives and children of the males exposed to AO. The range of breakage among the wives was 0.02–0.14 breaks per cell (mean 0.053 ± 0.037); one dicentric chromosome was observed. Among the four children studied, the mean chromosome breakage rate was 0.035 ± 0.034 breaks per cell (range 0.00–0.08). No structural rearrangements were observed in this group. Statistical analysis of these mean breakage rates (t-test) indicated a significant increase in the exposed

TABLE II. Chromosome Damage Observed in Ten Males Exposed to Agent Orange[1]

Individual No.	Chromosome damage				
	Gaps	Breaks		Rearrangements	Breaks/cell
		Chromatid	Isochromatid		
1	6	8	0	0	0.16
3	2	5	2	0	0.14
5	1	4	2	0	0.12
7	2	4	2	2 (Dic)[2]	0.20
10	4	5	3	0	0.16
12	7	6	0	1 (Dic)	0.16
13	4	4	0	0	0.08
17	6	6	0	0	0.12
20	1	1	0	0	0.02
22	3	2	0	0	0.04
Total	36	45	9	3	

[1]Analysis based on 50 cells per individual. $\bar{X} \pm SD = 0.120 \pm 0.057$ breaks/cell.
[2]Dicentric.

TABLE III. Chromosome Damage Observed in Nine Wives and Four Children Not Exposed to Agent Orange[1]

Individual No.		Chromosome damage			
		Breaks			
	Gaps	Chromatid	Isochromatid	Rearrangements	Breaks/cell
Unexposed wives[2]					
2	4	3	0	0	0.06
4	3	2	0	0	0.04
6	2	1	0	0	0.02
8	3	2	0	0	0.04
11	3	4	0	0	0.08
14	4	2	0	0	0.04
18	3	2	3	1 (Dic)	0.14
21	2	2	0	0	0.04
23	3	1	0	0	0.02
Total	27	19	3	1	
Unexposed children[3]					
9	3	2	0	0	0.04
15	2	1	0	0	0.02
16	3	0	0	0	0.00
19	3	3	1	0	0.08
Total	12	6	1	0	

[1]Analysis based on 50 cells per individual.
[2]$\overline{X} \pm S.D. = 0.053 \pm 0.037$.
[3]$\overline{X} \pm S.D. = 0.035 \pm 0.034$.

males when compared to unexposed wives ($t = 4.28$ df $= 17$; $P < 0.001$) and children ($t = 4.75$ df $= 12$; $P < 0.001$). However, no significant difference between the mean chromosome breakage rates between the groups of children and their mothers ($t = 1.3$; df $= 11$; $P < 0.02$) was seen.

Table IV lists the SCE data from the three groups of individuals studied. The observations are presented as SCE frequencies per cell and per chromosome. Since some metaphases scored for SCE contained less than 46 chromosomes, the frequency of SCE/chromosome is probably the more useful parameter. Similar statistical evaluation (t-test) between the mean values of the groups showed no significant differences in SCE frequencies, regardless of the basis for calculation, ie, SCE per cell or per chromosome. Non-significant correlation coefficients between chromosome breakage and SCE frequencies, both on a per cell and a per chromosome basis, were obtained for the entire population of 23 individuals studied ($r_{per\ cell} = -0.12$; $r_{per\ chromosome} = -0.02$). This result supports the view that two different mechanisms are responsible for the induction of chromosome breaks and SCE's.

DISCUSSION

From studies of AO performed before 1970, it is unclear whether the observed effects resulted from 2,4,5-T, the contaminant dioxin, or a combination of the two compounds [Grant, 1979], since all commercial formulations of 2,4,5-T contained varying amounts of dioxin [Galston, 1971]. Both 2,4,5-T and dioxin have been

TABLE IV. Frequencies of Sister Chromatid Exchanges (SCE) Observed Among the 23 Individuals Examined

	SCE per cell			SCE per chromosome		
No. SCE	Mean	Range	No. cells	Mean	Range	No. chromosomes
Exposed males						
214	9.72	4–14	22	0.214	0.089–0.435	1,000
177	8.04	3–18	22	0.180	0.075–0.391	983
137	5.70	0–12	24	0.127	0.000–0.293	1,081
175	9.21	1–17	19	0.201	0.033–0.415	872
217	8.03	1–20	27	0.177	0.032–0.445	1,226
177	8.43	2–20	21	0.184	0.050–0.435	962
199	9.05	0–15	22	0.197	0.000–0.429	1,011
49	6.12	3–7	8	0.144	0.086–0.189	339
130	7.64	1–10	17	0.174	0.025–0.357	748
307	12.28	4–27	25	0.276	0.095–0.688	1,111
$\bar{X} \pm$ SEM = 8.42 $\pm$ 0.589				$\bar{X} \pm$ SEM = 0.187 $\pm$ 0.013		
Unexposed wives						
145	7.63	0–12	19	0.169	0.000–0.471	857
169	7.35	3–18	23	0.165	0.083–0.391	1,027
225	10.23	2–18	22	0.232	0.045–0.529	971
151	6.86	3–13	22	0.155	0.086–0.321	975
187	7.48	1–12	25	0.160	0.038–0.316	1,170
143	8.41	2–14	17	0.186	0.053–0.400	770
284	10.52	2–15	27	0.235	0.079–0.458	1,210
137	8.56	2–12	16	0.193	0.071–0.381	710
337	14.04	0–29	24	0.312	0.000–0.600	1,081
$\bar{X} \pm$ SEM = 9.01 $\pm$ 0.757				$\bar{X} \pm$ SEM = 0.200 $\pm$ 0.017		
Unexposed children						
228	7.53	1–16	30	0.162	0.022–0.348	1,392
256	8.25	1–16	31	0.175	0.027–0.372	1,428
202	8.86	2–20	23	0.194	0.043–0.444	1,049
265	9.81	1–18	27	0.217	0.022–0.500	1,214
$\bar{X} \pm$ SEM + 8.61 $\pm$ 0.483				$\bar{X} \pm$ SEM = 0.188 $\pm$ 0.011		

implicated as clastogens in plants and animals [Jackson, 1972; Greig et al, 1973; Buu-Hoi et al, 1972], as mutagens in insects [Zetterberg, 1978] and mammals [Khera and Ruddick, 1973], and as teratogens in mammals [Giavini et al, 1983]. Dioxin has been associated with adverse effects on reproductive capacity [Khera and Ruddick, 1973] and is a potent inducer of microsomal enzymes [Berry et al, 1977], and a possible carcinogen in animals [Green et al, 1977].

Animals exposed to dioxin develop chromosome breaks in bone marrow cells [Muranyi-Kovacs et al, 1976], but sister chromatid exchange frequency is not altered [Lamb et al, 1981]. Studies of workers engaged in producing or spraying 2,4,5-T showed an increased number of chromatid aberrations [Yoder et al, 1973]. However, data resulting from investigation of a manufacturing accident in Seveso, Italy, are ambiguous and difficult to interpret [Pocchiari et al, 1979]. The authors refer to a "slight increase of dispersion of total cell aberration frequency" in the exposed population, but differences between controls and exposed individuals were not significant.

Field and Kerr [1979] suggested a teratogenic effect of dioxin by reporting a linear correlation between the use of 2,4,5-T in the previous year in Australia and an increase in neural tube defects. This correlation disappeared during the 2 years that 2,4,5-T production was monitored in order to keep its dioxin content below 0.1 parts per million. Likewise 2,4,5-T has been circumstantially implicated in an almost twofold increase in stillbirths in the Alsea Basin in Oregon, though the epidemiologic evidence has been judged inadequate to support such a conclusion.

The claims of abnormalities among Vietnam veterans exposed to AO and increased frequencies of birth defects among their children have received much attention. However, no well-designed epidemiologic studies are available, perhaps because of the very difficult task of correct data collection. Of the ten exposed males evaluated in the present investigation, eight were referred because of one or more abnormal children, and two had pregnant spouses who were anxious concerning the birth of a child with congenital defects. The abnormalities of these children (Table I) showed no consistent pattern. While eight of the ten couples studied had children with birth defects, the sample is self-referred because of abnormal pregnancy history or parental concern and, hence, highly biased. There are no data that support or refute an increased incidence of birth defects, or an increase of specific anomalies in children of Vietnam veterans exposed to AO.

While six of the ten fathers studied had increased chromosome breakage when compared with their unexposed relatives, all the offspring studied had normal frequencies of chromosome breakage. Therefore, it is not possible to assume a causal relationship between chromosome damage in fathers and the nonspecific anomalies observed in the children. Furthermore, AO exposure occurred many years prior to conception of the children and subsequent chromosome analysis. If indeed there is a relationship between AO exposure and chromosome breakage, the mechanism responsible must be of a latent nature and capable of bridging long periods of time.

At least two possible explanations may account for long-lived persistence of chromosome alterations years after toxic exposure. Those lymphocytes possessing chromosome damage induced by an external agent may remain in the non-dividing state for many years, only to manifest the aberrations when stimulated by PHA. The observation of chromosome damage in lymphocytes of patients treated with x-rays for ankylosing spondylitis years after treatment supports this possibility [Buckton et al, 1962]. Similar findings have been observed after whole-body radiation exposure [Bloom et al, 1967], and in fetuses exposed in utero [Bloom et al, 1968].

Secondly, dioxin has been shown to be lipophilic and is detectable in beef fat [Anonymous, 1975]; it has also been found in fish and crustacia in Vietnam many years after AO spraying [Westing, 1973]. It is, therefore, possible that dioxin is bound in the adipose tissue of exposed individuals and constitutes a source of chronic exposure. Therefore, the observed chromosome breakage in exposed individuals may reflect a response to dioxin released from tissue storage over a long period of time.

While there is no doubt that these preliminary results in the AO-exposed individuals indicate an increased frequency of chromosome breakage, a mechanism explaining these findings is unclear. The possibility that paternal exposure to AO may be in some way related to an abnormal pregnancy outcome is disconcerting. In man, any association between dioxin and birth defects and/or chromosome breakage is, at best, tenuous and, presently, difficult to document; and further evaluation of a well-designed epidemiological study of this "at risk population" is essential.

ACKNOWLEDGMENT

This study was supported in part by grants from the Chicago Foundlings Home and The National Institute of Dental Research (PHS DE 2872-11).

REFERENCES

Anonymous: EPA has found unsafe levels of TCDD in half of beef fat samples. Chem Engng News 53(34):10, 1975.

Berry DL, et al: Transplacental induction of mixed function oxygenasis in extrahepatic tissues by 2,3,7,8-tetrachlorodibenzo-para-dioxin. Biochem Pharmacol 26:1383–1388, 1977.

Bloom AD, Neriishi S, Archer PG: Cytogenetics of the in utero exposed of Hiroshima and Nagasaki. Lancet ii:10–12, 1968.

Bloom AD, et al: Chromosome aberrations in leukocytes of older survivors of the atomic bombings of Hiroshima and Nagasaki. Lancet ii:802–805, 1967.

Buckton KE, et al: A study of the chromosome damage persisting after x-ray therapy for ankylosing spondylitis. Lancet ii:676–682, 1962.

Buu-Hoi NP, et al: Organs as targets of dioxin intoxication. Naturwissenschaften 59:174–175, 1972.

Cohen MM, Hirschhorn K, Frosch WA: In vivo and in vitro chromosome damage induced by LSD-25. New Engl J Med 277:1043–1049, 1967.

Epstein SS: Teratological hazards due to phenoxyherbicides and dioxin contaminants. Environ Sci Res 2:708–729, 1973.

Field B, Kerr C: Herbicide use and incidence of neural tube defects. Lancet i:1341–1342, 1979.

Galston AW: Some implications of the widespread use of herbicides. Bioscience 21:891–892, 1971.

Giavini E, Prati M, Vismara C: Embryotoxic effects of 2,3,7,8 tetrachlorobenzo-p-dioxin administered to female rats before mating. Environ Res 31:105–110, 1983.

Grant FW: The genotoxic effects of 2,4,5-T. Mutat Res 65:83–229, 1979.

Green S, Moreland F, Shen C: Cytogenetic effects of 2,3,7,8-tetrachlorodibenzo-para-dioxin on rat bone marrow cells. FDA Bylines, No. 6:292–294, 1977.

Greig JW, et al: Toxic effects of 2,3,7,8-tetrachlorodibenzo-para-dioxin. Food Cosmet Toxicol 11:585–595, 1973.

Jackson WT: Cytological effects of 2,4,5-trichlorophenoxyacetic acid and of dioxin contaminants in 2,4,5-T formulation. J Cell Sci 10:15–20, 1972.

Khera KS, Ruddick JA: Polychloro-dibenzo-para-dioxins: Perinatal effects and dominant lethal tests in Wistar rats. Adv Chem Ser 70:72, 1973.

Lamb JC, et al: Male fertility, sister chromatid exchange, and germ cell toxicity following exposure to mixtures of chlorinated phenoxy acids containing 2,3,7,8-tetrachlorodibenzo-p-dioxin. J Toxicol Environ Health 8:825–834, 1981.

Majumdar SK, Goha JK: Mutation test of 2,4,5,-trichlorophenoxyacetic acid on Drosophila melanogaster. Can J Genet Cytol 16:465–466, 1974.

Muranyi-Kovacs I, Rudah G, Imbert J: Bioassay of 2,4,5-trichlorophenoxyacetic acid for carcinogenicity in mice. Br J Cancer 33:626–633, 1976.

Perry P, Wolff S: New Giemsa method for the differential staining of sister chromatids. Nature 251:156–158, 1974.

Pocchiari F, Silvano V, Zampieri A: Human health effects from accidental release of TCDD at Seveso, Italy. Ann NY Acad Sci 320:311–320, 1979.

Wasson JS, Huff JE, Loprieno N: A review of the genetic toxicology of the chlorinated dibenzo-para-dioxins. Mutat Res 47:141–160, 1978.

Westing A: AAAS Herbicide Assessment Commission. Science 179:1278–1279, 1973.

Yoder J, Watson M, Benson WW: Lymphocyte chromosomal analysis of agricultural workers during extensive occupational exposure to pesticides. Mutat Res 21:335–340, 1973.

Zetterberg G: Genetic effects of phenoxy acids on microorganisms. In Ramel C (ed): "Chlorinated Phenoxy Acids and Their Dioxins, Mode of Action, Health Risks and Environmental Effects." Stockholm: Ecol Bull, Vol 27, 1978, pp 193–204.

Dental Maturation in Hemifacial Microsomia

Hannelore T. Loevy and Scott W. Shore
Department of Pediatric Dentistry, University of Illinois College of Dentistry, Chicago

Hemifacial microsomia (HFM) is a congenital syndrome in which the mandible shows a spectrum of severity of malformation. The malformation is generally unilateral but may be bilateral, and if so, is then usually asymmetrical. Eighty-nine patients (58 males and 31 females) with unilateral HFM were evaluated for mandibular tooth development using the technique of Demirjian and Goldstein [1976]. According to Pruzansky's classification of severity of malformed mandibles in HFM [1969], the study sample consisted of 57 grade I cases, 26 grade II cases, and 6 grade III cases. Tooth development patterns of the affected and non-affected sides were compared with one another using 45° oblique cephalometric radiographs. Eight cases were studied separately, since three showed bilateral congenital absence of the second premolar, three showed unilateral congenital absence of the second premolar on the affected side, and two had the first permanent molar extracted. In spite of the difference in severity of mandibular anomalies in each group, 45.7% (37) of the patients showed symmetry of tooth maturation. Of the 54.3% (44) patients showing asymmetric tooth maturation, 54.4% (24) showed more advanced dental maturation on the affected side and 45.5% (20) showed more advanced dental development on the non-affected side. These findings suggest that the mandibular deformity associated with HFM does not have an effect on dental maturation when compared with the antimere of the non-affected side.

Key words: tooth development, hemifacial microsomia, maxillofacial abnormalities, maxillofacial development, mandible abnormalities, ear abnormalities, microtia

INTRODUCTION

Hemifacial microsomia (HFM) is a congenital malformation characterized by deformities of the mandible and the ear. There is progressive asymmetric growth of structures derived from the first and second branchial arches. The condition is predominantly unilateral, but bilateral cases occur.

There is considerable diversity in the manifestations of HFM. Other structures also derived from the first and second branchial arches may be involved, such as the maxilla, malar bones, zygomatic arch, pterygoid process of the sphenoid bone, facial nerve, and muscles of mastication and facial expression. Some authors feel that

EDITORS' NOTE: Dr. Pruzansky contributed to the research reported in this paper and was listed as a co-author prior to his death.

Part of this material was presented at the meeting of the International Association for Dental Research, March 14–18, 1984, Dallas, Texas.

Address reprint requests to Hannelore T. Loevy, Dept. of Pediatric Dentistry, College of Dentistry, University of Illinois at Chicago, P.O. Box 6998, Chicago, IL 60680.

Goldenhar syndrome, in which defects of the eye, eyelid, and vertebral anomalies are also manifested is a variation of HFM; others consider the Goldenhar, Treacher Collins, and Hallerman Streiff syndromes as separate clinical entities [Grabb, 1965; Poswillo, 1973].

HFM is usually sporadic, but autosomal dominant and autosomal recessive modes of inheritance have been suggested in some cases [Rollnick and Kaye, 1983; Taysi et al, 1983]. Teratogenic agents such as thalidomide have also been implicated by some investigators in man [Smithells and Leek, 1963] and in experimental animals [Poswillo, 1973].

Clinically, the appearance of these patients is dominated by facial asymmetry of greater or lesser intensity. The mandibular anomaly is classified into three types, depending on the skeletal anatomy of the ramus and the temporomandibular joint [Pruzansky, 1969]. In grade I deformity, the mandible and the temporomandibular joint are present but hypoplastic. Grade II deformity is characterized by a small, abnormally shaped ramus and an underdeveloped displaced temporomandibular joint. In grade III deformity, the ramus and the glenoid fossa are absent. The skeletal abnormality is not predictably related to the abnormalities of the facial soft tissues or to the appearance of the external ear [Figueroa and Pruzansky, 1983].

Since normal mandibular growth is affected in HFM, it was considered of interest to evaluate dental development in a series of cases and compare the dental maturation of the affected and the non-affected sides of these patients.

METHODS AND MATERIALS

Patients evaluated in this study were selected from a large number of cases under treatment at the Center for Craniofacial Anomalies at the University of Illinois at Chicago. Subjects were selected in whom only one side was affected at the time of the mixed dentition. Only those cases in which good radiographic data were available were chosen. In almost all instances, oblique radiographs were used, since panoramic radiographs were available in only a small number. The sample consisted of 58 boys and 31 girls, mostly Caucasian. Patients were classified according to the severity of the deformity as grade I, II, or III following the classification of Pruzansky [1969] (Table I). The age of the patients ranged from 3 years 3 months to 13 years with an

TABLE I. Distribution of HFM Patients According to Sex, Race, and Grade of Mandibular Deformity

Sex/race[1]	Grade I	Grade II	Grade III	Total
M/C	29	19	4	52
M/B	1		1	2
M/H	4			4
F/C	19	6	1	26
F/B	1			1
F/H	3	1		4
Total	57	26	6	89

[1]M = male; F = female; C = Caucasian; B = black; H = Hispanic.

average of 7 years 8 months. If more than one oblique radiographic survey was available, the earliest was used. In no case was the same patient evaluated more than once.

A control series of normal white children with no systemic disease was also investigated. This group of patients from a suburban private office consisted of 51 boys and 49 girls randomly selected. The purpose of evaluating this group was to determine differences in dental maturation between the left and right sides in normal healthy children. Panoramic radiographs were used for this purpose.

Tooth maturation was determined using the method described by Demirjian and Goldstein [1976]. Each side of the mandible was used for evaluation. The first and second molars and both premolars on each side of the mandible were evaluated in all children. The stage of development of each tooth was given a maturity score. A maturity score for each side is defined as the sum of the scores of the individual teeth on that side. This total is then converted to dental age for the side, girls and boys being evaluated separately using tables for each sex provided by Demirjian and Goldstein [1976]. In an earlier study we compared the distribution of dental age of 202 Chicago white children to Demirjian's series of French Canadian children and found that Chicago white children had more advanced dental maturity [Loevy, 1983]. Therefore, we used this group of Chicago white children to compare the distribution of dental maturity with that of HFM patients. The data were analyzed using the chi square test for goodness of fit [Conover, 1971].

RESULTS

Of 89 patients with HFM studied, 8 were evaluated separately. In two cases the first permanent molar had been extracted; in three cases the second premolars were congenitally absent on both sides, and in three cases the second premolars were congenitally absent on one side only. In the last three cases the absence was on the affected side of the mandible.

Of the 81 cases in which all teeth were present, 37 cases had the same maturation pattern on both sides. In 44 cases there was an unequal maturation pattern. Of these, the affected side was more advanced in maturation in 24 cases, while in 20 cases the non-affected side was more advanced. The dental maturation appeared to be independent of the severity of the mandibular defect. Of the 100 suburban children, dental maturation was the same on both sides in 99 of the 100 cases.

The comparison of dental maturation in both our Chicago white patients and our suburban group demonstrated a significant advancement in maturation when compared to Demirjian's French Canadian group. Of our two groups, the suburban group was more advanced than the Chicago group. It was therefore considered that the Chicago group was a good standard for evaluation of dental maturity in our patients with HFM. When all patients with HFM were compared to the Chicago white children, it was noted that there was slight retardation in dental maturation in the HFM group as a whole with the non-affected side developing somewhat more slowly (Table II). When this was broken down further into the three groups of equal maturation on both sides, advanced maturation on affected side, and advanced maturation on the non-affected side, a statistically significant difference from the Chicago white children in any group could not be described (Table III).

TABLE II. Comparison of Distribution of Dental Maturation of HFM Patients (81) With Chicago White Normal Children

Percent	Expected	Affected side observed*	Non-affected side observed**
3	3.2	3	3
3–10	7.6	5	12
10–50	24.0	31	22
50–90	22.4	27	29
90–97	13.6	14	13
97	10.0	1	2

*$0.025 < P < 0.05$.
**$P = 0.05$.

TABLE III. Dental Maturity Findings: 89 Patients With Hemifacial Microsomia (HFM)

	Grade I	Grade II	Grade III	Total
Sides equal	27 + 1[1]	9	1	37 + 1[1]
Affected side advanced[2]	10	5	1	16
Affected side advanced[3]	3 + 1	3	2	8 + 1[1]
Non-affected side advanced[2]	8	3	0	11
Non-affected side advanced[3]	5	3	1	9
Congenitally missing teeth				
Bilateral	3	0	0	3
Unilateral	1	1	1	3
Total	59	24	6	

[1]First molar extracted.
[2]Less than 10%—advancement.
[3]More than 10%—advancement.

DISCUSSION

Hemifacial microsomia is primarily a descriptive term for a large group of congenital deformities without proper understanding of the etiologic factors involved. While there is undoubtedly involvement of one or more structures derived from the first and second branchial arches, these structures are not uniformly affected in different patients. Figueroa and Pruzansky [1982] demonstrated that a severely malformed external ear does not necessarily indicate a severely malformed mandible, on the same side or vice versa. While most cases do not seem to have a genetic basis, families with several cases have been documented and reported [Rollnick and Kaye, 1983]. However, in families in which familial occurrence has been reported, there has been great variability in the degree of phenotypic expression. Moreover, at least four examples of monozygotic twins discordant for hemifacial microsomia have been reported [Setzer, 1981; Burck, 1983; Grabb, 1965].

Prenatal vascular disruption has also been described as a possible etiologic factor. In mice examined by Poswillo [1973], hematoma formation was considered responsible for lack of proper development. Timing, extent, and location of hematoma formation may explain the wide spectrum of clinical findings.

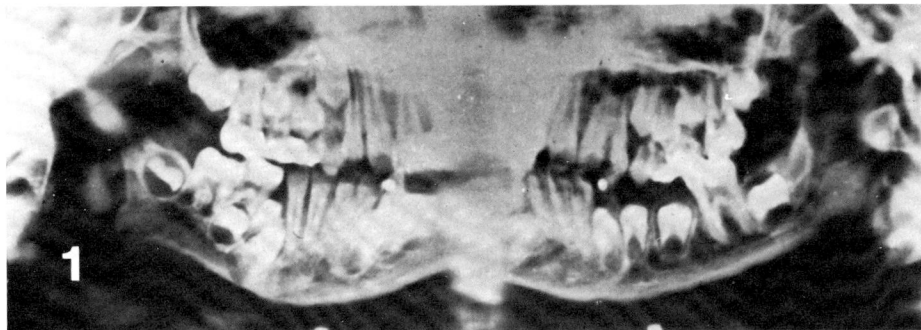

Fig. 1. Panoramic radiograph of a boy aged 8 years, 6 months. Compare the difference in dental maturation of the premolars and particularly of the molars of both sides.

In addition to the great clinical variability, associated anomalies [Cohen, 1971], etiologic heterogeneity, and postnatal growth differences among patients have been reported [Rune et al, 1983]. Since the final outcome of the growth and development process is based in part on the interaction of developing structures, tissues such as bone, muscle, connective tissue, and cartilage exert an influence on adjacent structures so that the end result depends to a large extent on functional environmental conditions. These considerations may explain the large diversity of findings in patients with HFM and the difficulty in classifying cases into a small number of types.

The dental findings are no exception to this diversity. Of the 81 cases, 44 patients showed an unequal maturation pattern. Of these 44 cases, there were 24 with more advanced maturation on the affected side and 20 with more advanced maturation on the non-affected side. As we have noted, of the 100 control cases, only one showed a slight difference in dental maturation between the left and right sides. It must be kept in mind that only dental maturation was studied, not dental eruption, in which another set of environmental factors would have to be analyzed. It is interesting to note that in all three cases of congenital unilateral absence of the second premolar this anomaly was on the affected side of the mandible.

When the HFM cases were compared with the Chicago white control group, we could not ascertain which group was responsible for the statistically significant retardation of maturation in our group of HFM taken as a whole. We can only assume that there were small non-significant differences in each subgroup that added up to borderline significance in the whole series.

It can be concluded that while there were definite differences in maturation when sides were compared, the findings suggest that the mandibular deformity associated with HFM does not have a statistically significant effect on dental maturation when antimeres are compared.

ACKNOWLEDGMENTS

The authors wish to thank Dr. I.M. Rosenthal and Miss A. Kowitz for their interest and assistance and Mrs. E. Rosenthal for her statistical analysis of the data. We also thank Ms. B. Adamick for her help with the manuscript.

This investigation was supported in part by grants from the National Institutes of Health (DE 02872).

REFERENCES

Burck U: Genetic aspects of hemifacial microsomia. Hum. Genet 64:291–296, 1983.

Cohen MM Jr: Variability versus "incidental findings" in the first and second branchial arch syndrome: Unilateral variants with anophthalmia. Birth Defects, 7(7):103–108, 1971.

Conover WJ: "Practical Non-parametric Statistics." New York: Wiley, Chapter 4, 1971, pp 186–194.

Demirjian A, Goldstein H: New systems for dental maturity based on seven and four teeth. Ann Hum Biol 3:411–421, 1976.

Figueroa AA, Pruzansky S: The external ear, mandible and other components of hemifacial microsomia. J Maxillofac Surg 10:193–266, 1983.

Grabb WC: The first and second branchial arch syndrome. Plast Reconstr Surg 36:485–508, 1965.

Loevy H: Maturation of permanent teeth in Black and Latino children. Acta Odontol Pediatr 4:59–62, 1983.

Poswillo D: The pathogenesis of the first and second branchial arch syndrome. Oral Surg 36:302–328, 1973.

Pruzansky S: Not all dwarfed mandibles are alike. Birth Defects 5(2):102–129, 1969.

Rollnick BR, Kaye CI: Hemifacial microsomia and variants: Pedigree data. Am J Med Genet 15:233–253, 1983.

Rune R, Sarnas KV, Selvik G, Jacobsson S: Roentgen stereometry with the aid of metallic implants in hemifacial microsomia. Am J Orthod 84:231–247, 1983.

Setzer ES, Ruiz-Castaneda N, Severn C, Ryden S, Frias JL: Etiological heterogeneity in the oculo-auriculo-vertebral syndrome. J Pediatr 98:88–90, 1981.

Smithells RW, Leek I: The incidence of limb and ear defects since the withdrawl of thalidomide. Lancet 1:1095–1097, 1963.

Taysi K, Marsh JL, Wise DM: Familial hemifacial microsomia. Cleft Palate J 20:47–53, 1983.

Association of Duane Retraction Syndrome With Craniofacial Malformations

Marilyn T. Miller

Department of Ophthalmology, University of Illinois College of Medicine, Eye and Ear Infirmary, Chicago

> Specific forms of ocular motor disturbances, such as Duane syndrome, occur with sufficient frequency in certain syndromes that the timing, location, and nature of the developmental disturbance may be established. The presence of this characteristic type of strabismus in a number of cases of hemifacial microsomia, especially the Goldenhar variants, may provide insight into the developmental disturbances of this large, complex group of patients. Evaluation of specific abnormalities of affected patients from the perspective of one discipline may further aid in the "lumping" or "splitting" process.

Key words: Duane syndrome, hemifacial microsomia, Wildervanck syndrome, Goldenhar syndrome, craniofacial anomalies, restrictive strabismus, developmental ocular muscle anomalies

INTRODUCTION

There are few noncomitant forms of eye motility disturbance that manifest limitation of ocular rotation in predictable fields of gaze and also have findings that separate them from ocular motor imbalances noted in common cranial nerve palsies. Duane retraction syndrome is the most usual type of congenital restrictive ocular motility disturbance in this group. There may be a neurologic motor component to the etiology, but also there are additional concurrent manifestations that result in a distinctive type of strabismus. Duane retraction syndrome represents about 1% of all strabismus cases examined, making it an unusual but not rare type of ocular motor disturbance [Kirkham, 1970]. While Duane retraction syndrome frequently occurs as an isolated, sporadic entity, familial patterns have been observed in 5-10% of the reported cases. Moreover, there is heightened awareness of its increased frequency in certain craniofacial syndromes and systemic anomalies. This syndrome also has been reported in association with various ocular diseases.

The classic clinical picture of retraction syndrome was described by Duane in 1905, although a number of cases predated his report [Smith, 1977]. A few forms of Duane syndrome have been classified according to the degree of limitation on abduction and adduction and the type of horizontal deviation in primary position [Huber, 1974]. The most frequent type shows an abnormality in motility consisting of (1) limitation on abduction, (2) narrowing of the palpebral fissure and retraction of the globe on attempted adduction, and (3) variable degrees of limitation on adduction

---

Address reprint requests to Marilyn T. Miller, M.D., Dept. of Ophthalmology, University of Illinois at Chicago, Eye and Ear Infirmary, 1855 West Taylor Street, Chicago, IL 60612.

© 1985 Alan R. Liss, Inc.

(Figs. 2C, 3A, 4). Another characteristic finding is the marked upshoot or downshoot of the eye in medial rotation. The syndrome may be bilateral but more frequently is unilateral, with a predilection for females and involvement on the left side [Kirkham, 1970].

Congenital structural anomalies of the muscle and tendons were initially postulated to be the cause of this unusual motility disturbance. An examination of the muscles in a few affected patients support this theory. However, more recent electromyographic data suggest that there is paradoxical innervation in many cases of Duane syndrome [Yarbrough et al, 1964; Hoyt and Nachtigaller, 1965]. Breinin [1957] believed that the observed co-contraction of medial and lateral rectus muscles in adduction was responsible for the retraction of the globe. One explanation for the unusual restriction imbalance in eye motility is that the oculomotor nerve sends fibers to the lateral rectus muscle. When affected patients attempt to adduct the eye, there is fixing of both the medial and lateral recti, causing retraction of the globe [Huber, 1974]. This theory is supported electromyographically and clinically; one patient with clinical bilateral Duane syndrome on examination at autopsy had no observable abducens nerve but had partial innervation of the lateral rectus muscle from branches of the oculomotor nerve [Hotchkiss et al, 1980]. That more than one etiologic factor may be responsible for the clincial picture of the retraction syndrome seems to be a tenable conclusion at this time.

CRANIOFACIAL ANOMALIES ASSOCIATED WITH DUANE SYNDROME

Duane syndrome has been reported with both systemic anomalies and other types of ocular conditions including ocular dermoids, astigmatism, colobomas of the globe, nystagmus, and a variety of rare malformations [Cross and Pfaffenbach, 1972; Pfaffenbach et al, 1972; Smith, 1977].Astigmatism in these cases is thought to be secondary to a difference in corneal curvature in different meridians (ie, not to lens-induced astigmatism) and may represent a derived complication owing to abnormal tension produced by the restrictive ocular motility rather than an associated anomaly.

Amblyopia also is a complication occurring in about 25% of all patients with Duane syndrome [Kirkham, 1970]. Contributing factors of amblyopia are high refractive errors, especially if asymmetric (anisometropia); other ocular disease; and strabismus in primary position [Kirkham, 1970]. Ocular disorders other than refractive errors or amblyopia appear to occur sporadically and are not frequently concurrent with craniofacial disorders. The notable exceptions are epibulbar dermoids and/or lipodermoids. These two types of dermoids are frequently associated with Duane syndrome and are reported in patients with systemic disease. In fact, it is rare if patients with these sets of ocular problems do not manifest some type of external or internal ear condition and, to a lesser extent, cervical spinal malformations. The craniofacial findings may be subtle, requiring radiologic evaluation or a careful history to detect the presence of ear tags that were removed in infancy.

Many series in the literature indicate a number of skeletal anomalies in patients with Duane syndrome [Aleksic et al, 1976; Baum and Feingold, 1973; Cross and Pfaffenbach, 1972; Ellis et al, 1981; Pfaffenbach et al, 1972]. In a review of 186 cases of Duane syndrome seen at the Mayo Clinic, Pfaffenbach et al [1972] noted congenital hearing and ear anomalies in 14 patients (7.5%). While this series may be biased toward syndrome patients, the distribution of pathologic conditions is notewor-

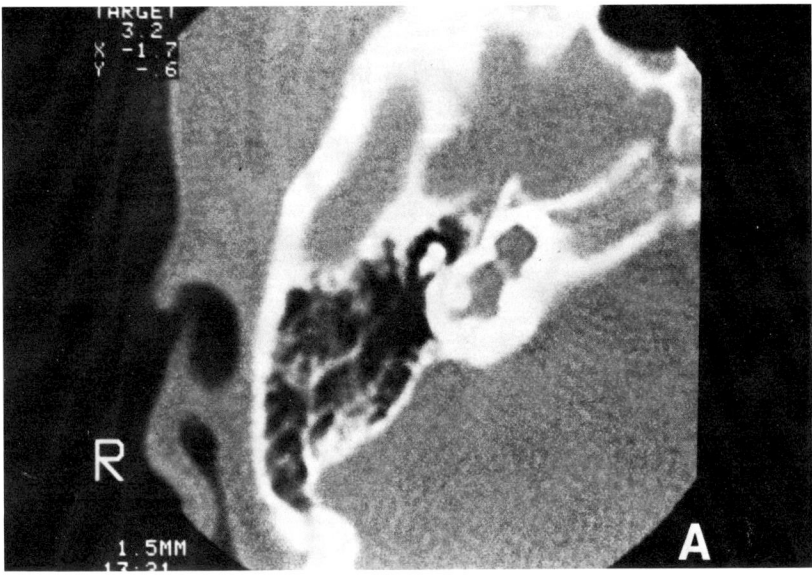

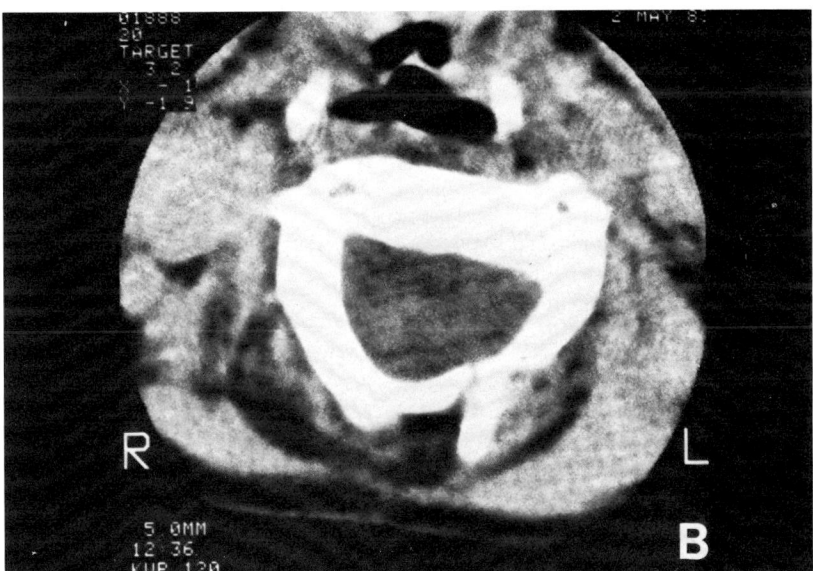

Fig. 1. Patient with sensorineural deafness, unilateral Duane syndrome and Klippel-Feil anomaly of the neck. A. Computed tomogram of inner ear; B. Computed tomogram of cervical spine.

thy. They also found radiologic evidence of spinal abnormalities in 16% of patients studied. After reviewing the literature, the authors suggested that patients with Duane syndrome are 10 to 20 times more at risk for skeletal anomalies of the ear than the general population [Pfaffenbach et al, 1972].

Looking at the problem from the perspective of patients with hearing defects, in a survey of 500 deaf children, Alexander [1973] noted seven cases of Duane syn-

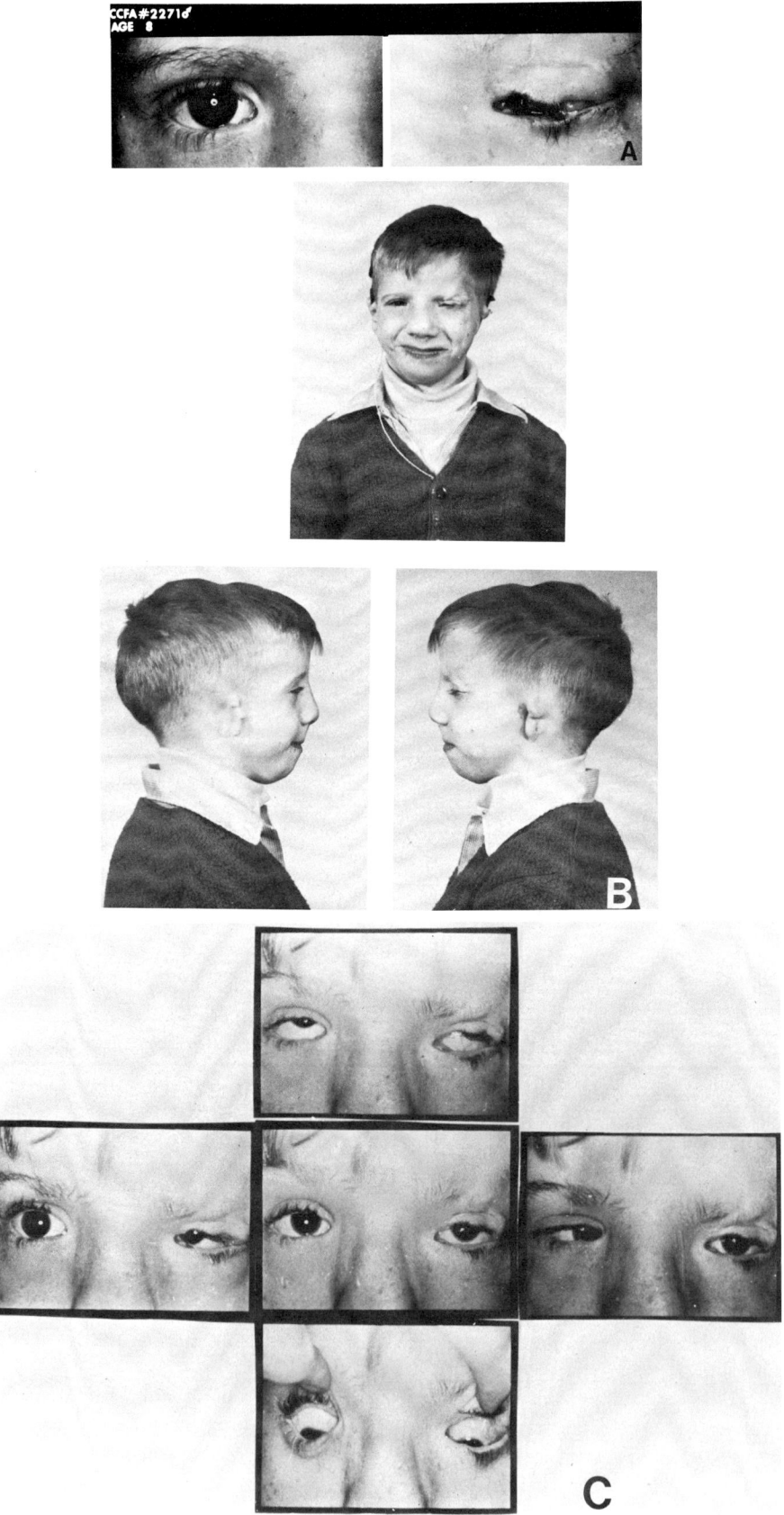

drome. Four additional patients demonstrated restriction of horizontal movement of all four horizontal muscles, which probably represents a less common form of Duane syndrome.

Although Duane syndrome occurs with malformations such as macrostomia, microstomia, cleft palate, oral, and systemic anomalies, an analysis of individual case reports suggests that this association is most often noted in two conditions—Wildervanck syndrome and hemifacial microsomia, particularly the Goldenhar variant. The triad of Duane syndrome associated with Klippel-Feil anomalies of the spine and sensorineural deafness has been designated cervico-oculo-acoustic syndrome by Wildervanck [Evenberg et al, 1963; Fraser and MacGillivray, 1968; Wildervanck, 1960]. Although the frequency of the isolated forms of Duane syndrome is higher in females (60–70%), there is almost complete predominance of females in Wildervanck syndrome, leading some authors to suggest X-linked dominant inheritance with lethality in males. Often patients manifest only part of the syndrome. Kirkham [1970] postulated autosomal dominant inheritance, incomplete penetrance, and variable expressivity with partial sex limitation. He reviewed 112 cases of Duane syndrome and noted 12 cases with perceptive deafness, five with Klippel-Feil anomaly, and only two with the complete triad. Wildervanck [1960] also observed variable expressivity of this syndrome and suggested that only two characteristics of the triad are needed to make the diagnosis. Interestingly, one patient in his original report had epibulbar dermoids.

In Fraser and MacGillivray's [1968] review of the literature, dermoids were noted in four case reports. They concluded that intermediate forms exist between cervico-oculo-acoustic syndrome and other first arch conditions such as Goldenhar syndrome. However, the strong familial pattern and very strong preponderance of females in Wildervanck syndrome are significantly different from hemifacial microsomia.

The deafness noted in Wildervanck syndrome is often secondary to a congenital inner ear anomaly, although mixed forms have been described. Regular and computed tomography of otologic structures have demonstrated frequent abnormalities of the middle ear structures and semicircular canals [Evenberg et al, 1963] (Fig. 1). Although not necessarily present in all cases, Duane syndrome is a diagnostic characteristic of Wildervanck syndrome. The association is much weaker between Duane syndrome and hemifacial microsomia, but it is still significant. More than 20 cases of this association are cited in the literature, and since the diagnosis is somewhat difficult unless made by an ophthalmologist, the number is probably underreported [Baum and Feingold, 1973; Budden and Robinson, 1973; Cross and Pfaffenbach, 1972; Ellis et al, 1981; Pfaffenbach et al, 1972; Smith, 1977; Wildervanck, 1960].

"Hemifacial microsomia" is the descriptive term used by Gorlin and others [1976] to characterize a group of patients who manifest a spectrum of malformations of the ear, mandible, mouth, eye, and often cervical spine. It occurs unilaterally in most but not all patients [Gorlin et al, 1963]. Goldenhar syndrome (oculo-auriculo-vertebral dysplasia) has been proposed by Gorlin and others [1963] to represent a variant of this entity. Goldenhar described the combination of epibulbar dermoids,

---

Fig. 2. Goldenhar-type patient. A. Note bilateral external and inner ear anomalies, and repaired left upper lid coloboma. B. Bilateral microtia. C. Duane syndrome. This composite depicts eye positions in various test fields of ocular muscle action. Note the straight eyes in primary position; limitation of abduction in attempted gaze right and narrowing of left palpebral fissure on adduction; limitation of abduction of left eye on attempted gaze left with narrowing of right palpebral fissure; no vertical limitation.

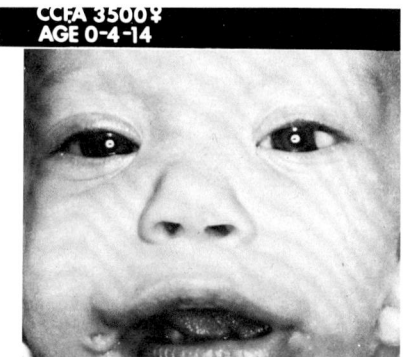

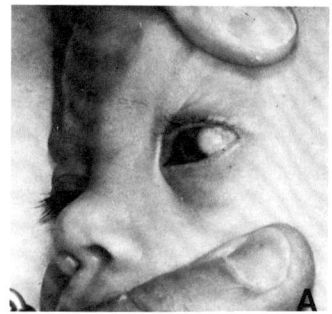

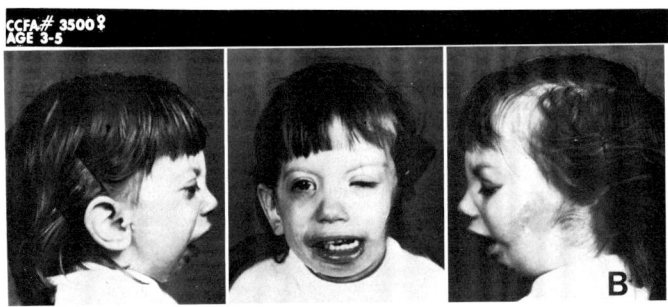

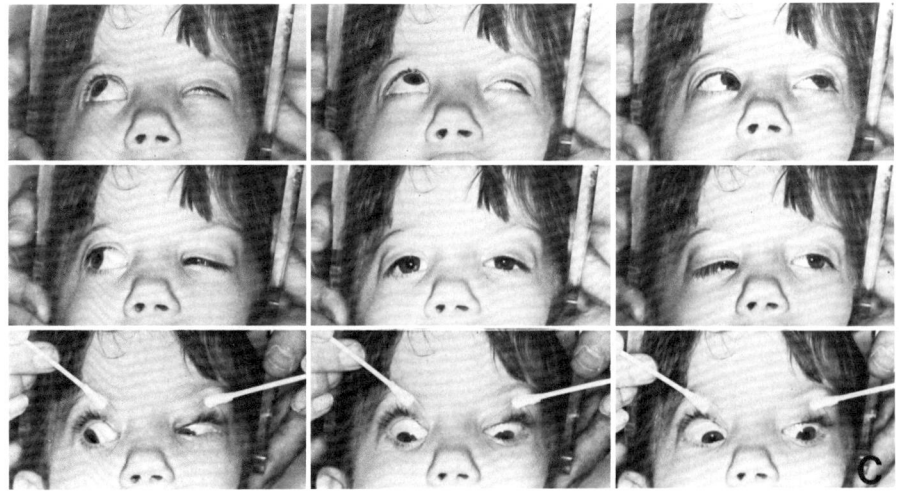

lipodermoids, and preauricular skin tags and fistulas. Later the association with upper lid coloboma and vertebral anomalies became well documented. In a review of this syndrome, Gorlin [1963] noted that the dermoids and ear anomalies were often bilateral but that the upper lid colobomas were usually unilateral. Duane syndrome has been reported both bilaterally (even in cases showing unilateral hypoplasia of facial bones) and unilaterally. Occasionally patients may exhibit unilateral Duane syndrome on the side contralateral to most of the other anomalies [Baum and Feingold, 1973; Velez, 1970]. When found in the hemifacial microsomia group, it appears that Duane syndrome occurs most frequently in the Goldenhar-type patient, who usually manifests epibulbar dermoids or lipodermoids [Aleksic et al, 1976; Baum and Feingold, 1973].

Poswillo [1973] has suggested from animal experiments that a hematoma at the time and site of stapedial artery development may be at least one etiologic factor for hemifacial microsomia. It could be speculated that disturbance of sixth nerve neurons by local hemorrhage followed by paradoxical reinnervation by the third nerve could result in various phenotypes of Duane syndrome. In the type of Duane syndrome with no abduction, it is postulated that the lateral rectus is functionally innervated only by a branch of the 3rd nerve, resulting in no abduction and co-contraction on attempted adduction. If the lateral rectus retains functional innervation by the sixth nerve, the eye could abduct to some degree but would show co-contraction and limitation on adduction.

Other types of paradoxical innervation that have been reported in patients with Duane syndrome might also represent innervational mistakes. One small group of Duane patients have demonstrated aberrant innervation of the lacrimal gland. These patients have inappropriate tearing, often called "crocodile tears", which occurs when sucking or eating [Brik and Athayde, 1973; Ramsay and Taylor, 1980; Regenbogen and Stein, 1968]. They may or may not have normal emotional tearing and also may show variable response to stimulation of the cornea (eg, by touch or with pungent fumes). Corneal hypoesthesia has been reported in a number of cases associated with Goldenhar syndrome [Baum and Feingold, 1973]. One interesting patient mentioned by Willshaw and Al-Ashikar [1983] has Goldenhar syndrome, Duane retraction syndrome, and ipsilateral jaw-winking syndrome. This could be an example of aberrant innervation of the lid.

Paradoxical innervation and inappropriate coinnervation of a structure, as seems to exist in some of these unusual patients, raise some neuro-developmental questions. In work done in adult carp by Marrotte and Mark [1970], the nerves to the ocular muscles were severed, and positional advantage for reinnervation was given to the abnormal cranial nerves. Abnormal (paradoxical) innervation was then observed in these fish. However, if normal innervation was also allowed to occur, it appeared to block the action of the incorrect connection, suggesting a strong local selectivity for appropriate matching. A different result was obtained by Scott [1975] in experiments performed on extraocular muscles of goldfish, in which he recorded physiologically functional reinnervational connections. The phenomenon of synaptic repression in different embryologic structures following nerve regeneration is important to under-

---

Fig. 3. Goldenhar-type patient in infancy showing macrostomia, severely deformed left ear displaced downward and epibulbar dermoid. B. Same patient at age 5. Note large epibulbar dermoid in left eye. C. Patient with Duane syndrome: test fields of gaze of ocular muscles. Note some limitation of abduction of left eye with marked narrowing of left palpebral fissure on adduction. There is a questionable mild Duane syndrome of the right eye.

stand the reparative sequence that follows damage to neurons in the developing embryo. The observations on the adult animal may not apply to the less differentiated but highly programmed embryo.

Although retraction of the globes on adduction is an identifying finding in Duane syndrome, it is not present in all cases that have the electromyographic characteristics of Duane syndrome. However, without retraction, the clinical diagnosis is difficult and patients appear to have gaze paresis. One such patient was reported to have Klippel-Feil anomaly, unilateral deafness, and cleft palate [Witzel, 1959]. We have examined a patient with Goldenhar syndrome who was unable to abduct and only slightly adduct either eye but who did not show retraction. Electromyography may give insight into unusual patients, but it could be reasonably speculated that all such patients have a form of Duane syndrome.

Duane syndrome has been noted in association with cleft palate in patients with Wildervanck-type syndrome [Cohney, 1963; Kirkham, 1970] and, infrequently, in those with hypertelorism [Awan, 1975]. One such interesting patient had median-facial cleft, Duane syndrome, lid coloboma, lipodermoid, and ear tags (Fig. 4).

The spinal anomalies reported in cases of Duane syndrome vary in type and degree from the severe Klippel-Feil anomaly of the Wildervanck syndrome to milder anomalies of cervical or thoracic vertebrae. In one unusual case, the typical motility disturbance had been associated with iniencephaly [O'Malley, 1982].

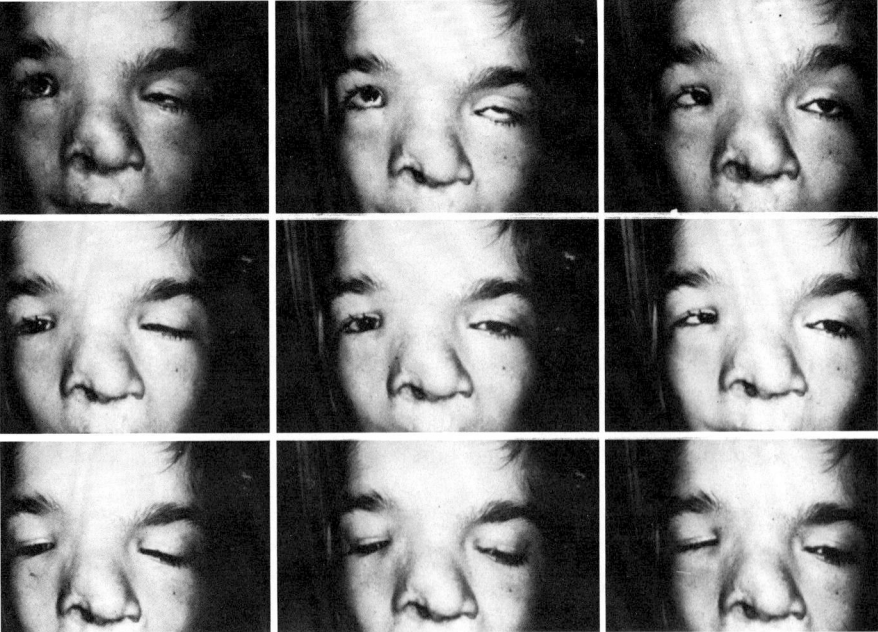

Fig. 4. Median facial cleft syndrome patient with Duane syndrome. Patient also had ear tags removed in infancy and had a small epibulbar dermoid of the right eye and lid notch.

SUMMARY

Because of the many interacting factors necessary to establish and maintain normal alignment and fusion, nonspecific ocular motor disturbances (ie, esotropia, exotropia) offer little diagnostic value in separating various craniofacial syndromes and carry no implication as to timing, location, and mechanism of the embryonic insult that produces a set of anomalies. On the other hand, specific forms, such as Duane syndrome, occur with sufficient frequency in certain syndromes to aid in establishing timing, location, and nature of the developmental disturbance. The presence of this very characteristic type of strabismus in a significant number of cases of hemifacial microsomia, especially the Goldenhar variant, may provide more insight into the developmental disturbance of this large, complex group of patients. Reevaluation of the specific abnormalities of such patients from the perspective of one discipline may further aid in either the "lumping" or "splitting" process.

This type of approach is also informative in understanding isolated anomalies. If a specific condition such as Duane syndrome normally occurs as a sporadic isolated anomaly but also exists with significant frequency with other specific malformations, analysis of the anomaly complex may narrow the time period of the embryonic disturbance and also give insight into the pathophysiology of its cause.

ACKNOWLEDGMENTS

I wish to thank Ms. Maxine Gere for her editorial assistance and Ms. Nydia Santiago for her excellent secretarial work.

This work was supported in part by Core grant EY 1792 from the National Eye Institute, Bethesda, Maryland, and the National Institute of Dental Research Grant #HHSMCFADEO 2872-15.

REFERENCES

Aleksic S, Budzilovich G, Choy A, et al: Congenital ophthalmoplegia in oculoauriculovertebral dysplasia-hemifacial microsomia (Goldenhar-Gorlin syndrome): A clinicopathologic study and review of the literature. Neurology 26:638, 1976.
Alexander J: Ocular abnormalities among congenitally deaf children. Can J Ophthalmol 8:428, 1973.
Awan KJ: Duane's retraction syndrome and hypertelorism. J Pediatr Ophthalmol 12:100, 1975.
Baum JL, Feingold M: Ocular aspects of Goldenhar's syndrome. Am J Ophthalmol 75:250, 1973.
Blodi FC, Van Allen WW, Yarbrough JC: Duane's syndrome: A brainstem lesion. Arch Ophthalmol 72:171, 1964.
Breinin GM: Electromyography—A tool in ocular and neurologic diagnosis. Part II. Muscle palsies. Arch Ophthalmol 37:165, 1957.
Brik M, Athayde A: Bilateral Duane's syndrome, paroxysmal lacrimation and Klippel-Feil anomaly. Ophthalmologica 167:1, 1973.
Budden SS, Robinson, C: Oculoauricular vertebral dysplasia. Am J Dis Child 125:431, 1973.
Cohney BD: The association of cleft palate with Klippel-Feil syndrome. Plast Reconstr Surg 31:179, 1963.
Cross HE, Pfaffenbach DD: Duane's retraction syndrome and associated congenital malformations. Am J Ophthalmol 70:442, 1972.
Evenberg G, Ratjen MD, Serenson H: Wildervanck's syndrome. Klippel-Feil's syndrome associated with deafness and retraction of the eyeball. Br J Radiol 36:562, 1963.
Fraser WI, MacGillivray RC: Cervico-oculo-acoustic dysplasia (the 'syndrome of Wildervanck"). J Ment Defic Res 12:322, 1968.

Gorlin RJ, Jue KI, Jacobson U, Goldschmidt E: Oculoauriculovertebral dysplasia. J Pediatr 63:991, 1963.

Gorlin RJ, Pindborg JJ, Cohen MM: "Syndromes of the Head and Neck." 2nd ed. St. Louis, MO: McGraw-Hill Book Co., 1976, p 546.

Hotchkiss MG, Miller NR, Clark AW, Green WR: Bilateral Duane's retraction syndrome: A clinical pathologic case report. Arch Ophthalmol 98:870, 1980.

Hoyt WF, Nachtigaller I: Anomalies of ocular motor nerves: Neuroanatomic correlations of paradoxical innervation. Duane's syndrome. Am J Ophthalmol 60:43, 1965.

Huber A: Electrophysiology of the retraction syndrome. Br J Ophthalmol 58:298, 1974.

Kirkham TH: Inheritance of Duane's syndrome. Br J Ophthalmol 54:323, 1970a.

Kirkham TH: Anisometropia and amblyopia in Duane's syndrome. Am J Ophthalmol 69:774, 1970b.

Kirkham TH: Duane's retraction syndrome and cleft palate. Am J Ophthalmol 70:209, 1970c.

Lemire RJ, Loeser JD, Leech RW, Alvord EC: "Normal and Abnormal Development of the Human Nervous System." Hagerstown: Harper and Row, 1975, p 306.

Marotte LR, Mark RF: The mechanism of selective reinnervation of fish eye muscle. I. Evidence from muscle functions during recovery. Brain Res 19:41, 1970.

O'Malley ER, Helveston EM, Ellis FD: Duane's retraction syndrome — Plus. J Pediatr Ophthalmol and Strab 19:161, 1982.

Pfaffenbach DD, Cross HE, Kearns TP: Congenital anomalies in Duane's retraction syndrome. Arch Ophthalmol 88:635, 1972.

Poswillo D: Pathogenesis at the first and second branchial arch syndrome. Oral Surg 35:302, 1973.

Ramsay J, Taylor D: Congenital crocodile tears: A key to the aetiology of Duane's syndrome. Br J. Ophthalmol 64:518, 1980.

Regenbogen L, Stein R: Crocodile tears associated with homolateral Duane syndrome. Ophthalmologia 156:353, 1968.

Scott S: Persistence of foreign innervation in reinnervated goldfish extraocular muscles. Science 189:644, 1975.

Smith A: Duane's syndrome. Ophthalmol Sem 2:33, 1977.

Velez G: Duane's retraction syndrome associated with Goldenhar's syndrome. Am J Ophthalmol 70:945, 1970.

Wildervanck LS: Een cervico-oculo-acusticus syndroom. Ned T Geneesk 104:260, 1960.

Willshaw HE, Al-Ashkar F: The branchial arch syndromes. Trans Ophthalmol Soc UK 103:331, 1983.

Witzel SH: Congenital paralysis of lateral conjugate gaze. Occurrence in a case of Klippel-Feil syndrome. Arch Ophthalmol 59:463, 1959.

The Dubowitz Syndrome: A Retrospective

Karlind T. Moller and Robert J. Gorlin
Cleft Palate Maxillofacial Clinic, (K.T.M.) and Department of Oral Pathology and Genetics (R.J.G.), University of Minnesota, Minneapolis

> The purpose of the article is to update information concerning Dubowitz syndrome. A review of the literature since the disorder was originally described in 1965 is presented. In addition, case reports are presented for two siblings described in 1971 describing speech and dental development and current clinical findings. Analysis of approximately 30 cases reveals prevalence of growth failure and delayed bone age, mild microcephaly, broad forehead with sparse frontal hair, telecanthus, blepharophimosis, abnormal pinnae, broad nose, and micrognathia. Overt cleft palate or submucous cleft palate is not a prevalent finding (16%). High-pitched and hoarse voice quality appears to be a constant feature. There is the suggestion of an association with leukemia, lymphoma, and neuroblastoma. Inheritance appears clearly autosomal recessive.

Key words: Dubowitz syndrome, microcephaly, growth failure, micrognathia, syndrome, blepharophimosis, cleft palate, high-pitched voice, autosomal recessive

INTRODUCTION

Dubowitz, in 1965, described sibs with intrauterine growth retardation, primordial short stature, microcephaly, mild mental retardation, and unusual facies. One child had an eczematous rash involving the face and flexures of the knees and elbows, the other did not. In his discussion, Dubowitz indicated that he believed that the children had Bloom syndrome. A few years later, R. Gorlin, in Minneapolis, and J. Opitz and F. Grosse, then in Madison, reported a single affected child, affected siblings, and a follow-up of one of the living sibs reported by Dubowitz. They suggested that the disorder was distinct from Bloom syndrome, that it appeared to have autosomal recessive inheritance, and that it should be called Dubowitz syndrome [Grosse et al, 1971]. In 1973, Opitz et al [1973] documented six new cases including two sets of sibs and presented a follow-up of the cases described earlier. Additional case reports followed [Fryns et al, 1979; Majewski et al, 1975; Muller et al, 1978; Opitz et al, 1973; Orrison et al, 1980; Sauer and Spelger, 1977; Wilroy et al, 1978].

The phenotype is becoming well defined. Wilroy et al [1978] analyzed all cases reported through 1977 and presented eight new examples.[1] We have reviewed cases

---

[1] We are hesitant to accept case 8 of Wilroy et al [1978] as a valid example of the disorder.

Address reprint requests to Karlind T. Moller, PhD., Director, Cleft Palate Maxillofacial Clinic, University of Minnesota, 515 Delaware Street S.E., Minneapolis MN 55455.

© 1985 Alan R. Liss, Inc.

published since 1977 and have reexamined the sibs reported by us in 1971 [Grosse et al, 1971].

CASE REPORTS

The siblings described by Grosse et al [1971] have been followed periodically in our Cleft Palate Maxillofacial Clinic regarding development, speech, hearing, and dental concerns.

Case 1 (Fig. 1)

Sib 1, a female, currently 18 years of age, had micrognathia, high-arched palate, short stature, talipes equinovarus, receding forehead, and sparse hair when first seen at age 4. At puberty, mild scoliosis (36) was diagnosed and corrected. She is now a high school graduate and plans to enter college. Academic performance has been average to above average.

Speech/hearing history and current observations. At 5 years, speech and language skills were judged to be delayed. Speech was intelligible if the listener knew the topic. Resonance was within normal limits but was difficult to assess in the presence of extremely high pitch and weak intensity. Articulation was characterized by multiple and inconsistent errors including substitutions, distortions, and omissions. Several errors were typically developmental, being observed in children approximately 3–4 years of age. Speech therapy was carried out. Approximately 1 year later, intelligibility improved considerably. Extremely high pitch remained, with overall weak intensity. Submucous cleft palate and bifid uvula were evident, but the velopharyngeal closure mechanism was judged adequate for speech at that time. Otological examination revealed a past history of otitis, but hearing was within normal limits. Partial visualization of the larynx indicated mild hypoplasia with no paralysis evident.

At 14 years, speech was generally intelligible but weak in intensity. Pitch remained high and voice quality was mildly hoarse. Resonance distortion was judged to be hypernasal, mild to moderate in severity. At 15 years, repair of the submucous cleft palate and a pharyngeal flap were performed.

Currently, speech is readily intelligible although intensity remains weak. Pitch, resonance, and articulation are judged to be within acceptable limits.

Dental findings. At 14 years, there was Class II malocclusion, severe crowding in the mandibular anterior area, and multiple diastemata. Missing teeth included the second premolar in each quadrant. The maxillary second molars were horizontally positioned. Orthodontic treatment was initiated and current occlusion is functionally and esthetically satisfactory.

Current clinical findings. Height is 150 cm (59 in) (3%ile) and head circumference 51.4 cm (-1.5 SD). Interorbital radiographic and clinical measurements were normal.

Case 2 (Fig. 2)

Sib 2, currently 14 years old, is the younger male sib originally diagnosed at age 10 months. He had dysmorphic pinnae, micrognathia, epicanthus, high-arched palate, pilonidal dimple, sparse hair, hypospadias, cryptorchism, and everted feet. He is currently enrolled in a learning disability program.

Speech/hearing history and current observations. At 21 months, his parents reported a two-word vocabulary. There was neither hypernasality nor evidence of food or liquid regurgitation into the nose. Bouts of otitis media were frequent. Neither

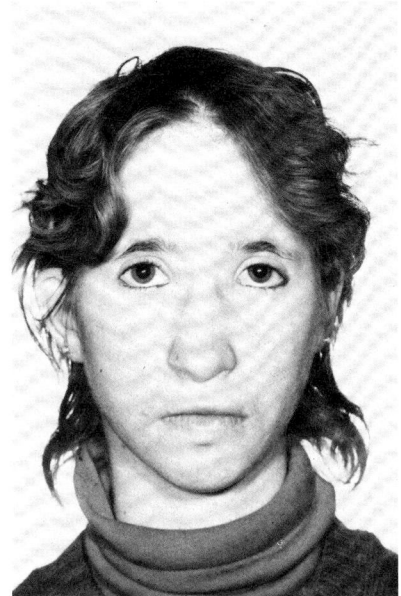

Fig. 1. Sib 1 at 18 years of age.

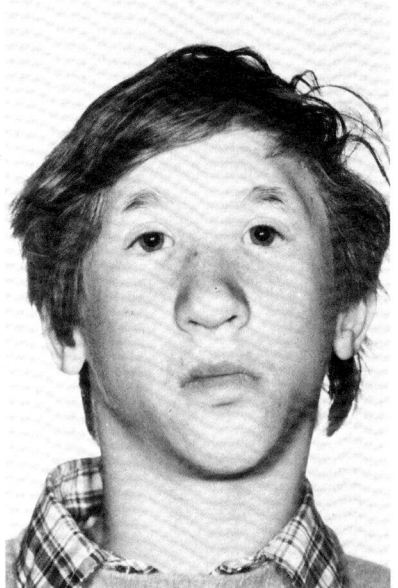

Fig. 2 Sib 2 at 14 years of age.

drainage nor hearing loss were evident at that time. At 10 years, speech was judged to be intelligible but there was hypernasal resonance distortion. Articulation was characterized by omission of medial and final consonants, distortions, and substitution of posterior sounds for more anterior sounds. Non-verbal performance (WISC-R) was normal but verbal performance was significantly reduced. He was enrolled in a special learning and behavior program. At 11 years, he was fitted with bilateral hearing aids and ventilating tubes were inserted. Oral pharyngeal examination showed bifid uvula and submucous cleft palate. The palate was repaired and a pharyngeal flap was performed at age 13. Current observations indicate mild to moderate hypernasality, sibilant distortions, inconsistent omission of final consonants, and harsh voice quality. A mild rising hearing loss in both ears was noted. Middle ear fluid was observed on otological examination.

Dental observations. At age 10, the two maxillary second molars were missing radiographically. There was hypoplasia of the maxilla and mandible and considerable anterior crowding in the lower arch. Full orthodontic treatment was initiated at age 12. Current observations indicate very acceptable occlusion.

Current clinical findings

Height is 148 cm (58 in) (3%ile) and head circumference is 50 cm. (-3 SD). Radiographic and clinical measurements indicate normal interorbital distance.

DISCUSSION

Analysis of the phenotype based on approximately 30 cases suggests that birth weight is about 2.25 kg and birth length approximately 45 cm. Prenatal growth failure has been evident in about 60% of all cases. Head circumference averages 30 cm at term. This persists and, in all cases, there is mild microcephaly, the degree of which is not correlated with mental retardation.

About one-third are poor feeders during infancy. About 35% also manifest frequent vomiting and chronic diarrhea. Motor milestones such as sitting and walking are reached at normal times. Evaluation of ten patients showed that while there is significant mental retardation in about 35%, most children were estimated to be in the dull normal range [Parrish and Wilroy, 1980]. Hyperactivity was manifested by approximately 40% [Parrish and Wilroy, 1980].

The more constant craniofacial features include microcephaly (100%), broad forehead with sparse frontal hair (90%), telecanthus (95%), ptosis/blepharophimosis (60%), abnormal pinnae (95%), broad nose (100%), and micrognathia (95%). Cleft palate and/or bifid uvula were found in only two patients and submucous cleft palate in three [Grosse et al, 1971; Opitz et al, 1973; Wilroy et al, 1978]. A high-pitched, hoarse voice is a constant feature.

Delayed bone age has been found in all cases.

Hypospadias and/or cryptorchoridism were found in about one-third of affected males. Eczema, originally included among the important stigmata, is mild but has been noted in about 65%. Variable minor soft tissue syndactyly of the toes has been documented in 40%.

Of considerable interest are reports that suggest an association with leukemia [Grobe, 1983], lymphoma [Sauer and Spelger, 1977], and neuroblastoma [Sauer and Spelger, 1977]. While there has been some suggestion that these patients have an immune defect, its precise nature has not been defined [Grosse et al, 1971; Majewski et al, 1975; Opitz et al, 1973; Sauer and Spelger, 1977]. Sauer and Spelger [1977] noted hypogammaglobulinemia in one sib and immunoglobulin A deficiency in another. However, both of these children had malignancies. [Dubowitz, 1965; Grosse et al, 1971; Opitz et al, 1973; Sauer and Spelger, 1977; Wilroy et al, 1978].

Affected sibs and identical twins [Wilroy et al, 1978] have been described by several authors, and consanguinity has been documented in at least one instance [Majewski et al, 1975]. An equal number of males and females have been affected. Inheritance is clearly autosomal recessive.

REFERENCES

Dubowitz V: Familial low birth weight dwarfism with an unusual facies and a skin eruption. J Med Genet 2:12–17, 1965.

Fryns JP, Fabry G, Willemyns F, van den Berghe H: The Dubowitz syndrome in a teenager. Am J Med Genet 4:345–347, 1979.

Grobe H: Dubowitz-Syndrom und akute lymphatische Leukämie. Mschr Kinderheilk 131:467–468, 1983.

Grosse R, Gorlin RJ, Opitz JM: The Dubowitz syndrome. Z Kinderheilk 110:175–187, 1971.

Majewski F, Michaelis R, Moosmann K, Biebrich JR: A rare type of low birth weight dwarfism: The Dubowitz syndrome. Z Kinderheilk 120:283–292, 1975.

Muller W, Frisch H, Gassner I, Kofler J: Seckel-Syndrom. Mschr Kinderheilk 126:454–456, 1978.

Opitz JM, Pfeiffer RA, Herrmann RPR, Kushnick T: The Dubowitz syndrome. Z Kinderheilk 115:1–12, 1973.

Orrison WW, Schnitzler ER, Chun RWM: The Dubowitz syndrome: Further observations. Am J Med Genet 7:155–170, 1980.

Parrish JM, Wilroy RS Jr: The Dubowitz syndrome: The psychological status of ten cases at follow-up. Am J Med Genet 6:3–8, 1980.

Sauer O, Spelger G: Dubowitz-Syndrom mit Immunodefizienz und malignem Neoplasma bei zwei Geschwistern. Mschr Kinderheilk 125:885–887, 1977.

Wilroy RS Jr, Tipton RE, Summitt RL: The Dubowitz syndrome. Am J Med Genet 2:275–284, 1978.

Hemifacial Microsomia and the Branchio-Oto-Renal Syndrome

Beverly R. Rollnick and Celia I. Kaye

Center for Craniofacial Anomalies, University of Illinois College of Medicine, Chicago (B.R.R., C.I.K.), and Lutheran General Hospital, Park Ridge, (C.I.K.), Illinois

Hemifacial microsomia (HFM) and the branchio-oto-renal syndrome (BOR) are both associated with malformations of the external ears; preauricular tags, pits, or sinuses; and conductive or mixed hearing loss. Other overlapping features have been described, including cervical appendages containing cartilage in HFM, and facial paresis in BOR; however, the significance of these findings has not been discussed by previous authors.

The purpose of this paper is to describe four additional propositi with overlapping features of BOR and HFM. In two cases there is a positive family history of either first and second branchial arch anomalies or malformation of the kidney. Two cases appear to be sporadic. The overlapping clinical features suggest that in some families HFM may constitute a component toward the severe end of the spectrum of the autosomal dominant BOR syndrome. The empiric recurrence risk for HFM was 3% in one study. If our interpretation of these reported cases is correct, genetic recurrence risks for individuals in these families may fall in the range of an autosomal dominant condition. Since expression of both conditions varies widely, and minor manifestations may be overlooked, the importance of careful evaluation of first- and second-degree relatives is emphasized.

Key words: hemifacial microsomia, branchio-oto-renal syndrome, BOR syndrome, genetic counseling, branchial cleft cartilage, branchial cleft sinuses/fistulas, preauricular pits/sinuses, microtia

INTRODUCTION

Differentiation between ear malformation syndromes with similar phenotypes can be difficult, especially if the propositus and family members exhibit variable expression of the condition. The purpose of this paper is to describe four propositi with overlapping clinical features of hemifacial microsomia (HFM) and the branchio-oto-renal syndrome (BOR) and to discuss the significance of these findings for purposes of genetic counseling.

The autosomal dominant BOR syndrome is associated with external ear malformations that include microtia, other structural defects of the pinna, preauricular appendages, and preauricular pits or sinuses. Other features of the syndrome include mixed hearing loss, branchial cleft fistulas, cysts, and/or cartilage, structural or

---

Address reprint requests to Beverly R. Rollnick, Center for Craniofacial Anomalies, University of Illinois College of Medicine, P.O. Box 6998, Chicago, IL 60680.

© 1985 Alan R. Liss, Inc.

functional renal anomalies, and aplasia of the lacrimal ducts. Expression varies widely. For the purposes of this paper, no distinction is made between the BO (*branchial* cleft and *otologic* anomalies) and BOR syndromes. External ear malformations associated with HFM also include microtia, preauricular appendages, and preauricular pits. Other features of the condition include conductive hearing loss, mandibular hypoplasia, facial paresis, epibulbar dermoids or conjunctival lipodermoids, and anomalies of the cervical spine. For the purposes of this paper we are treating HFM, Goldenhar syndrome, and oculoauriculovertebral dysplasia as a single entity on a spectrum of severity. A wide range of other anomalies may also be present in some individuals, suggesting phenotypic and etiologic heterogeneity. Some cases of HFM are familial, but the mode(s) of inheritance requires clarification [Rollnick and Kaye, 1983].

In addition to similar external ear malformations in BOR and HFM, there are other overlapping features. Gorlin et al [1976] and Smith [1982] illustrated cervical appendages containing cartilage in two individuals with HFM. Fraser [1978] noted facial paresis associated with the BOR syndrome. As an example of the BOR syndrome, Melnick [1976] cites Bourguet's family, in which the mother and her six offspring had branchial arch anomalies, hearing loss, and facial paresis.

We now present four additional propositi with overlapping features of HFM and BOR. These individuals were identified from 288 patients with HFM-Goldenhar-oculoauriculovertebral dysplasia at the Center for Craniofacial Anomalies—Illinois (CCFA).

CASE REPORTS
Case 1

Case 1 (CCFA# 6032), a Caucasian female, was seen at the age of 4 months with a left grade III microtia and preauricular pit, a right preauricular pit, a left grade I

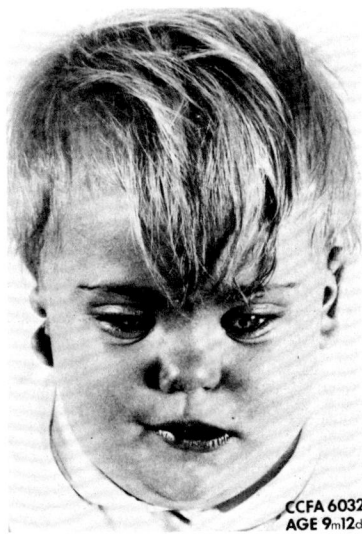

Fig. 1. Case 1, CCFA# 6032, a Caucasian female with left grade 1 mandibular hypoplasia.

mandibular hypoplasia, and a left maximal conductive hearing loss (Fig. 1,2). Height, weight, and head circumference were between the 50th and 75th percentile for age. There were no other physical or developmental abnormalities. The pedigree for the family is shown in Figure 3.

Case 1a (CCFA# 6144; pedigree# III-5), the male sibling of case 1, exhibited bilateral preauricular pits on the anterior helices (Fig. 4). Intraoral examination was normal as were cephalometric x-rays. Audiometry revealed normal hearing sensitivity.

Case 1b (CCFA# 6145; pedigree# II-6), the mother of case 1 and case 1a, had bilateral pits on the anterior margins of the helices and a discharging left branchial cleft sinus (Fig. 5). Hearing sensitivity was normal. In addition, the left mandibular ramus was discovered to be 4 mm shorter than the right on lateral cephalometric x-rays (Fig. 6).

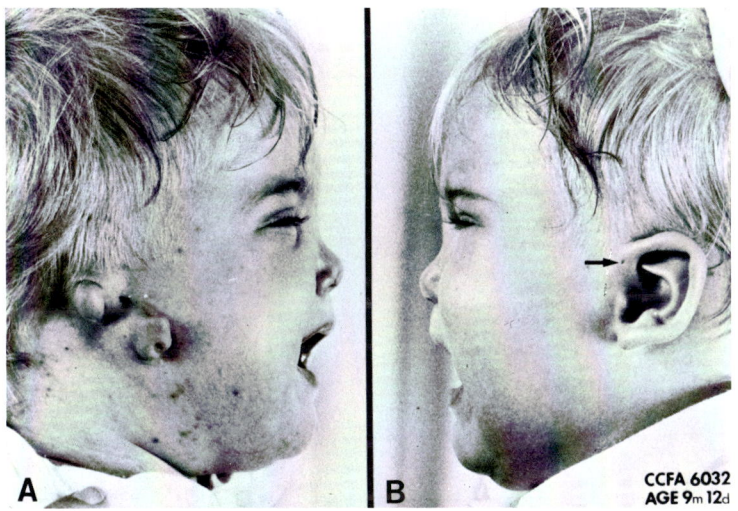

Fig. 2. Case 1, CCFA# 6032, illustrating (A) left grade III microtia and preauricular pit and (B) a right preauricular pit (arrow).

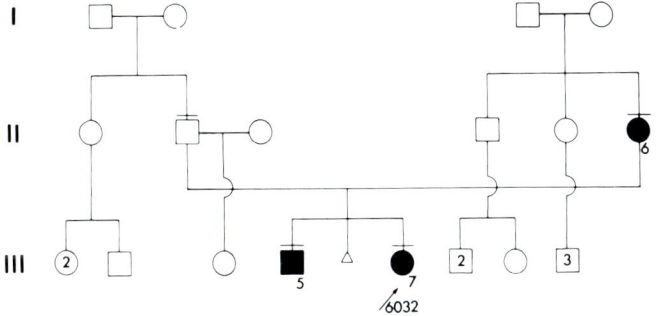

Fig. 3. Pedigree for case 1, CCFA# 6032.
↗, proband, CCFA# 6032; □,○, unaffected male, female; ■̄,○̄, examined by staff; ②,②, 2 males, females; ■,●, affected male, female; △, spontaneous abortion; II-6 bilateral preauricular pits, left branchial cleft sinus, left mandibular ramus shorter than right; III-5 bilateral preauricular pits; III-7 left Gr III microtia, left Gr I mandible, bilateral preauricular pits.

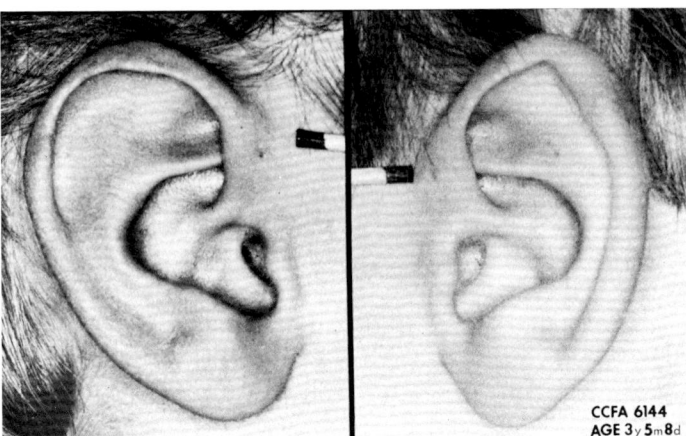

Fig. 4. Case 1a, CCFA# 6144, the Caucasian male sibling of Case 1 (CCFA# 6032) illustrating bilateral preauricular pits on the anterior helices.

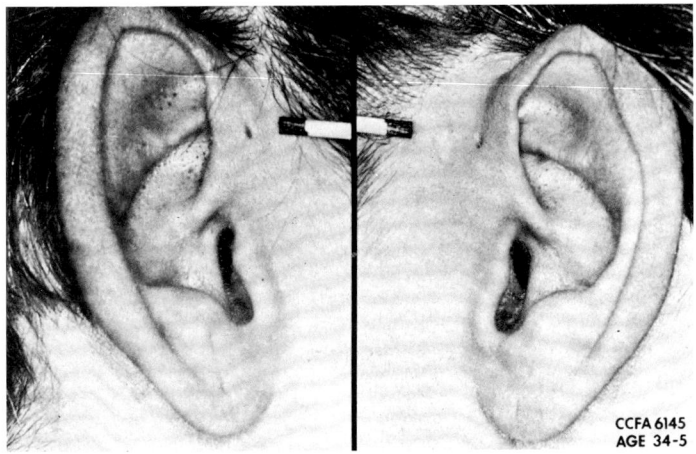

Fig. 5. Case 1b, CCFA# 6145, the Caucasian mother of Case 1 and 1a, illustrating bilateral pits on the anterior margins of the helices.

Case 2

Case 2 (CCFA# 5194), a Caucasian male, exhibited a left grade III microtia with agenesis of the external auditory canal, left grade II mandibular hypoplasia, and left macrostomia. The mandible deviated to the left during function. There was persistent branchial cartilage and an epidermal tag in the left cervical region (Fig. 7). Intraoral examination revealed soft palatal elevation to the right side only during phonation. Height, weight, and head circumference were of approximately the 97th percentile for age. Audiometry demonstrated bilateral conductive hearing loss. Cephalometric x-rays showed retrognathia with asymmetry of the mandibular borders. The left mastoid was less developed than the right. Intravenous pyelography was normal in infancy. Temporal bone tomography revealed inner ear structures to be unremarkable. There was agenesis of the left external auditory canal with a bony plate in the lateral

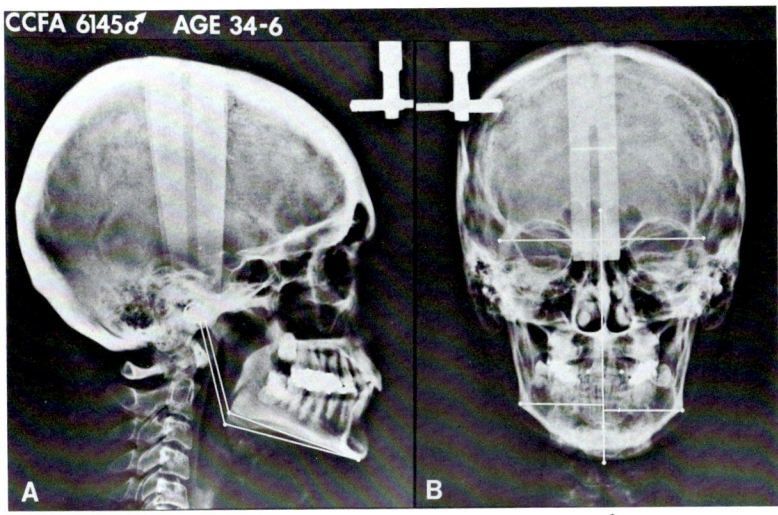

Fig. 6. Lateral (A) and A-P (B) cephalometric x-rays of case 1b (CCFA# 6145) showing the left mandibular ramus to be 4 mm shorter than the right.

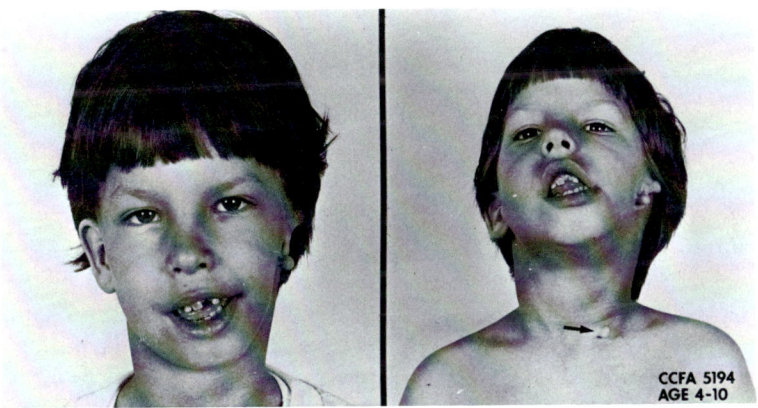

Fig. 7. Case 2, CCFA# 5194, a Caucasian male with left grade III microtia, left grade II mandibular hypoplasia, and persistent branchial cartilage (arrow) in the left cervical region.

wall of the middle ear cavity. The tympanic cavity was hypoplastic, but the antrum was nearly normal in size. The mastoid antrum was small and partially aerated. The ossicular mass was fused and fixed to the atretic plate. The pedigree for this family is shown in Figure 8.

Case 2a (pedigree# II-2), the father of case 2, had an ectopic left kidney detected on intravenous pyelography. The ears were of normal shape and there was no hearing loss.

Case 3

Case 3 (CCFA# 6431), a Caucasian male, presented in the first year of life with bilateral incomplete cleft lip, a left cleft of the secondary palate, a left grade II

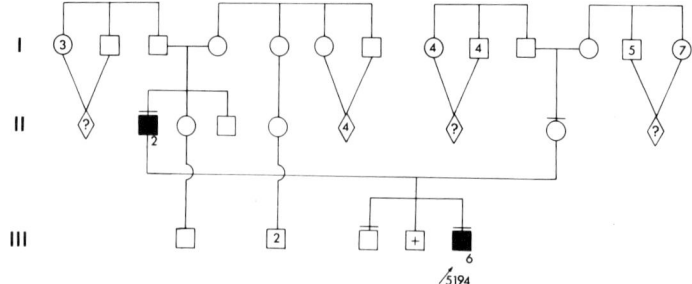

Fig. 8. Pedigree for case 2, CCFA# 5194.
↗, proband, CCFA# 5194; □,○, unaffected male, female; ②,③, 2 males, 3 females; ⊞, male, deceased; ◇, unknown number of males, females; ☐,○̄, male, female, examined by staff; ■, affected male; II-2 ectopic kidney; III-6 bilateral microtia, mandibular hypoplasia, branchial cleft cartilage.

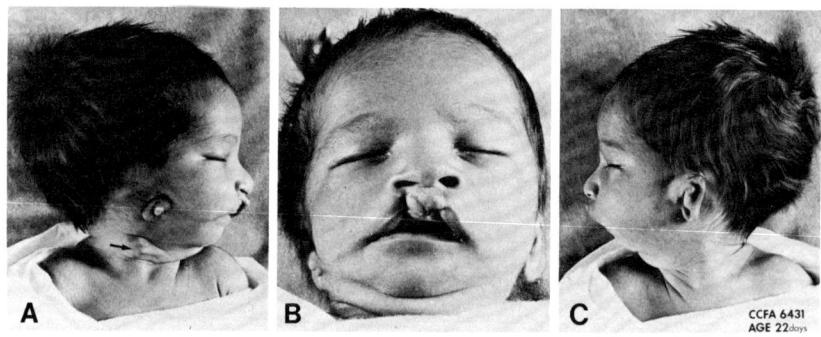

Fig. 9. Case 3, CCFA# 6431, a Caucasian male with (A) a left cervical cartilaginous appendage (arrow), (B) bilateral incomplete cleft lip, and (C) bilateral grade II microtia and hypoplastic left mandible.

microtia with a lowset and atretic canal, and a right grade II microtia with an abortive canal. The left mandible was hypoplastic, and there was a left cervical cartilaginous appendage (Fig. 9). Height and weight were below the 3rd percentile for age. The head circumference was at the 50th percentile for age. There were no other physical abnormalities except a grade II/VI harsh midsystolic ejection heart murmur. Echocardiogram was normal. The chromosomes were 46, XY normal. Audiometry revealed a moderate bilateral conductive hearing loss. At the age of 15 months, the Bayley Scale indicated a mental developmental index of 67, consistent with a 4–5-month delay. Family history was negative. The mother was found to have no anomalies on physical examination by CCFA staff.

Case 4

Case 4 (CCFA# 6451), a Caucasian female, exhibited bilateral microtia, hypoplasia of the left mandible, bilateral preauricular tags, and a right cervical fistula (Fig. 10). The left external auditory canal was absent, and there was maximum conductive hearing loss of the left ear. Speech evaluation revealed moderate to severe articulatory and vocal abnormalities at the age of 3 years. A bifid uvula was present. An intravenous pyelogram was normal. Growth parameters were at the 25th percentile for age. Family history was negative by report.

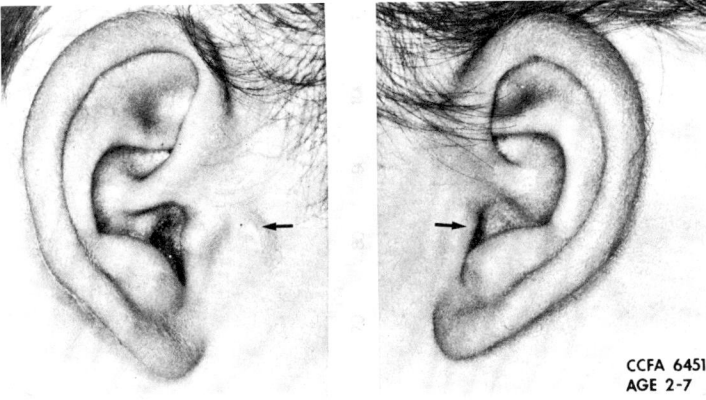

Fig. 10. Case 4, CCFA# 6451, bilateral preauricular tags in a Caucasian female.

DISCUSSION

Several factors complicate the process of distinguishing between HFM and BOR; for example, the overlapping branchial arch anomalies, some common elements in embryogenesis, and widely varying clinical expression. The overlapping features of HFM and BOR include malformed auricles, preauricular appendages and/or pits, hearing loss, and branchial cleft cartilage [Smith, 1982; Gorlin et al, 1976]. Facial paresis may also be a feature of both conditions [Fraser, 1978; Melnick, 1976]. Clinical expression of both disorders varies widely, and affected individuals may manifest only minor features such as preauricular pits.

Minor ear malformations occur relatively frequently in the general population. For example, preauricular tags occur in 0.2% of live births; branchial cleft sinuses in 0.02%; and preauricular pits or sinuses in 0.8%. Nonsyndromic preauricular pits or sinuses occur approximately 8½ times more frequently in blacks than in whites. The other ear malformations occur with equal frequency in both races [Melnick, 1980]. Therefore, an isolated minor ear anomaly in a first-degree relative of a patient with an ear malformation syndrome may be difficult to interpret, since the finding may be either syndromic or nonsyndromic and not associated with the patient's condition.

We have observed four propositi with features of both HFM and BOR, including preauricular pits, branchial cleft fistulas, and branchial cleft cartilage. Gorlin et al [1976] and Smith [1982] described two individuals with HFM who had branchial cleft cartilage, a common finding in the BOR syndrome. To our knowledge, there are no data on the frequency of this finding in patients with HFM. Fraser [1978] and Melnick [1976] reported facial paresis in association with the BOR syndrome. Facial paresis is a frequent manifestation of HFM. We know of no data on the frequency of this finding in patients with the BOR syndrome. These overlapping features suggest that in some families HFM may constitute a component toward the severe end of the spectrum of the BOR syndrome. Support for this hypothesis is provided by the two positive family histories reported here (cases 1 and 2).

In case 1, the Caucasian propositus has the HFM phenotype (microtia and mandibular hypoplasia) combined with bilateral preauricular pits. Her mother manifests bilateral preauricular pits, a draining branchial cleft sinus, and a 4-mm discrepancy in the lengths of the ramii. Her brother manifests bilateral preauricular pits. Renal studies were recommended but not completed. Our interpretation of these findings is that the members of this family exhibit variable expression of the same autosomal dominant condition, possibly the BOR syndrome. One alternative explanation is that the propositus has both HFM (microtia and mandibular hypoplasia) and BOR (bilateral preauricular pits), and her mother and brother have the BOR syndrome. Since this explanation requires that the patient be affected with two separate disorders of the branchial arch system, it is less plausible to us. A second alternative explanation is that the branchial arch anomalies exhibited by the propositus are unrelated to those exhibited by her mother and brother. Because these anomalies are embryologically related, this explanation also does not seem plausible to us.

In case 2, the Caucasian propositus has the HFM phenotype with bilateral microtia and mandibular hypoplasia, combined with branchial cleft cartilage and an epidermal tag on the neck. An intravenous pyelogram (IVP) in infancy revealed no renal anomalies. An IVP on the father of the propositus revealed an ectopic kidney. This individual has no malformations of the external ear or hearing loss. For the reasons cited above, our interpretation is that the anomalies in this father and son may be etiologically related and constitute manifestations of BOR. Alternatively, the propositus may be affected with HFM in association with branchial cleft cartilage, and his father's renal anomaly may be an unrelated finding.

Two of our propositi have no known positive family history and may represent sporadic cases; however, renal studies and audiograms were not done on family members. These two individuals have overlapping features of HFM and BOR, including branchial cleft cartilage (case 3) and a branchial cleft fistula (case 4).

Many authors report that most cases of HFM are sporadic with low recurrence risks, although pedigrees consistent with autosomal dominant and autosomal recessive transmission have been recorded. The complex is also seen in association with numerous chromosomal malformation syndromes. Etiologic heterogeneity in HFM has been reviewed by Rollnick and Kaye [1983]. While attention has been called to minor manifestations of the condition, such as preauricular appendages and pits, in first- and second-degree relatives, there are few systematic family studies. Many case studies of HFM do not report either the presence or absence of minor manifestations in close relatives. Therefore, such manifestations may have gone undetected. In one large study of 97 pedigrees [Rollnick and Kaye, 1983], members of four families were found to have positive histories of preauricular pits in the absence of other anomalies of the branchial arches. The propositi all had HFM. In one Caucasian family, paternal first-, second-, and third-degree relatives had isolated preauricular pits. In one Caucasian family, a first-degree relative had a preauricular pit. In one black family, two second-degree relatives and one third-degree relative had preauricular pits. In one family the Caucasian propositus and his mother had HFM; the maternal grandmother had a preauricular pit. In all, 8% of the first-degree relatives (35/433) and 6% (11/176) of sibs were found to have manifestations of HFM. The empiric recurrence risk was 3%. The pattern (s) of inheritance requires clarification, and both etiologic and phenotypic heterogeneity are likely.

In contrast, the BOR syndrome is an autosomal dominant condition with a recurrence risk of 50% for individuals who carry the gene. If there is an association between the HFM phenotype and the BOR syndrome in some families, then genetic counseling for recurrence risks for HFM would be significantly different. These risks may be as high as 50%. Since expression of both conditions varies widely, and minor manifestations may be overlooked, the importance of careful evaluation of first- and second-degree relatives is emphasized. In this way additional data could be obtained to refute or lend support to our interpretation.

ACKNOWLEDGMENTS

The authors thank Drs. Alvaro Figueroa and Hans Friede for cephalometric analysis and Joann Darrow for typing the manuscript.

This work was supported in part by grants from the National Institutes of Health (DE 02872) and Maternal and Child Health Services, Department of Health and Human Services.

REFERENCES

Fraser FC, Ling D, Clogg D, Nogrady B: Genetic aspects of the BOR syndrome-branchial fistulas, ear pits, hearing loss, and renal anomalies. Am J Med Genet 2:241–252, 1978.

Gorlin RJ, Pindborg JJ, Cohen MM Jr: "Syndromes of the Head and Neck," 2nd ed. New York: McGraw Hill Book Co., 1976, pp 546–552.

Melnick M, Bixler I, Nance WE, Silk K, Yune H: Familial branchio-oto-renal dysplasia: A new addition to the branchial arch syndromes. Clin Genet 9:25–34, 1976.

Melnick M: The etiology of external ear malformations and its relation to abnormalities of the middle ear, inner ear, and other organ systems. Birth Defects-OAS, XVI (4): 303–331, 1980.

Rollnick BR, Kaye CI: Hemifacial microsomia and variants: Pedigree data. Am J Med Genet 15:233–253, 1983.

Smith: "Recognizable Patterns of Human Malformation," 3rd ed. Philadelphia: W.B. Saunders Co., 1982, pp 497–500.

VI. EXPERIMENTAL ANIMAL STUDIES

The Significance of Receptor Physiology for Corticosterone-Induced Cleft Palate in A/J Mice

Kenneth S. Brown and Robert M. Hackman

Laboratory of Developmental Biology and Anomalies, National Institute of Dental Research, National Institutes of Health, Bethesda, Maryland

Mean plasma corticosterone levels of A/J mice rise from nonpregnant levels of 20.4 μg% to 40.6 μg% on day 11 and 167.11 μg% on day 14 of pregnancy. These changes in mean steroid levels are associated with proportionally increased diurnal swings. This suggests that the control mechanisms for diurnal swings respond in a proportional, rather than an absolute, way in regulating plasma hormone levels. Large diurnal hormone swings may be teratogenic or facilitate teratogenesis. The rules of receptor physiology may have wide application to the understanding of teratogenic risk.

Key words: Cleft palate, corticosterone, receptor physiology, animal teratogens, mice, glucocorticoid

INTRODUCTION

Plasma glucocorticoid levels exhibit diurnal fluctuation [Haus and Halberg, 1970]. The mechanism of control for this rhythmic change and the sensory system that monitors the levels are unknown. Data presented here suggest that the control system for diurnal hormone fluctuation shares a basic physiological feature with many other receptor-mediated sensory systems. If this is true, the control system properties may be important in understanding teratogenesis.

Many of the external sensory systems, ie, vision, hearing, touch, taste, and smell respond with decreasing sensitivity as the basal level of stimulus is increased. When stimulus levels are high, large changes of stimulus are required to elicit responses that are elicited by small changes when the stimulus levels are lower [Brown, 1973]. For example, a subject trying to maintain a constant sound intensity will allow greater fluctuations of a loud sound than of a soft sound.

Data from studies reported here indicate that the amplitude of the diurnal changes in plasma levels of corticosterone, the major glucocorticoid of rodents, in A/J mice, shows a similar relationship to the mean plasma level. When the mean for the 24-

---

Robert M. Hackman, PhD, is now at the College of Human Development and Performance, University of Oregon, Eugene, OR 97403.

Address reprint requests to Kenneth S. Brown, M.D., Laboratory of Developmental Biology and Anomalies, National Institute of Dental Research, National Institutes of Health, Building 30, Room 414, Bethesda, MD 20205.

© 1985 Alan R. Liss, Inc.

hour period is low, the diurnal variation is low, and when the mean plasma level is high, large diurnal swings occur. This suggests that the sensory system for diurnal responses to serum corticoid levels is similar in response pattern to other senses.

The objectives of this study were to determine and compare the magnitude and duration of changes in plasma corticosterone levels in A/J mice, a strain known to be sensitive to the teratogenic effect of exogenous glucocorticoids, during pregnancy and to determine whether changes in diurnal pattern occur as a result of changes in physiological state during gestation. Such data are needed to evaluate adequately the teratogenic effects of exogenous glucocorticoids during pregnancy.

MATERIALS AND METHODS

Plasma corticosterone levels were analyzed from samples collected at intervals over a 24-hour period in nonpregnant A/J females and from pregnant females on the 11th and 14th day after the observation of a vaginal plug (plug day 0). All females were caged in groups of six or less in an artificially lighted air-conditioned colony with clock regulated light on from 6:00 A.M. to 6:00 P.M. with food and water ad libitum.

Pregnant females were bled on the 11th or 14th day of gestation at either 10:00 A.M., 2:00 P.M., 6:00 P.M., 10:00 P.M., or 10:00 A.M. of the following day. Nonpregnant females were bled at the same time along with each group. Bleeding was done by suborbital puncture with a heparinized capillary tube. No more than 280 μl of blood was drawn from each animal. Each bleeding was completed within 3 minutes from the time the lid was removed from the cage in order to prevent elevation of plasma corticosterone levels owing to handling or stress [Gross et al, 1972]. Blood samples were centrifuged, and the plasma was separated and frozen until day of assay. Corticosterone was determined by radioimmunoassay [Gross et al, 1972], and individual values were calculated by a computer program [Rodbard and Frazier, 1973], as micrograms percent (micrograms of corticosterone per 100 ml of plasma).

RESULTS

Figure 1 shows the values of corticosterone for a 24-hour period in nonpregnant and in pregnant day 11 and day 14 mice. The y-axis is scaled in $\log_{10} \mu g$ in order to normalize the variation within time groups and for spatial convenience. The mean value for all plasma samples on nonpregnant animals was 20 μg% (N = 90; SD, 12.6). The range of means at each time was 9.7 μg%, and the diurnal pattern was similar to those reported for other mice and rats [Cheifetz, 1971, Ader et al, 1967].

On day 11 of pregnancy the 24-hour plasma mean was 40.6 μg% (N = 38; SD, 21.7) and the range was 24 μg% between 10:00 A.M. and 10:00 P.M. with the level at 10:00 A.M. on day 12 significantly higher than that at 10:00 A.M. on day 11. On day 14 the mean for 24 hours was 167 μg% (N = 33, SD, 89.4) with a range of 106 μg% between 10:00 A.M. and 10:00 P.M. of day 14 and 148 μg% between 10:00 P.M. day 14 and 10:00 A.M. day 15.

Although large changes in mean plasma corticosterone levels occurring between day 10 and 14 of gestation [Barlow et al, 1974] complicate the diurnal cycle, the ratios of the mean to the standard deviation and Figure 1 show that the range of diurnal

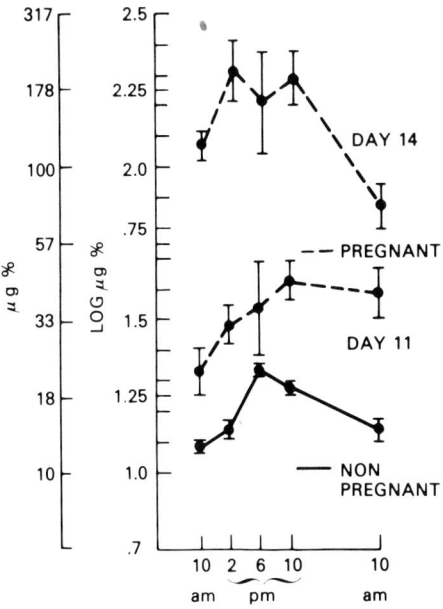

Fig. 1. Diurnal and secular changes in serum corticosterone levels of A/J mice during days 11 and 14 of gestation compared to changes in nonpregnant female A/J as plotted on a log scale. Bars are ± 2 standard errors of the mean log (μg/100 ml) from at least six individuals at each time. The linear scale is provided for reference.

variation increased proportionally with the 24-hour mean and roughly maintained the pattern of the nonpregnant diurnal cycle. The rapid rise in plasma corticosterone during day 11, previously reported [Barlow et al, 1974], accounts for the skewing of the diurnal pattern on that day. However, considering the deviation of the 10:00 A.M. point, there is still an increase in diurnal range over the nonpregnant value.

DISCUSSION

The two models of interaction between secular changes and diurnal changes (Fig. 2) have very different implications for the range of individual levels over any specific time. The data in Figure 1 seem to support the proportional model, which is based on standard receptor physiology [Brown, 1973]. This is in agreement with current biochemical evidence that suggests that glucocorticoids function physiologically, in part, by interaction with specific receptor proteins, and that glucocorticoids modify cell surface receptors for epidermal growth factor and insulin [Pratt et al, 1980]. Further, it has been shown that more glucocorticoid is bound to tissues in sensitive A/J than in resistant C57BL/6J fetuses [Pratt et al, 1981].

Treatment of pregnant mice with exogenous glucocorticoids during days 11 to 14 of pregnancy increases the rate of cleft palate in fetuses of several strains of mice [Kalter, 1965]. External maternal stimuli such as restraint [Rosenzweig and Blaustein, 1970; Barlow et al, 1975], water deprivation [Brown et al, 1974], and shipping [Brown et al, 1972] increase the rate of cleft palate in A/J. The implications of the

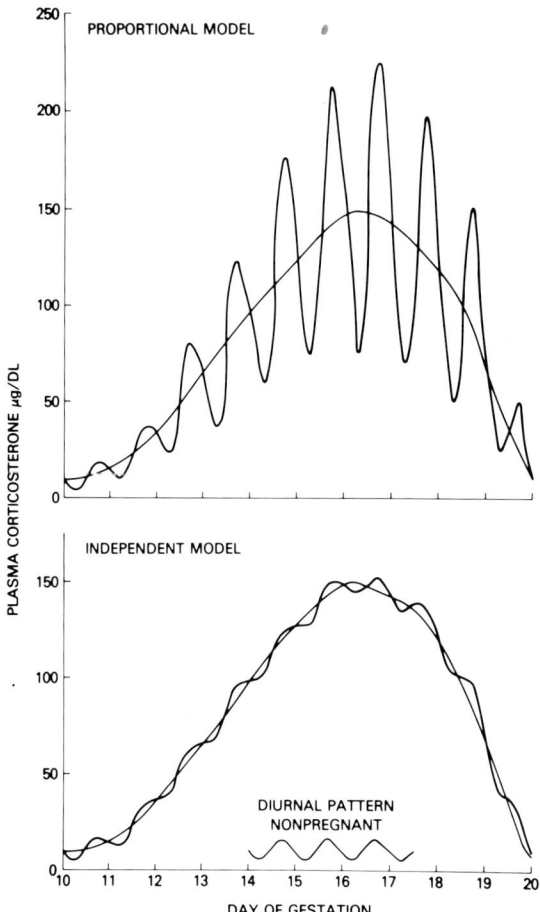

Fig. 2. Graphical representations of the expected plasma corticosterone concentration in μg/DL (mg%) using the pattern of daily mean changes reported by Barlow et al [1974] and the diurnal variation reported here. In the proportional model the diurnal variation amplitude maintains a constant proportion to the mean, while in the independent model the diurnal variation maintains a constant absolute range about the mean. The mean changes are similar for the two models that are plotted on a linear scale.

wide diurnal fluctuations in plasma corticosterone levels reported here for potential exposure of the fetus to very large and variable hormone concentrations may explain some of the intralitter variability. Also, the recognized relative retardation of development in A/J [Trasler, 1965] exposes morphologically younger fetuses that may be more susceptible to teratogenic effects to the higher glucocorticoid levels occurring after day 11 of pregnancy. The amplitude of diurnal plasma hormone variations may be one of the maternal factors that are recognized [Fraser et al, 1954; Kalter, 1954; Loevy, 1963] to be involved in the inheritance of susceptibility to malformation by glucocorticoids.

The diurnal peak levels observed here are similar to those reported for chronic stress [Barlow et al, 1975]. Chronic stress appears to cause suppression of the cycle with maintenance of peak levels for many hours [Barlow et al, 1975]. Thus, the effect of stress as a teratogen, and also the effect of exogenous glucocorticoid, may be through the prolongation of normal peak levels for long periods rather than through the very high acute levels.

All chemoreceptors that have been studied obey the Weber-Fechner "law" [Brown, 1973]. However, physiological conditions in the internal milieu suitable to test internal chemoreception responses—namely, that basal levels change over a wide range and there is secondary variation due to other stimuli—are unusual. The occurrence of large basal hormone level changes in pregnancy and the diurnal fluctuation of the same hormones owing to independent stimuli are relatively unique. These results indicate that the endocrine control of corticosterone plasma levels might exhibit similar physiological control mechanisms as have been found for external chemoreceptors.

Diurnal changes in the fetal growth of Wistar rats have been reported [Barr, 1973]. The mean dry weight of fetuses increased only half as much from 9:00 A.M. to 9:00 P.M. as it did from 9:00 P.M. to 9:00 A.M. during the last 3 days of gestation. The hours of decreased growth are thus associated with increased maternal glucocorticoid levels.

The glucocorticoid inhibition of RNA and protein synthesis in whole embryos and the sensitivity to induction of cleft palate in embryos by glucocorticoids are at a maximum on days 11 and 12 of gestation [Andrew et al, 1973]. These responses are greater in A/J than in C3H, a strain less sensitive to glucocorticoid-induced cleft palate [Andrew et al, 1973]. The quantity of receptor for glucocorticoid in fetal jaws has been shown to be correlated with the incidence of cleft palate after maternal hormone treatment in several mouse strains [Goldman et al, 1977]. The maxiumum difference between amounts of receptors in embryos of the sensitive A/J and resistant C57/BL/6J strain occurs on day 12 [Salomon et al, 1978].

The interaction between timing of the appearance of specific receptors in embryonic tissues and the timing of the increase of hormone in maternal plasma may be a factor in determining susceptibility to corticoid-induced defects. When plasma levels are high and receptors are present at an early stage of embryonic development, the potential for teratogenesis is maximized. Our observations suggest that large and variable diurnal swings may have an inherent teratogenic impact on genetically sensitive fetuses and facilitate anomaly production by exogenous agents.

The mechanisms by which regulation of serum levels of hormones and many other developmentally and teratogenically significant molecules is accomplished in most cases involves specific receptors. This is also true for the P450 system of xenobiotic metabolizing enzymes [Nebert and Bigelow, 1982]. The general significance of the rules of receptor physiology that apply to such systems for the teratogenic potential of agents that are active through specific receptors has not been considered.

The general implications of the decrease in regulatory sensitivity as a function of increase in level of general adaptation is that a much larger increase in a teratogenic metabolite or xenobiotic can exist before maternal regulation occurs when the mother is adapted to a high baseline level than when the maternal baseline is low. In the case of a toxic pollutant, for example, if the level is generally low, a small increase will be detected and maternal regulatory processes will occur, but if the general level is higher, there will be a decrease in sensitivity to an increase, and higher levels can occur before maternal regulatory mechanisms will modify them. Since this relation is a logarithmic one, the unregulated increases can be relatively great and might, at a critical period, pass some teratogenic threshold that would not have been exceeded had the lower base level and its greater regulatory sensitivity been present in the mother. This type of mechanism may be a component of "maternal effects," both genetic, with regard to the maternal regulatory system, and environmental, with regard to maternal exposures.

REFERENCES

Ader R, Friedman SB, Grota LI: "Emotionality" and adrenal function: Effects of strain, tests and the 24-hour corticosterone rhythm. Anim Behav 15:37–44, 1967.

Andrew FD, Bowen D, Zimmerman EF: Glucocorticoid inhibition of RNA synthesis and the critical period for cleft palate induction in inbred mice. Teratology 7:167–176, 1973.

Barlow SM, McElhatton PR, Sullivan FM: The relation between maternal restraint and food deprivation, plasma corticosterone, and induction of cleft palate in the offspring of mice. Teratology 12:97–104, 1975.

Barlow SM, Morrison PJ, Sullivan FM: Plasma corticosterone levels during pregnancy in the mouse: The relative contributions of the adrenal glands and foetal-placental units. J Endocrinol 70:473–483, 1974.

Barlow SM, Morrison PJ, Sullivan FM: Effects of acute and chronic stress on plasma corticosterone levels in the pregnant and nonpregnant mouse. J Endocrinol 66:93–99, 1975.

Barr M Jr: Prenatal growth of Wistar rats: Circadian periodicity of fetal growth late in gestation. Teratology 7:283–288, 1973.

Brown JL: Sensory systems. In: Brobeck JR (ed): "Physiological Basis of Medical Practice," 9th ed. Baltimore: Williams and Wilkins, Chapter 8, 1973, pp 8–165.

Brown KS, Johnston MC, Murphy PF: Isolated cleft palate in A/J mice after transitory exposure to drinking-water deprivation and low humidity in pregnancy. Teratology 9:151–158, 1974.

Brown KS, Johnston MC, Niswander JD: Isolated cleft palate in mice after transportation during gestation. Teratology 5:119–124, 1972.

Cheifetz PN: The daily rhythm of the secretion of corticotrophin and corticosterone in rats and mice. J Endocrinol 49:11–12, 1971.

Fraser FC, Kalter H, Walker BE, Fainstat TD: The experimental production of cleft palate with cortisone and other hormones. J Cell Comp Physiol 43 (Suppl 1):237–259, 1954.

Goldman AS, Katsumata M, Jaffe SY, Gasser DL: Palatalcytosol cortisol-binding protein associated with cleft palate susceptibility and H-2 genotype. Nature 265:643–645, 1977.

Gross HA, Ruder HJ, Brown K, Lipsett M: A radioimmunoassay for plasma corticosterone. Steroids 20:681–695, 1972.

Haus E, Halberg F: Circannual rhythm in level and timing of serum corticosterone in standardized inbred mature C-mice. Environ Res 3:81–105, 1970.

Kalter H: The inheritance of susceptibility to the teratogenic action of cortisone in Mice. Genetics 39:185–196, 1954.

Kalter H: Interplay of intrinsic and extrinsic factors. pp. 37–80. In: Wilson JG, Warkany J (eds): "Teratology: Principles and Technique." Chicago: The The University of Chicago Press, Chapter 3, 1965, pp 37–80.

Loevy H: Genetic influences on induced cleft palate in different strains of mice. Anat Rec 145:117–122, 1963.

Nebert DW, Bigelow SW: Genetic control of drug metabolism: Relationship to birth defects. Semin Perinatol 6:105–115, 1982.

Pratt RM, Yoneda T, Silver MH, Salomon DS: Involvement of glucocorticoids and epidermal growth factor in secondary palate development. In Pratt RM, Christiansen RL (eds): "Current Research Trends in Prenatal Craniofacial Development." New York: Elsevier/North Holland, 1980, pp 345–352.

Rodbard D, Frazier GR: National Technical Information Service Report No. PB217366 and PB217367, 1973.

Rosenzweig S, Blaustein FM: Cleft palate in A/J mice resulting from restraint and deprivation of food and water. Teratology 3:47–52, 1970.

Salomon D, Zubairi Y, Thompson EB: Ontogeny and biochemical properties of glucocorticoid receptors in midgestation mouse embryos. J Steroid Biochem 9:95–107, 1978.

Trasler, DM: Strain differences in susceptibility to teratogenesis: Survey of spontaneously occurring malformations in mice. In Wilson JG, Warkany J (eds): "Teratology Principles and Techniques." Chicago: The University of Chicago Press, 1965, pp 38–55.

Genetic Variation in Spontaneous and Diphenylhydantoin-Induced Craniofacial Malformations in Mice

Kenneth S. Brown, Mark I. Evans, and Leslie C. Harne

Laboratory of Developmental Biology and Anomalies, National Institute of Dental Research, National Institutes of Health, Bethesda, Maryland (K.S.B., L.C.H.); Section of Human Biochemical and Developmental Genetics, NICHD, (M.I.E.) and Department of Obstetrics and Gynecology, George Washington University Medical School, Washington, DC (M.I.E.)

The mouse strain CL/Fr has been produced by selection for high frequency of cleft lip. It is also sensitive to induction of cleft palate by glucocorticoids, as are its A strain relatives. "Star" strain is free of spontaneous clefts, and is resistant to glucocorticoid teratogenic effects. CL/Fr is also sensitive to toxic effects (80% death at 25 mg/kg) of diphenylhydantoin (DPH), whereas Star is not. Reciprocal crosses between CL/Fr and Star parents were followed for three generations of back-crossing to CL/Fr, with treatment by chronic subcutaneous (SC) DPH injection (20 mg/kg daily from day 0 of pregnancy). Two patterns of response were observed for facial clefts. Primary palate clefts (CL, CLP, lip scars) were not affected by DPH treatment, and showed a regression on % CL/Fr genome suggestive of a two- or three-locus recessive effect with the sensitive alleles from CL/Fr. Secondary palate clefts and open eyelids, considered as a group as relatively late developmental defects, showed a pattern suggestive of a dominant gene which increases risk of malformation in DPH-treated embryos, expressed in the crosses, but not in the absence of treatment or in the presence of the full "Star" genome.

Key words: CL/Fr mice, Star mice, animal studies, craniofacial malformations, diphenylhydantoin, cleft lip and palate

INTRODUCTION

Many studies have shown an epidemiologic association between prenatal administration of anticonvulsant therapy with diphenylhydantoin (DPH) and an increased rate of congenital malformations [Elshove and Van Eck, 1971; Spadel and Meadow, 1978; Monson et al, 1973; Shapiro et al, 1976]. An estimated 2% of all babies in the general population suffer from serious defects; however, approximately 6% of babies born to epileptic mothers taking DPH have some defect [Low, 1973]. The spectrum varies from major craniofacial structural defects such as cleft lip and palate (approxi-

---

Mark I. Evans's current address is Department of Obstetrics and Gynecology, Wayne State University School of Medicine, Detroit, MI 48201.

K.S.B. and M.I.E. are participants in the NIH Interinstitute Medical Genetics Program.

Address reprint requests to Kenneth S. Brown, Laboratory of Developmental Biology and Anomalies, National Institute of Dental Research, National Institutes of Health, Bethesda, MD 20205.

© 1985 Alan R. Liss, Inc.

mately 0.2%) to the less severe and more commonly occurring "hydantoin syndrome"—microcephaly, growth retardation, digital hypoplasia, and mental deficiency [Smith, 1977]. There has been some confusion as to whether epilepsy per se, or DPH, is primarily responsible for the increased risk of malformation [Shapiro et al, 1976; Low, 1973]. Unfortunately, there is no reliable or ethical way to perform a random cohort study to test the teratogenic affects of DPH on epileptics in pregnancy. Studies of existing data suffer from an inability to equate populations who were taking DPH and those who were not—either because of poor compliance or lack of diagnosis.

The need for animal models to study DPH effects and susceptibilities is paramount. Several fine studies have investigated the teratogenicity of DPH and some of its metabolites in rodents [Harbison and Becker, 1972, 1975]; others have attempted to define the pathogenesis of DPH-related lesions [Sullivan and McElhatton, 1975; Keith and Gallop, 1979; Millicovsky and Johnston, 1981; Millicovsky et al, 1982]. However, attempts to quantify susceptibility in terms of genetic predisposition have been limited. Thus, the purpose of this study was to attempt to define genetic variation of DPH teratogenicity among animal strains independent of epilepsy, to provide a basis for future biochemical investigations that could study the pathogenesis of DPH-related congenital malformations.

MATERIALS AND METHODS

The mouse strain CL/Fr has been selected to have high ($\pm 20\%$) frequency of cleft lip [Brown, 1980; Juriloff, 1980]. It was inbred for over 20 generations after cross of A/J to a stock with migratory spot lesion, and subsequent back-crosses to A/J with selection for high cleft lip and palate (CLP) frequency [Staats, 1980]. In preliminary studies, CL/Fr has been found to be sensitive to DPH-induced cleft palate [Hetzel and Brown, 1974, 1975], in contrast to "Star" strain mice. "Star" strain was raised by Gottschewski since 1948 by brother-sister mating after occurrence of the gene Cat (dominant cataract), which is homozygous in the strain. The parent stock was sent by Bittner to Gottschewski in 1938. Star is resistant to DPH-induced cleft palate, and does not have any spontaneous cleft lip. Preliminary studies had shown that CL/Fr had 80% fetal death at 25 mg/kg DPH, although Star fetuses showed no increased mortality at that dose.

Reciprocal crosses between CL/Fr and Star, and reciprocal back-crosses from the F_1 offspring of CL/Fr × Star to CL/Fr, were carried out for three generations (Fig. 1). Untreated and DPH-treated pregnancies were examined for each mating type. The treatment group received 20 mg DPH/kg SC (diphenylhydantoin sodium injection, Parke-Davis, 1/10 with isotonic saline) daily starting at day 0 of gestation. All animals were housed in standard shoe box cages with NIH-07 diet and water ad libitum. The quarters were air-conditioned, and artificial light was on from 6:00 A.M. to 6:00 P.M.

For each pregnancy, determined by observation of a vaginal plug on day 0, weights of females at mating and on day 17 were recorded. The uterine contents were examined and the implantation sites counted. Among living fetuses the examination was limited to facial traits, which were examined under a dissecting microscope. Unilateral or bilateral cleft of the lip, scar of the site of fusion of the lip, isolated cleft of secondary palate, and open eyelid were recorded when present. Primary epithelial closure defects (PECD), ie, the lip clefts and associated defects, were considered in one group as occurring before day 11. Secondary epithelial closure defects (SECD),

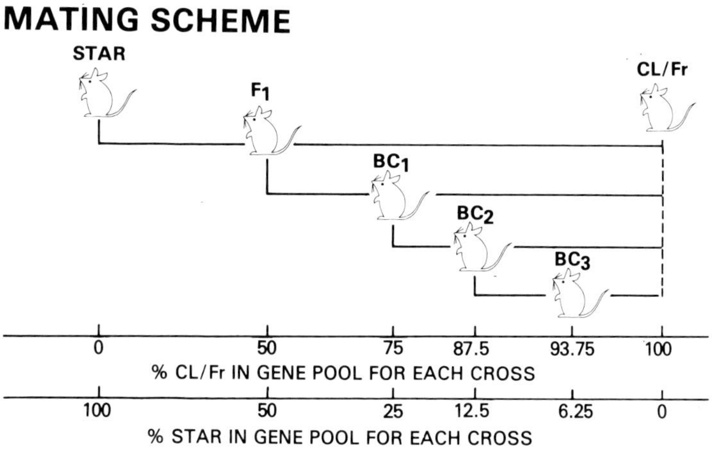

MATING SCHEME

Fig. 1. Mating scheme for analysis of response to DPH and spontaneous defects. Percentages at bottom reflect proportions of genetic contribution from each parent strain for growth crosses.

ie, isolated cleft palate and failure of eyelid closure, which occur after day 14, were included in a second group.

Two-way analysis of variance was employed to assess differences between DPH and control groups and among the various purebred and hybrid genotypes. Since a significant difference could not be demonstrated between reciprocal hybrids for maternal intrauterine environment, the data were pooled for further analysis of malformation rates. Goodness of fit of prospective genetic models was assessed by the X^2 test. Pearson product moment correlations and least-square fits were used to develop regression lines.

RESULTS

A total of 5,878 fetuses from 634 litters were examined. In all hybrid strains, the fertility of the hybrid strain was consistently greater than that of the purebred mother (Tables I, II). DPH mothers also demonstrated more implantation sites than did control mothers, but initial maternal weights and weight increases were non-contributory.

The incidence of PECD was unrelated to DPH. However, there were significant differences across genotypes ($F = 22.45$, $p < .01$). Minimum susceptibility was found in Star, with increasing incidence as the percentage of CL/Fr genotype in the gene pool increased in back-crosses to CL/Fr (Fig. 2).

Control mice (not exposed to DPH) developed cleft palate and/or open eyelid (SECD) at a rate independent of genetic constitution (Fig. 3). With exposure to DPH, however, the purebred Star and CL/Fr strains had incidences of SECD of 18% and 13%, respectively. Paradoxically, the F_1 generation had 28% SECD. With back-crosses to CL/Fr, the incidence of SECD malformations decreased as the gene pool approached that of CL/Fr.

GENETIC INTERPRETATION

The measured breeding performance of hybrid males mated to inbred susceptible females (CL/Fr) is a sample of the genetic constitution of the males. The differences

TABLE I. Fertility of Mice in Reciprocal Hybrids (Litter Size)

Purebred parents	Hybrid parents[1]		
	F_1	BC_1	BC_2
CL/Fr ♂	8.9	9.8	10.7
CL/Fr ♀	7.5	7.5	7.6

[1]Two-way analysis of variance. Homozygous vs heterozygous mother: $F = 21.32$ $p < .01$.
Genotype of hybrid: F = not significant.

TABLE II. Fertility and Survival in DPH and Control Mice

	DPH	Controls
Mean number of implantation sites per litter	9.60 (n = 3,762)	8.62 (n = 2,086) $p < .01$
% Live fetuses per site	87.1	85.6 NS[1]

[1]Not significant.

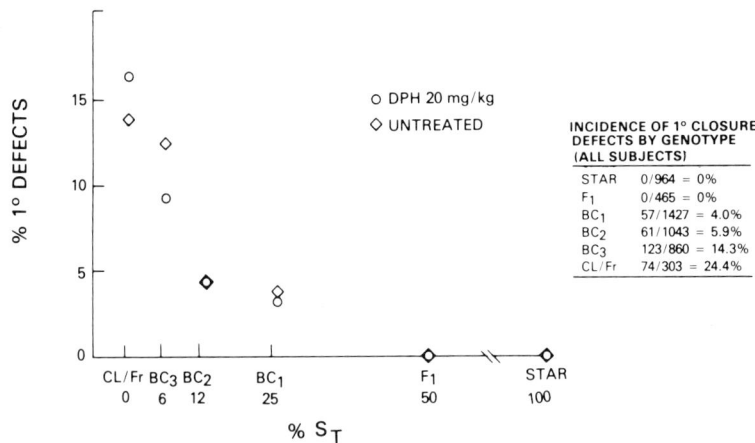

Fig. 2. Incidence of primary (PECD) closure defects for all crosses in DPH and control mice. The incidence of PECD appeared unrelated to DPH exposure.

in malformation rates from generation to generation reflect changes in paternal genotype.

The data for PECD suggest an epistatic autosomal recessive model for differences in malformation rates between the two strains. Using the higher strain (CL/Fr) as 100% effect and the lower strain as 0%, observed values for back-crosses with intermediary genotypes can be plotted as in Figure 4. To correctly estimate the pattern of genetic change, the loss of genes at each generation owing to the lethal effects of

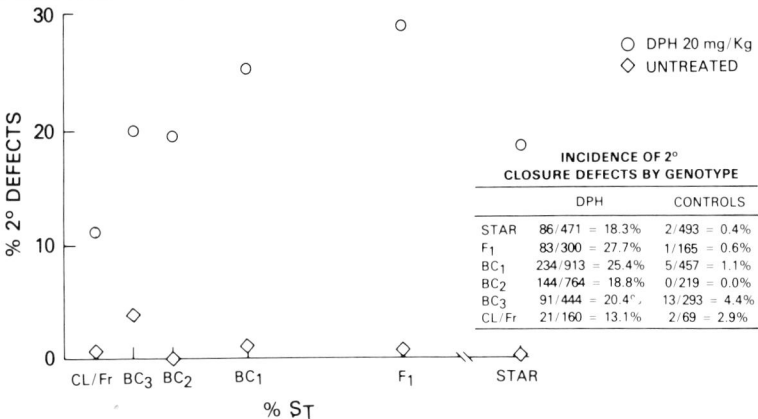

Fig. 3. Incidence of secondary (SECD) closure defects for all crosses of DPH treated and control mice. For control mice SECD incidence was independent of genotype. DPH-induced SECD, however, varied markedly by genotype and paradoxically the highest incidence was in the F_1 generation with obscuring incidence in back-crosses.

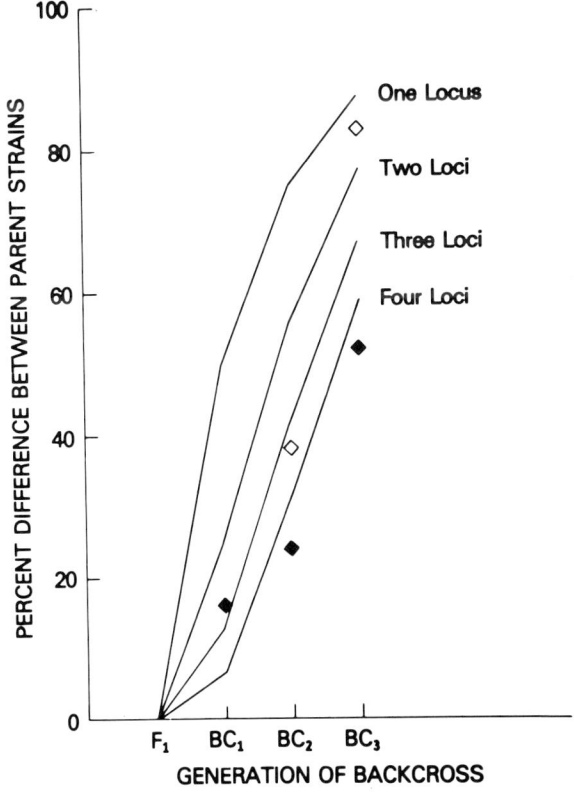

Fig. 4. Proposed genetic model for PECD. An autosomal recessive model is suggested. In the figure the predictions of models using 1–4 loci are shown. The observed data are shown as open figures for BC_2 and BC_3; the solid figure data points show predictions taking into account changing gene pools because of genetic load. With the corrected values, the data are compatible with an epistatic autosomal recessive model of two or three loci. This is a redundancy model in which several loci are acting in parallel so that all loci must be "inactive" in order for the defect to be expressed.

the craniofacial malformations must be considered. When this genetic load is incorporated in the calculations, the data are compatible with a model with at least two loci that are mutually epistatic.

The data for SECD, in which the F_1 rate was the highest, suggest a model in which the gradual decrease in malformation rates with back-crosses toward CL/Fr is explained by the changing gene pool. The loci in CL/Fr become increasingly homozygous recessive with successive back-crosses. The specifics of the model are detailed in Figure 5. The predicted model was compared against the known data by X^2. The model could not be rejected. Simpler models deviated from the data significantly. More complex models could be designed to fit the data.

DISCUSSION

The delineation of genetic differences in teratogenicity of prenatal administration of DPH among mouse strains can be correlated to human studies of teratogenicity in

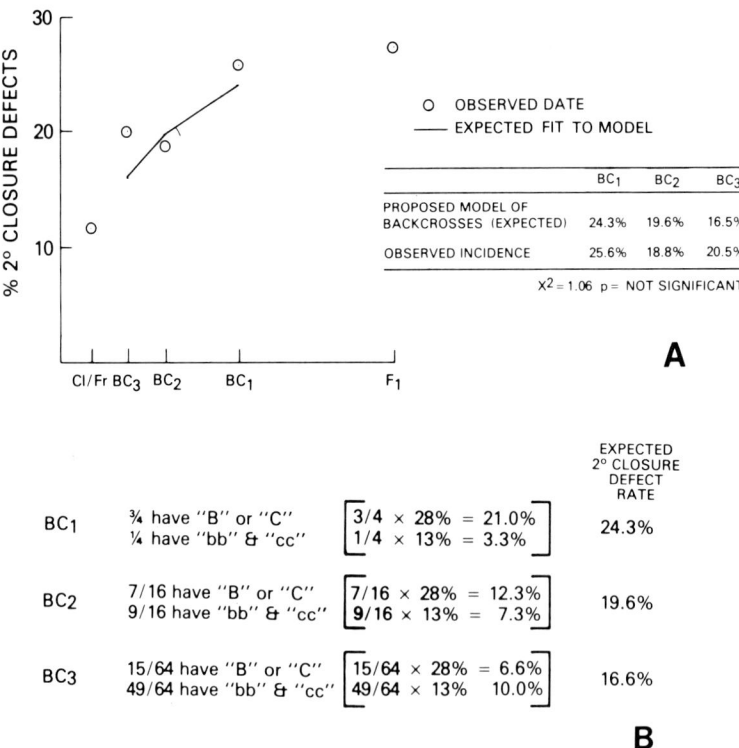

Fig. 5. A. Proposed genetic model for DPH-induced SECD. The changing gene pool with decreasing frequency of SECD with back-crossed CL/Fr is compatible with a two-loci model for increasing resistance to DPH with increasing homozygous recessive genes. The F_1 generation is heterozygous at both loci, confering maximum susceptibility. With back-crosses, the percentage of heterozygotes decreased. B. Using the F_1 rate (28%) and the CL/Fr rate (13%) expected, rates were calculated as in B and shown as line in A.

several areas. The establishment of reproducible differences in susceptibility by genetic constitution provides a basis for investigation of biochemical mechanisms yielding such differences. Several authors have suggested enzymatic alterations in DPH-induced malformations that might potentially correlate with altered absorption, serum concentration, clearance rates, or quantities and proportions of various metabolites [Keith and Gallop, 1979, Millicovsky and Johnston, M81]. The establishment of a baseline malformation rate along a regression plotted by genotype allows a careful inspection of changing parameters that can then be correlated with changing incidence of malformation.

There is a striking difference in drug response between PECD, which showed no teratogenic response, and SECD, which was clearly influenced by drug treatment. The differences in genetic behavior and teratogen sensitivity of the early events (PECD) as compared to the later (SECD) events may be due to differences in exposure to drug related to the changes of placentation between 9 and 15 days, to accumulation of DPH, to changes in fetal liver function during development, or to different types of biological processes involved in the PECD and SECD. Some effects of DPH treatment, for example, increased serum copper and ceruloplasmin [Massie et al, 1980], require several days after start of treatment. Since copper is a cofactor for many enzymes processing collagens, changes in tissue copper may play an important role in teratogenesis.

The data also suggest potential differences in congenital susceptibility to DPH as a function of the genotype of the father. Such paternal influence (ie, to the fetal genotype) suggests the importance of fetal input to susceptibility of drug teratogenicity. The fit of a model with relatively few genetic variables suggests that there are a limited number of metabolic processes controlling the difference between susceptibility or resistance to the teratogenic effect on the DPH-treated fetus. This suggests that a biochemical identification might be feasible. With such an identification might come a rationale for the study of similar processes in human development [Brown and Hetzel, 1977]. Hopefully, it will be possible to identify patients who are at greater risk for DPH teratogenicity, and thus allow the most appropriate titration of DPH dosage for such patients.

REFERENCES

Brown KS: Isolated cleft palate in domestic and laboratory mammals. pp. 403–427, In: Pratt RM, Christiansen RL (eds): "Current Trends in Prenatal Craniofacial Development." New York: Elsevier/North Holland, 1980, pp 403–427.
Brown KS, Hetzel SC: The fetal hydantoin syndrome in mice. Birth Defects XIII(3D):273, 1977.
Elshove J, Van Eck JAM: Congenital malformations, particularly cleft lip with or without cleft palate in children of epileptic mothers. Ned Tijdschr Geneeskd. 115:1371-1971.
Hetzel S, Brown KS: Effects of chronic diphenylhydantoin on pregnant mice. J Dent Res, 53:190, 1974.
Hetzel S, Brown KS: Facial clefts and lip hermatoma in mouse fetuses given diphenylhydantoin. J Dent Res 54:83, 1975.
Harbison RD, Becker BA: Diphenylhydantoin teratogenicity in rats. Toxicol Appl Pharmacol 22:193, 1972.
Harbison RD, Becker BA: Comparative embryotoxicity of diphenylhydantoin and some of its metabolites in mice. Teratology 10:237, 1975.
Juriloff DM: The genetics of clefting in the mouse. In: Melnick, Bixler, Shields (eds): "Etiology of Cleft Lip and Cleft Palate." New York: Alan R. Liss, 1980, pp 39–71.
Keith DA, Gallop PM: Phenytoin, hemmorhage, skeletal development and vitamin K in the newborn. Med Hypotheses 5:1247, 1979.

Low CR: Congenital malformations among infants born to epileptic women. Lancet 1:9,1973.
Massie HR, Colacicco JR, Aiello VR: Phenytoin-induced serum copper and ceruloplasmin in C57BL/6J mice of different ages. Age 3:33–37, 1980.
Millicovsky G, Ambrose JH, Johnston MC: Developmental alterations associated with spontaneous cleft lip and palate in CL/Fr mice. Am J Anat 164:29–44, 1982.
Millicovsky G, Johnston MC: Maternal hyperoxia reduces the incidence of phenytoin-induced cleft lip and palate in A/J mice. Science 212:671–672, 1981.
Monson RR, Rosenberg L, Hartz SC, Shapiro S, Heinonen OP, Slone D: Diphenylhydantoin and selided congenital malformations. N Engl J Med 281:1049, 1973.
Shapiro S, Slone D, Hartz SC, Rosenberg L, Siskind V, Monson RR, Mitchell AA, Heinonen OF, Idanpaan-Heikkila J, Haro S, Saxen J: Anticonvulsants and parental epilepsy in the development of birth defects. Lancet 1:272, 1976.
Smith DW: Distal limb hypoplasia in the fetal hydantoin syndrome. Birth Defects 13:355, 1977.
Spadel BD, Meadow SR: Maternal epilepsy and abnormalities of the fetus and newborn. Lancet 2:829, 1978.
Staats J: Standardized nomenclature for inbred strains of mice. Seventh Listing Cancer Res 40:2083–2128.
Sullivan FM, McElhatton PR: Teratogenic activity of the antiepileptic drugs phenobarbitol phenytoin and primidone in mice. Toxicol Appl Pharmacol 34:271, 1975.

Blebs and Hematomas in the Lips of CL/Fr and A/J Mice

Kenneth S. Brown, Suzanne C. Hetzel, Leslie C. Harne, and Sally Long

Laboratory of Developmental Biology and Anomalies, National Institute of Dental Research, National Institutes of Health, Bethesda, Maryland (K.S.B., S.C.H., L.C.H.) and Department of Anatomy, Medical College of Wisconsin, Milwaukee (S.L.)

> Newborn-CL/Fr mice have ± 20% frequency of cleft lip with or without cleft palate (CLP) depending on environment. However, examination of early fetal development from days 12 to 15 disclosed an increased number of hematomas or fluid-filled blebs in the regions of maxillary process fusion. The earliest stages do not appear to involve the blood supply directly but separate the epithelium from underlying mesenchyme by clear blebs. Similar defects were found in untreated A/J mice. These findings suggest that osmotic and hemodynamic abnormalities may be part of the mechanism of cleft lip formation in these related strains and that these defects may result from a biochemical defect of the connective tissue matrix in regions of process fusion.

Key words: CL/Fr mice, A/J mice, cleft lip and palate, animal studies, maxillary process

INTRODUCTION

The pathogenesis of cleft lip in humans can only be estimated from the observation of fetuses and newborns at stages much after the occurence of the actual failure of the fusion of the primary palate processes except in rare cases of abortion [Nishimura and Okamoto, 1976]. Much secondary modification of the histological detail of the region of fusion has occurred that obscures the nature of the event directly involved. The same is true for newborn and late gestation mouse fetuses, to a lesser extent because of the much shorter time between normal palate closure and birth, ie, 10 days compared to 32 weeks in man [Smith, 1976].

In the course of examination of gross and histological studies of two mouse strains that have spontaneous cleft palate we have made a sequence of observations that suggest that in mice of these strains there is an underlying defect in mesenchyme-epithelial adhesion expressed in the region of the fusion of the primary palate processes. These observations are consistent with a pattern of consequences following the expression of one primary abnormality.

Address reprint requests to Kenneth S. Brown, Laboratory of Developmental Biology and Anomalies, National Institutes of Health, Bethesda, MD 20205.

© 1985 Alan R. Liss, Inc.

MATERIALS AND METHODS

Our initial observations were made independently in the course of other teratological studies on the two related strains A/J and CL/Fr. Preliminary observations have been reported as abstracts [Long, 1971; Hetzel and Brown, 1975; Brown and Hetzel, 1977].

The A/J mice fetuses were collected on days 14 or 15 from a colony with 10% spontaneous cleft lip. They were classified by the morphological rating system [Trasler, 1965]. Histological sections of the nasal capsule and lip were stained with toluidine blue. CL/Fr fetuses were collected from timed matings as part of the control of other experiments in which observation of the plug was considered to be on day zero and mating was assumed to be at midnight, so that 8 A.M. was day 0, 8 hours. The colony had 17% facial clefts of various types and combinations or lip scars, as previously reported [Brown, 1980]. Selected fetuses were photographed at time of removal. Serial sections of the lip and nasal capsule were cut in frontal plane from specimens with different combinations of abnormality at days 12, 14, 15, and 17 of development. They were stained with hematoxylin and eosin. Some specimens were injected with India ink intracardially and then cleared in alkali and methylsalicylate to expose the pattern of the vessels of the snout.

RESULTS

The distribution of phenotypes among the faces of newborn CL/Fr in our colony at NIDR is shown in Table I. About two thirds of the malformed newborn have bilateral clefts of the lip with cleft palate. There are three times as many unilateral left cleft lips with cleft palate as there are right unilateral clefts with cleft palate. In contrast there are twice as many right cleft lips as there are left cleft lips. This pattern suggests that left cleft lips have a much lower threshold for secondary cleft palate or, conversely, that right cleft lips with normal left sides have a relatively good chance of secondary palate closure. Nearly 25% of the malformed had cleft of the secondary palate without cleft of the primary palate. Among these, six showed scars of the lip representing secondary fusion of a primary lip cleft. More than half of the lip scars observed were associated with secondary palate clefts. Not recorded in these observations were the presence of hematomas or enlarged vessels in the lip.

TABLE I. Phenotypic Frequencies of Lip and Palate Abnormalities in Live Newborn CL/Fr Mice in 1,586 Litters

	Number	%
Normal	7,988	82.64
Bilateral cleft lip and cleft palate	1,190	12.31
Right cleft lip and cleft palate	107	1.10
Left cleft lip and cleft palate	322	3.33
Bilateral cleft lip	5	0.05
Right cleft lip	4	0.04
Left cleft lip	2	0.02
Cleft palate	35	0.36
Cleft palate with lip scar	6	0.06
Lip scar	5	0.05

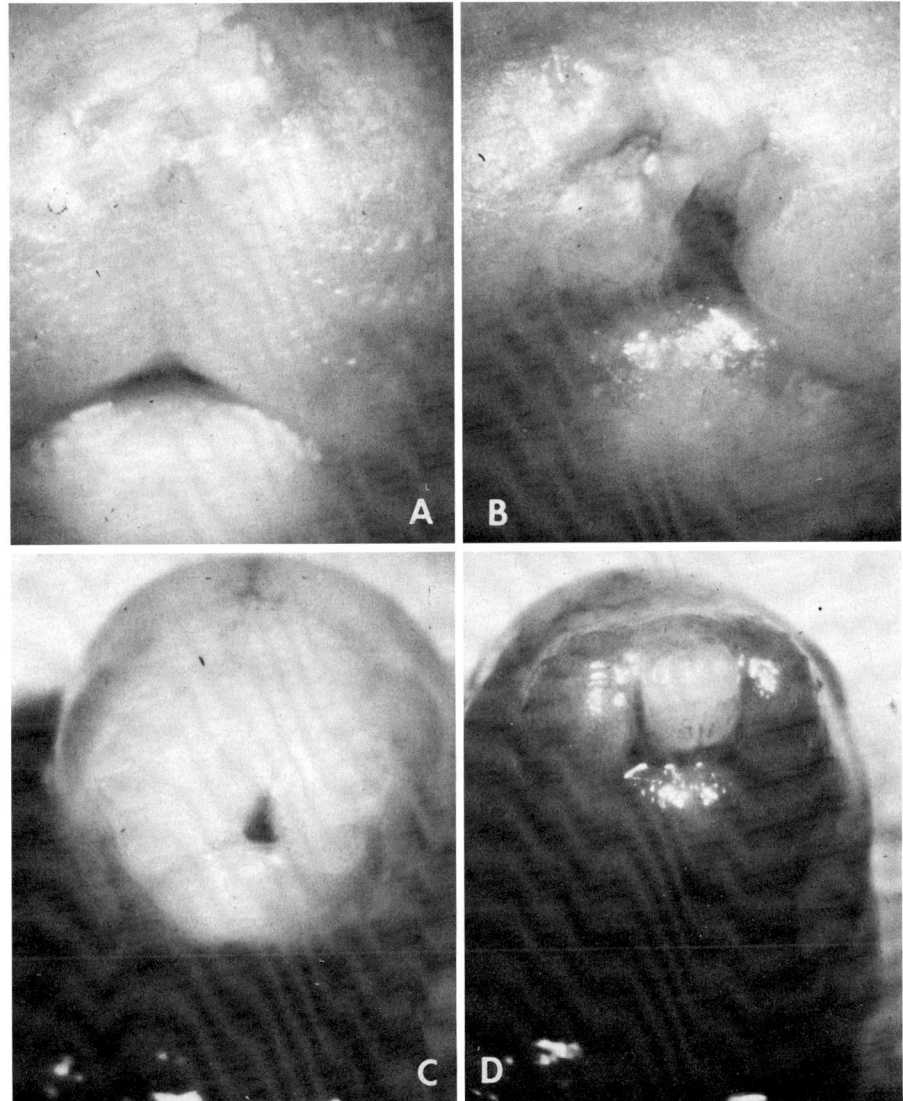

Fig. 1. Variations in lip form form in CF/Fr day 17 fetuses. A) normal. B) Unilateral right cleft lip with skin flap and scar on left side. C) Bilateral lip scars with deep hematoma in right seam line. D) Bilateral cleft lip.

Figures 1 and 2 illustrate the variety of lip forms seen in CL/Fr fetuses in late gestation. Figure 1B shows a structural disorganization with a flap of skin crossing the cleft, suggestive of a secondary rupture or tear instead of the smooth surface cleft associated with failure of primary fusion of the lip processes as seen in 1D. Figures 1C and 2 demonstrate deep and superficial hematomas or engorged vessels.

Histological sections of fetuses showing evidence of hematoma (Figs. 3, 4) revealed three types of blood-filled spaces, enlarged vessels with endothelial lining, blood-filled spaces in the tissues without lining but showing compression of adjacent

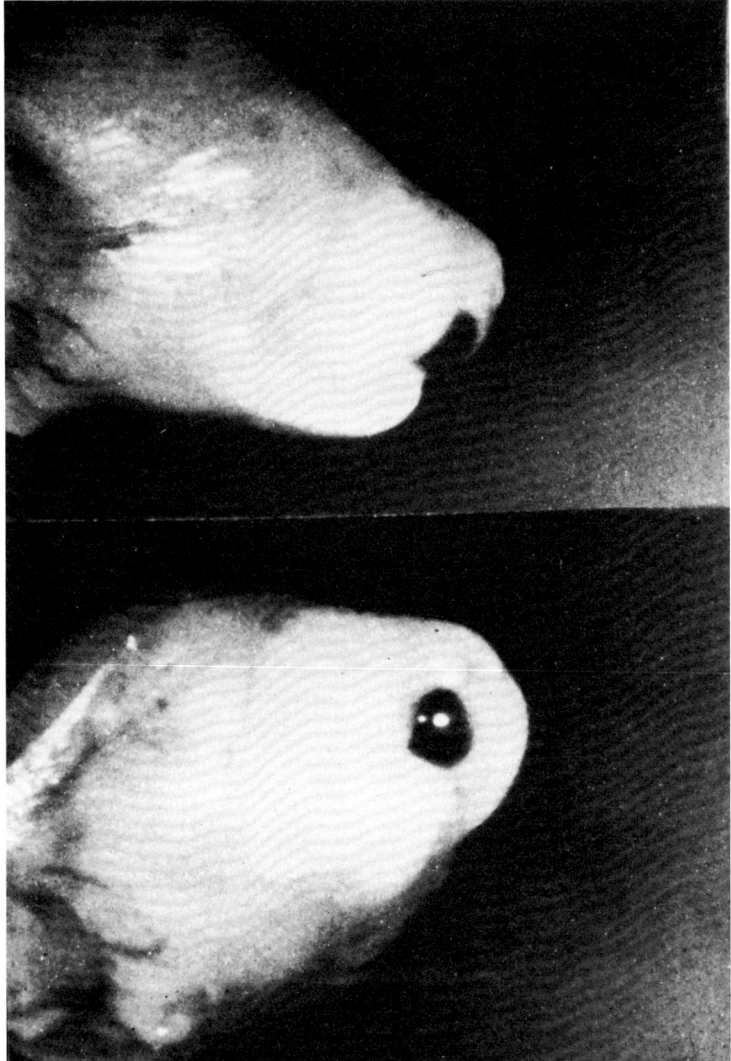

Fig. 2. Enlarged superficial vessel in right seam and midline of day 17 CL/Fr fetus from side (top) and ventral view.

tissues, and, at earlier stages (Fig. 5), clear spaces in the junctions of the fusing processes separating the two processes (Fig. 6).

Injection of India ink into the vessels of fetuses showing obvious hematomas at day 17 (Fig. 7) showed the vascular connections of the blood-filled spaces at this stage. These large vessels suggest a relatively high flow of the arteriovenous fistula type.

The early stages of the lesion, as seen on day 12 (Fig. 7), show separation of the epithelium from the underlying mesenchyme by red cell-free spaces of rounded shape, suggesting relatively high internal pressure located in the regions where fusion of processes to form the lip is taking place (Fig. 7A,B). In some cases there appears to

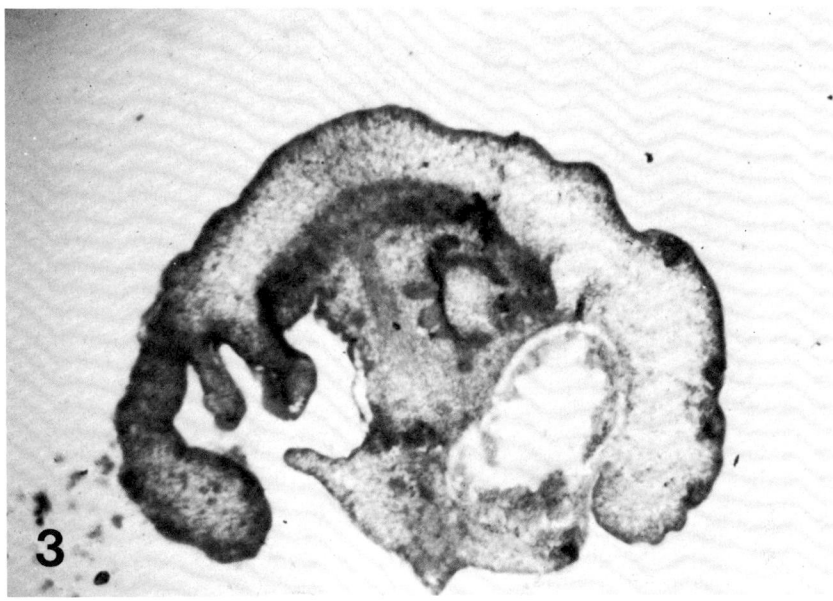

Fig. 3. Large right side hematoma which deforms the nasal capsule in a day 14 CL/Fr fetus cleft on left side.

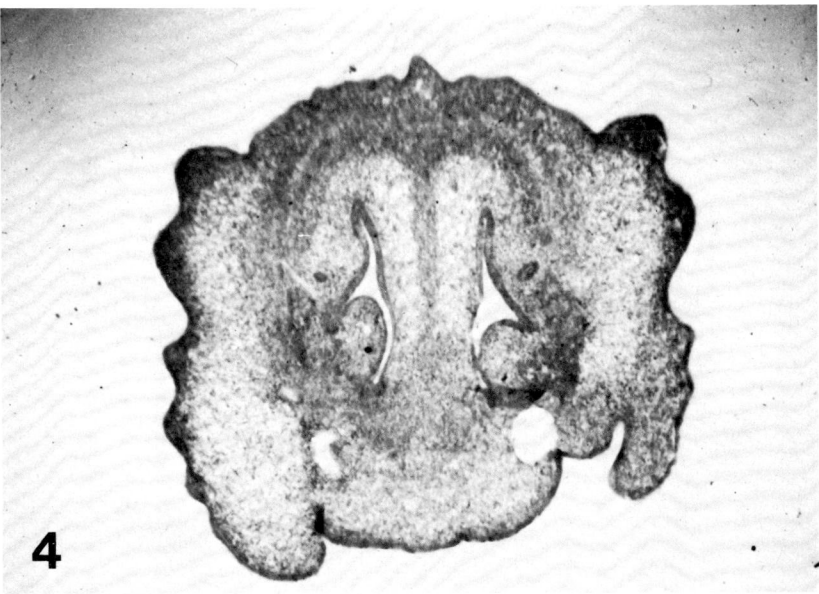

Fig. 4. Hematoma on left and clear distended space on right in the line of the primary palate fusion of maxillary and nasal processes in a day 13 CL/Fr fetus.

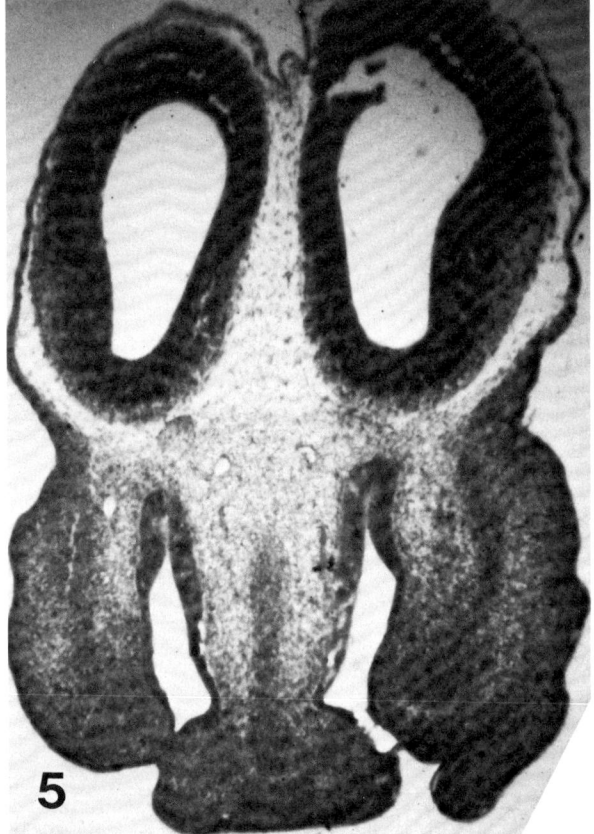

Fig. 5. Day 12 CL/Fr embryo showing fluid-filled bleb in the seam on the right and normal closure of the seam on the left.

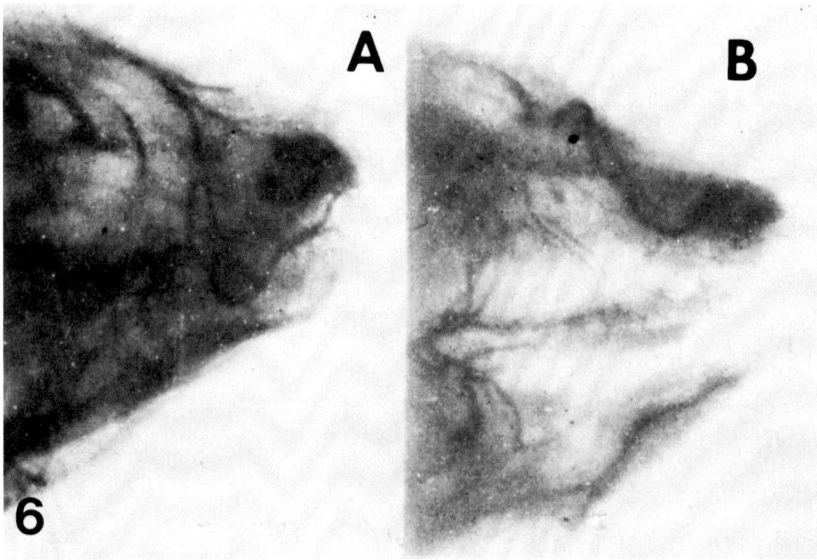

Fig. 6. Cleared day 17 CL/Fr fetus after India ink injection through the left heart demonstrating major vessel connecting to the large hematoma in the right lip. A) From side; B) from below, showing left cleft of lip and cleft palate.

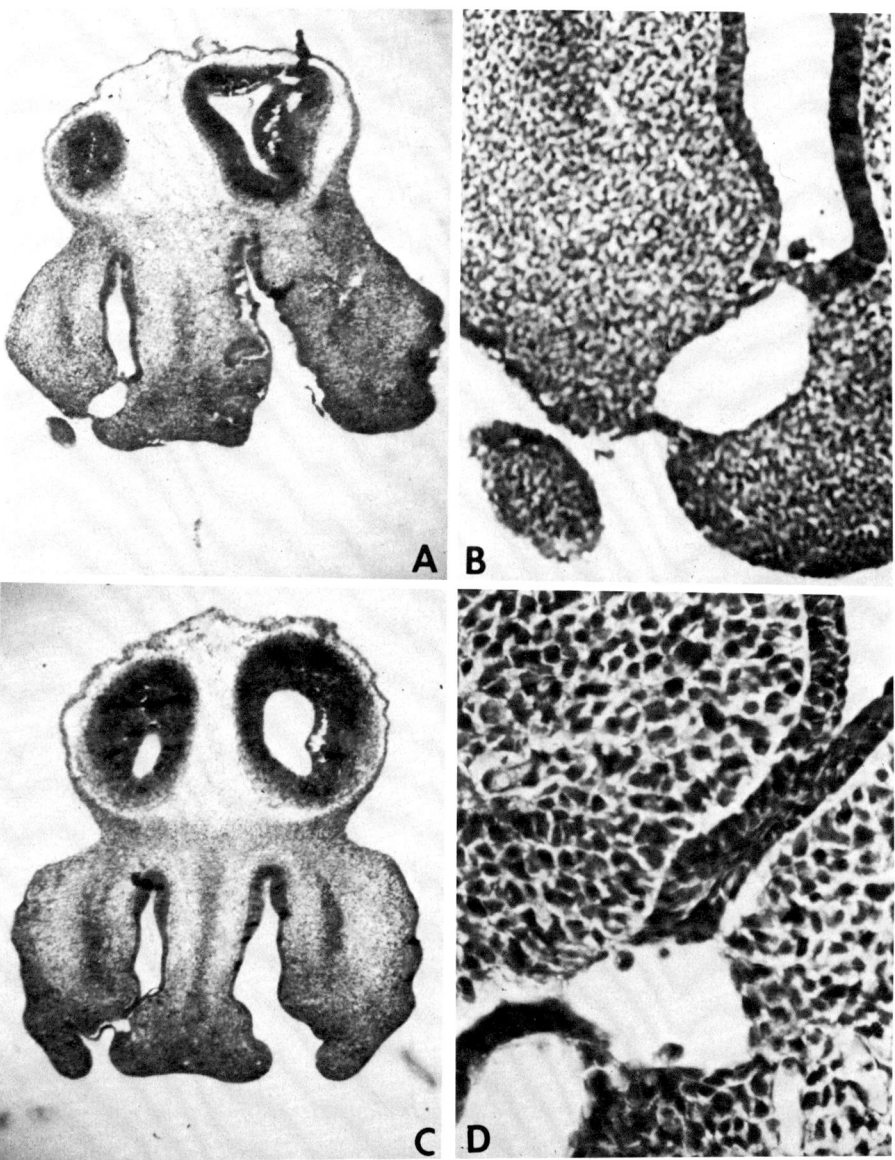

Fig. 7. Day 12 CL/Fr fetuses showing fluid-filled blebs in the region of primary palate process fusions at ×6 and ×25 for two specimens (A, B) and (C, D) stained with hematoxylin and eosin.

be dissection of adjacent epithelium (Fig. 7C,D). These lesions are not present in other regions of epithelial attachment and are not easily seen on direct examination by dissecting microscope due to lack of hemoglobin in the space.

The pattern of enlarged vessels in the upper lip of A/J mice is similar to that of CL/Fr in that these are not seen or are very rare in newborn or late fetal stage normal animals. They do occur in normal animals of A/J associated with the period of secondary palate closure (Table II) but later disappear. The A/J fetuses with cleft lip appear to have them prior to the period of secondary palate fusion, and they persist.

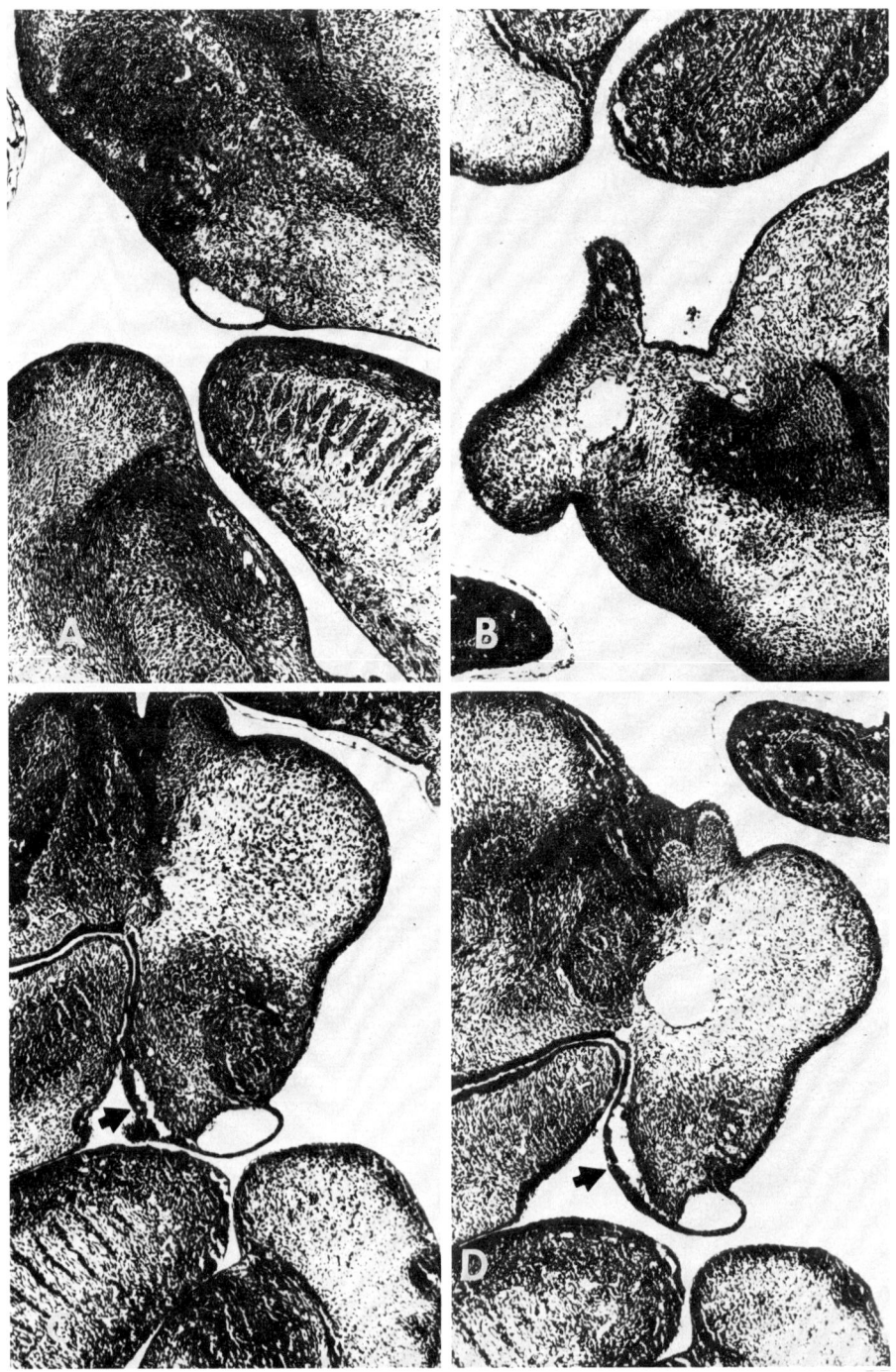

Fig. 8. Frontal sections through anterior palate and lip of days 14 and 15 A/J fetuses. A) No cleft lip; B, C, D) cleft lip. Subepithelial separations and adjacent to enlarged vessel (arrows) are seen in C and D.

TABLE II. The Rate of Occurence of Superficial Vascular Enlargement or Hematoma in the Upper Lip of Normal and Cleft Lip A/J Mouse Fetuses at Different Stages of Development

Morphological rating	Normal		Cleft Lip	
	Number	%	Number	%
7	1	0	1	100
8	7	100	2	100
9–10	22	77	8	100
11–12	24	36	5	100
13–14	18	17	3	100
15–16	16	0	7	100
17–18	15	0	2	100
19–20	5	0	0	—

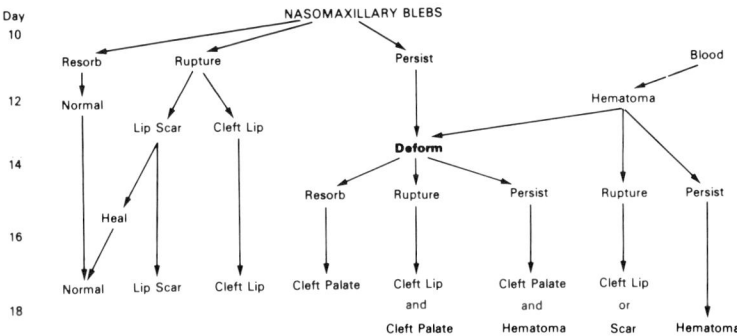

Fig. 9. A schematic diagram of the pedigree of events following from the present of nasomaxillary blebs in CL/Fr mice. All the consequences are actually seen in newborn animals as shown in Table I and Figures 1–8.

Histologically, the enlarged vessels seen in A/J lips are similar to CL/Fr in that they are in the region of fusion of the primary palate and many are at the epithelial mesenchyme junction (Fig. 8). They differ in that all seem to be lined with endothelium although there seem to be some with adjacent dissection between epithelium and underlying tissue. As seen in CL/Fr, there are associated large vessels. There is some difficulty in distinguishing between endothelium and compressed adjacent mesenchyme in these preparations as in CL/Fr.

DISCUSSION

The available descriptive data on CL/Fr and A/J can be assembled into a pattern that appears to account for all the observed phenotypes with only two primary events (Fig. 9). First is the occurence of nasomaxillary blebs which separate mesenchyme from overlying epithelium in the regions of presumptive process fusion. Second is the invasion of these spaces by the vascular tree with stasis and hemolysis causing expansion or rupture. As displayed in Figure 9, this cascade of sequential events can be put on a time scale which makes some sense when matched against the observations in both A/J and CL/Fr. Since secondary palate fusion may very well be associated with the same kinds of processes of cell death and autolysis of tissues that occur in regions of primary palate fusion, there may be an expected increased risk for a repeat of the biochemical events that underlie them if the involved enzymes enter the circulation.

The basis for the blebs and their localization must be in some weakness of the connective tissues underlying the epithelium. This is similar to some of the human collagen diseases of the Ehlers Danlos syndrome [Pinnell and Murad, 1983]. Some support for this analogy is the observation by Robey [1979] that A/J mice contain less collagen in their skin than Swiss Webster mice and synthesize collagen more rapidly. When treated with steroids, A/J have a greater reduction in collagen synthesis. This suggests that the A/J strain mice have a "collagen disease" which expresses itself as poor tissue growth and sensitivity to localized developmental enzymatic changes that are involved in tissue remodeling the growth. Clearly this is a relatively mild syndrome compared to the collagen disease of mice with defects at the mottled locus which have copper transport problems resulting in defects of collagen processing, which result in aortic anurisms or intrauterine death in hemizygous males [Green, 1981].

The new DNA technology may soon allow an examination of these mice for defects of collagen genes as has been done for osteogenesis imperfecta [Byers and Bonadio, 1984], and the examination may reveal similar high degrees of genetic heterogeneity. Even closely related strains such as CL/Fr and A/J may have differences at the single locus level on DNA. These may account for the heterogeneity of A/J and CL/Fr in regard to spontaneous cleft lip rate.

REFERENCES

Brown KS: Isolated cleft palate in domestic and laboratory mammals. In: Pratt RM, Christiansen RL (eds): "Current Research Trends in Prenatal Craniofacial Development." New York: Elsevier-North Holland, 1980, pp 403–421.

Brown KS, Hetzel SC: The fetal hydantoin syndrome in mice (Abstract). Birth Defects XIII:3D, 1977.

Byers PH, Bonadio JE: Lethal mutations in type I collagen: Structure-function relationships in the type I collagen molecule. In: Brown KS, Salinas CF (eds): "Craniofacial Mesenchyme in Morphogenesis and Malformation." Birth Defects: Original Article Series 20 (3), New York: Alan R. Liss, 1984, pp 65–78.

Green MC (ed): "Genetic Variants and Strains of the Laboratory Mouse," Mo lucus. New York: Gustav Fisher, 1981, pp 162–165.

Hetzel S, Brown KS: Facial clefts and lip hematoma in mouse fetuses given diphenylhydantoin. J Dent Res 54:83, 1975.

Long S: The nasal capsule in A/J mice with spontaneous cleft lip. Teratology 4:493, 1971.

Nishimura H, Okamota N: "Sequential Atlas of Human Congenital Malformations." Baltimore: University Park Press, 1976, pp 86–91.

Pinnell SR, Murad S: Disorders of collagen. In: Stanbury JB, et al (eds): "The Metabolic Basis of Inherited Disease," 5th ed. New York: McGraw Hill, 1983, pp 1425–1499.

Robey PG: Effect of dexamethasone on collagen metabolism in two strains of mice. Biochem Pharmacol 28:2261–2266, 1979.

Smith DW: "Recognisable Patterns of Human Malformation," 2nd ed. Philadelphia: W.B. Saunders, 1976.

Trasler DG: Strain differences in susceptibility to teratogenesis: Survey of spontaneously occurring malformations in mice. In: Wilson JG, Warkany J (eds): "Teratology, Principles and Techniques." Chicago: University of Chicago press, 1965, pp 38–55.

Experimental Fusion of the Naturally Cleft, Embryonic Chick Palate

Mark W.J. Ferguson and Lawrence S. Honig

Department of Basic Dental Sciences, Turner Dental School, The University of Manchester, Manchester, England (M.W.J.F.) and Laboratory for Developmental Biology, Andrus Gerontology Center, University of Southern California, Los Angeles (L.S.H.)

The palatal shelf medial edges of day 8 (Hamburger-Hamilton [HH] stages 32–33) and day 9 (HH stage 35) embryonic chicks were surgically disrupted in ovo and in vitro in an attempt to discover if the naturally cleft chick palate could be induced to fuse experimentally. At HH stages 32–33 (day 8) the chick palatal shelves were apart at the time of in ovo operation. Consequently, their medial edges did not fuse but rather underwent embryonic wound healing with re-epithelialisation (which often formed needle track invaginations), but no signs of inflammation or scar or scab tissue formation. Conversely, at HH stage 35 (day 9) the palatal shelves are in contact at the time of in ovo operation and so underwent fusion. The extent of palatal fusion depended upon the extent of initial medial edge epithelial disruption. Fusion did not spread from the operated sites to adjacent unoperated areas, where the palatal shelves were in contact with each other. Occasional epithelial seams were formed, but these persisted and did not undergo cell death. There was no evidence of inflammation or scar or scab tissue at the operated sites. Abnormal bony and muscular blastemae appeared in the continuity zones of these experimentally intact chick palates. Mortality was high for embryos operated upon in ovo. Palatal shelves explanted from HH stages 32, 33, and 35 chick embryos and cultured in vitro with their medial edges in contact did not fuse unless their medial edge epithelia were surgically disrupted, in which cases fusion always occurred regardless of the stage of the explanted shelves. The present experiments document the ability of chick palatal shelves to fuse, and the reason for natural cleft palate in this species is postulated to reside in failure of the mesenchyme to effectively signal medial edge epithelial cell death. Further ultrastructural, biochemical, and experimental investigations are suggested. Moreover, the naturally cleft chick palate is suggested as a suitable model to study embryonic wound healing and cleft palate surgery. Embryonic wound healing in the chick palate closely resembles that seen in fetal monkey skin and rat oral mucosa. Embryonic operations appear to be advantageous as scar tissue and secondary deformations are reduced.

Key words: palate development, cleft palate, chick, embryonic surgery, embryonic wound healing, epithelial mesenchymal interactions, medial edge epithelia, palate fusion, palate evolution

Dr. L.S. Honig is now at the Department of Anatomy, R-304, University of Miami, School of Medicine, P.O. Box 016960 Miami, FL 33101.

Address reprint requests to Professor Mark W.J. Ferguson, Head of Department of Basic Dental Sciences, Turner Dental School, University Dental Hospital of Manchester, Higher Cambridge Street, Manchester M15 6FH, England.

© 1985 Alan R. Liss, Inc.

INTRODUCTION

It is well known that the palates of most birds (particularly the schizognathous species) are naturally cleft, with a midline choana connecting the oral and nasal cavities [Bellairs and Jenkin, 1960; McLelland, 1979]. Morphological studies of the developing chicken embryo have revealed that although the palatal shelves approximate and contact each other around day 9 (Hamburger-Hamilton [HH] stage 35) they do not fuse; rather, the medial edge epithelial cells keratinise, resulting in cleft palate [Shah and Crawford, 1980; Koch and Smiley, 1981]. The developmental mechanisms that produce the naturally cleft avian palate are unknown. In mammals, palatal shelf contact is followed by fusion of the medial edge epithelial cells to form an epithelial seam, which then degenerates so establishing mesenchymal continuity across the intact palate [Greene and Pratt, 1976; Shah, 1979].

In the mammalian system, factors such as inadequate shelf size, excessive head width, or excessive intraoral movements, which prevent the palatal shelves from being in close and quiescent contact at the appropriate developmental time, all produce cleft palate [Poswillo, 1975; Trasler and Fraser, 1977]. Such factors, therefore, represent possible normal developmental mechanisms causing the naturally cleft chick palate; excessive shelf movement is a particularly likely mechanism as it is known that the avian palate consists mostly of muscle [Bellairs and Jenkin, 1960; McLelland, 1979] and that explanted chick palatal shelves spontaneously contract when cultured *in vitro* [Koch and Smiley, 1981; Ferguson et al, 1984]. To investigate these possibilities, we designed experiments in which the medial edge epithelia of day 8 and 9 (HH stages 33-35) embryonic chick palatal shelves were surgically disrupted in ovo and in vitro. Predictions from our hypothesis indicate that if the palatal shelves fused under these experimental conditions, then factors such as shelf movement have probably little to do with the genesis of natural cleft palate in chicken embryos. Conversely, if the palatal shelves re-epithelialised, as in mammalian fetal wound healing [Sopher, 1975, Goss, 1977a,b] and the palate did not fuse, then such factors may well be important. Moreover in crocodilians, eg. *Alligator mississippiensis*, the closest living phylogenetic relatives of birds, it is known that the palatal shelves progressively close in an anteroposterior direction. In contrast to mammals, crocodilian palatal closure involves only limited anterior epithelial cell death, and fusion is achieved mainly as a result of progressive migration of epithelial cells out of the closure zone in a postero-nasal direction [Ferguson, 1981a,b, 1982, 1984, 1985]. We therefore wished to investigate whether embryonic avian palatal shelves, which were surgically lacerated anteriorly and perhaps induced to fuse, would show medial edge epithelial cell migration and progressive antero-posterior palatal closure, in a fashion comparable to their crocodilian relatives.

MATERIALS AND METHODS

As outlined in Figure 1 the experimental strategy was to perform operations both on living chicken embryos in ovo and also on explanted chick palatal shelves cultured in vitro. Fertile Rhode Island red chick eggs were purchased from Redwing Hatchery (Los Angeles, CA) and artificially incubated. All eggs were windowed on the appropriate incubation day, and only those embryos falling within the requisite Hamburger-Hamilton (HH) [1951] stage were used.

In ovo operations were performed on 42 chick embryos at HH stage 32 (day 8) and on 71 chick embryos at HH stage 35 (day 9). Surgical access was obtained by

EXPERIMENTAL SCHEME

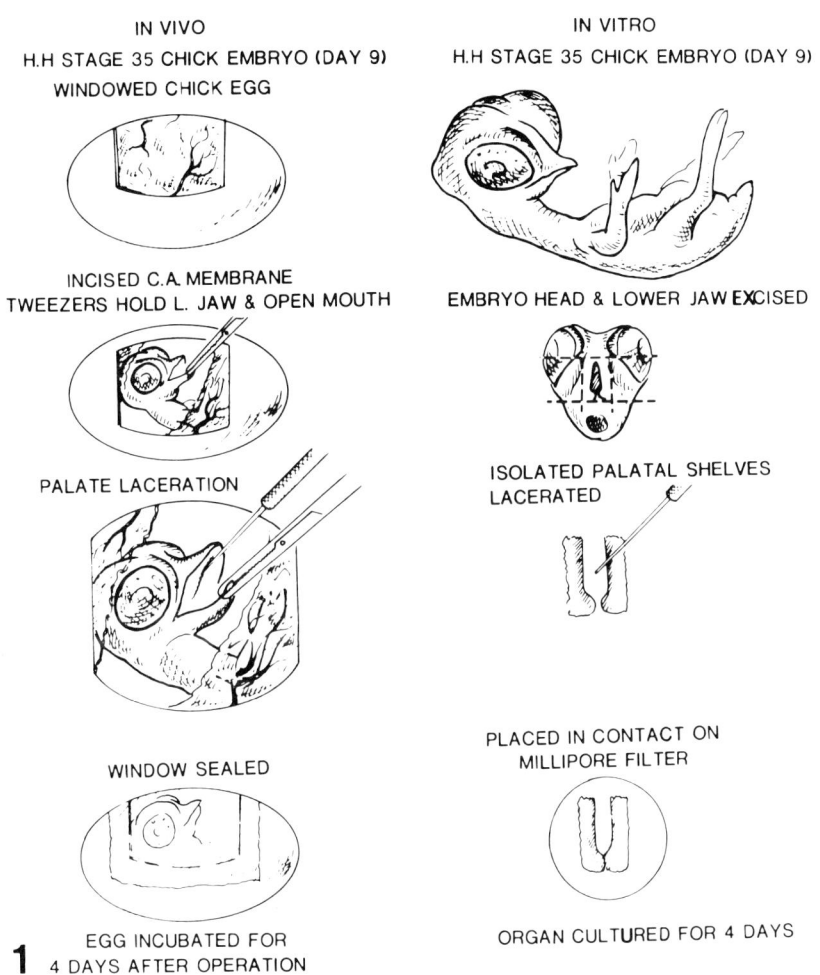

Fig. 1. The experimental scheme for the in vivo and in vitro experiments.

windowing the egg (Fig. 1). Under a dissecting microscope the chorio-allantoic membrane and the amnion were incised separately at non-vascular sites, using sharp forceps. The lower jaw was located and held with blunt, flattened forceps both to stabilise the embryo and to hold the mouth open (Fig. 1). Preliminary trials had shown that Meckel's cartilages are sufficiently developed at this stage to permit the embryo to be held in a stable position. Care was taken to minimise damage to the lower jaw, as the latter is known to influence upper jaw and general craniofacial development at this stage [Wouterlood and Van Pelt, 1979, Wouterlood and Dullemeijer, 1979]. Holding the lower jaw, and with the embryonic chick head at the level of the eggshell window, several different operations were performed on the palate using electrolytically sharpened tungsten needles. In the simplest operation the medial edge epithelia of each palatal shelf were surgically lacerated along the entire shelf length by inserting the tip of the needle anteriorly and dragging it posteriorly. In other operations only restricted lengths (anterior, middle, or posterior) of the medial edges of opposing palatal shelves were lacerated, whilst the remainder were left intact, in an attempt to discover if closure would occur at the surgical site and spread to non-operated areas. In other operations, the medial edge epithelia of both shelves were stained in ovo, using a dilute solution of nile blue sulphate A, and carefully dissected off the underlying mesenchyme. Control embryos were sham operated in a manner identical to that described above except that no manipulations of the palatal medial edge epithelia were performed. In all embryos the lower jaws were then released and closed, the embryonic chick heads, returned to their positions within the egg and the window sealed with sellotape. Eggs were incubated at 37°C and optimal humidity for four days, at which time the eggs were reopened and the embryos removed, staged, and fixed in either 10% buffered formal saline for light microscopy or Karnovsky's glutaraldehyde/paraformaldehyde fixative for scanning electron microscopy. The heads were removed from the bodies of the fixed embryos to facilitate further processing.

Comparable experiments were conducted in vitro. Palatal shelves were aseptically explanted from day 8 (HH stage 32) and day 9 (HH stage 35) chick embryos, and placed in pairs with their medial edges touching on discs of Millipore filters. Their medial edge epithelia were exposed to operative procedures similar to those described for the in ovo experiments. Control explants had no treatment to their medial edge epithelia. The discs of Millipore filter and attached chick palatal shelf pairs were then placed on a wire grid over 500 μl of media in Falcon Organ Culture Dishes. The media was chemically defined and consisted of Eagle's minimum essential medium at pH 7.4 supplemented with 0.56 mM ascorbic acid, 0.66 mM glycine, 2.05 mM L-glutamine, 15 mM Hepes buffer and 1% antibiotic-antimycotic (Gibco, New York). Ferguson et al [1984] have shown that this media and culture technique are permissive for embryonic palatal differentiation in chicks, mice, and alligators; and the reader is referred to this publication for further details of technique. The explants were cultured in air at 100% humidity, the media being changed daily, at which time macroscopic observations were made with a stereo-dissecting microscope. After 2, 3, and 4 days in culture, explants were fixed in either buffered formal saline or Karnovsky's fixative.

Details of the numbers of embryos or explants in each experimental treatment, their stages at operation and termination, the percentage mortality, and the results of the operative procedures are given in Table I.

The palatal shelves of all specimens were inspected and photographed macroscopically under a stereo zoom dissecting microscope. Those for light microscopy were decalcified in 10% trichloroacetic acid (end point determined by radiography), dehydrated through ascending grades of alcohol, cleared in xylene, embedded in Fibrowax (Raymond A Lamb, London), serially sectioned in the frontal plane at 8 μm and alternate sections stained with Harris iron haematoxylin, eosin, and alcian blue; Weigert iron haematoxylin, Unna's variation of van Gieson and alcian blue; Mallory trichrome; Gomori trichrome; and Linder nerve stain. Specimens for scanning electron microscopy (SEM) were dehydrated through ascending grades of acetone, critical-point-dried from amyl acetate and CO_2, sputter-coated with gold, and viewed in a Cambridge S180 Stereoscan.

TABLE I. Details Concerning the Types of Operation, the Embryonic Stages at Operation and Termination, the Mortality Rate, and the Palatal Appearance After Termination for Both the In Ovo and In Vitro Experiments

Type of operation	HH stage (days) at operation	Total number of embryos	HH stage (days) at termination	Number of dead embryos/explants (% mortality)	Number of living embryos/explants with unfused palates, ie, natural cleft palate (% of living embryos)	Number of living embryos/explants with partially fused palates (% of living embryos)	Number of living embryos/explants with completely fused palates (% of living embryos)
In ovo							
Laceration of the entire medial edges of both palatal shelves	32–33 (day 8)	20	37–38 (days 11–12)	11 (55%)	8 (88%)	1 (12%)	0 (0%)
	35 (day 9)	30	38–39 (days 12–13)	20 (66%)	0 (0%)	1 (10%)	9 (90%)
Laceration of a restricted length of the medial edge of both palatal shelves	32–33 (day 8)	5	37–38 (days 11–12)	3 (60%)	2 (100%)	0 (0%)	0 (0%)
	35 (day 9)	14	38–39 (days 12–13)	10 (71%)	0 (0%)	4 (100%)	0 (0%)
Staining and removal of the medial edge epithelia of both palatal shelves	32–33 (day 8)	8	36–38 (days 10–12)	3 (37%)	5 (100%)	0 (0%)	0 (0%)
	35 (day 9)	17	38–39 (days 12–13)	11 (65%)	0 (0%)	1 (16%)	5 (84%)
Control sham operation	32–33 (day 8)	9	36–38 (days 10–12)	3 (33%)	6 (100%)	0 (0%)	0 (0%)
	35 (day 9)	10	38–39 (days 12–13)	3 (30%)	7 (100%)	0 (0%)	0 (0%)
In vitro							
Laceration of the entire medial edges of both palatal shelves	32–33 (day 8)	8	after 2–4 days in culture	0 (0%)	0 (0%)	0 (0%)	8 (100%)
	35 (day 9)	10	after 2–4 days in culture	0 (0%)	0 (0%)	0 (0%)	10 (100%)
Laceration of a restricted length of the medial edges of both palatal shelves	32–33 (day 8)	5	after 2–4 days in culture	0 (0%)	0 (0%)	5 (100%)	0 (0%)
	35 (day 9)	10	after 2–4 days in culture	0 (0%)	0 (0%)	10 (100%)	0 (0%)
Staining and removal of the medial edge epithelia of both palatal shelves	32–33 (day 8)	5	after 2–4 days in culture	0 (0%)	0 (0%)	0 (0%)	5 (100%)
	35 (day 9)	10	after 2–4 days in culture	0 (0%)	0 (0%)	0 (0%)	10 (100%)
Control explants	32–33 (day 8)	6	after 2–4 days in culture	0 (0%)	6 (100%)	0 (0%)	0 (0%)
	35 (day 9)	10	after 2–4 days in culture	0 (0%)	10 (100%)	0 (0%)	0 (0%)

RESULTS

Survivorship of Embryos and Explants

Embryonic mortality was high for experimental operations on the palate (approximately 60%) and for control operations (approximately 30%) performed in ovo (Table I). Analysis of the dead embryos revealed that nearly all had died within a few hours of the operation. There was a significant difference between the mortality rates achieved by each of the two operators. Operation on the relatively inaccessible oral cavities of chick embryos of these late stages are technically difficult to perform without either excessive bleeding from or trauma to the embryo and its related membranes. The reason experimental operations had a higher mortality than controls likely derives from the longer operative time and greater embryonic trauma (eg, bleeding from the palate) involved in the former. Nonetheless, there was a significant improvement in mortality rate as the experiment progressed, suggesting that with operative practice the percentage of embryos surviving could be increased.

There was no mortality in vitro, demonstrating the permissive conditions of our culture technique [Ferguson et al, 1984].

Starting Material and Control Embryos

At HH stages 32-33 (days 7-8) the bilateral horizontal palatal shelves did not contact each other in the midline. Approximation commences around HH stage 34, and by HH stage 35 the medial edges of the palatal shelf pairs were in contact throughout their entire lengths (Figs. 2,3). Following fixation and processing, however, an artefactual (shrinkage) space was observed between the palatal shelves at HH stage 35 and later (Figs. 3, 5-7); such a space was not present in fresh embryos.

No physical connection was demonstrated histologically between the medial edge epithelia of opposing palatal shelves at any stage. The oral and medial edge epithelia differentiated into keratinised stratified squamous and the nasal into pseudostratified ciliated columnar epithelia (Figs. 3, 5-7). The lateral nasal walls became crenelated with marked infoldings of the epithelium (Figs. 5-7). Presumably these allowed for changes in shape as the palatal shelves contracted in response to palatal muscular activity [White, 1968]. Epithelial ingrowths for small salivary glands were present on the oral and medial edges of the palatal shelves at HH stage 38 (Figs. 5-7). A distinct subepithelial connective tissue stroma was present at HH stage 35, particularly beneath the oral and medial edges of the palate (Fig. 3). This was rich in glycosaminoglycans and collagen (as evidenced by staining with alcian blue and Mallory) but relatively avascular. The stroma became more marked as development progressed (Figs. 5-7). Elsewhere, in the more central regions of the palatal shelves, differentiation and growth of the bony anlage for the maxillae and palatines together with the palatal muscular anlage advanced significantly from HH stage 35 (Fig. 3) to stage 38 (Figs. 5-7).

Day 8 Operations in Ovo

Following experiments at HH stages 32-33 (day 8), almost no embryo exhibited signs of palatal closure, regardless of the type of operation performed (Table I). A variety of appearances were evident histologically at HH stages 37-38 (days 11-12). In most the medial edges of the palatal shelves exhibited epithelial tracks in the

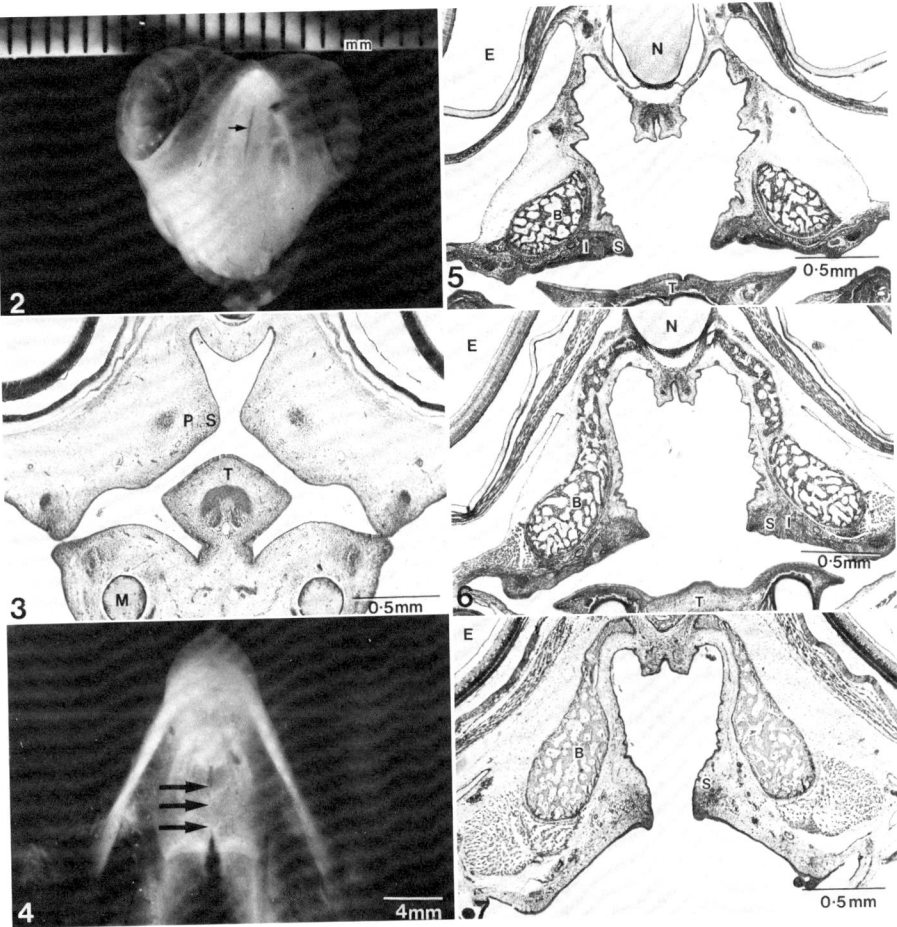

Fig. 2. Intra-oral view of the palate of a day 9 (HH stage 35) chick embryo. The palatal shelves are in contact in the midline but the palate is cleft (arrowed).

Fig. 3. Transverse section through the head of a HH stage 35, day 9 chick embryo. The space between the palatal shelves is an artefact. M = Meckel's cartilage; P = palatal shelves; S = subepithelial connective tissue stroma; T = tongue. (H&E) Haematoxylin and eosin and alcian blue.

Fig. 4. Macroscopic view of the palate of a HH stage 38 (day 12) chick embryo that had been partially lacerated along the medial shelf edges at HH stage 35 (day 9). Fusion has occurred in the area of operation (arrowed) but has not spread, so that the palate is cleft anterior and posterior to this site.

Fig. 5. Transverse section through the palate of a normal (control) HH stage 38 (day 12) chick embryo. The space between the cleft palatal shelves is a shrinkage artefact. B = bony blastemae for the maxillae and palatines (Figs. 6,7); E = eye; I = invagination for palatal salivary glands; N = nasal septum; S = subepithelial connective tissue stroma; T = tongue. Mallory trichrome.

Fig. 6. Transverse section posterior to that in Figure 5. For abbreviations see Figure 5 legend. Mallory trichrome.

Fig. 7. Transverse section posterior to that shown in Figure 6. For abbreviations see Figure 5 legend. Weigert, iron haematoxylin, van Gieson, and alcian blue.

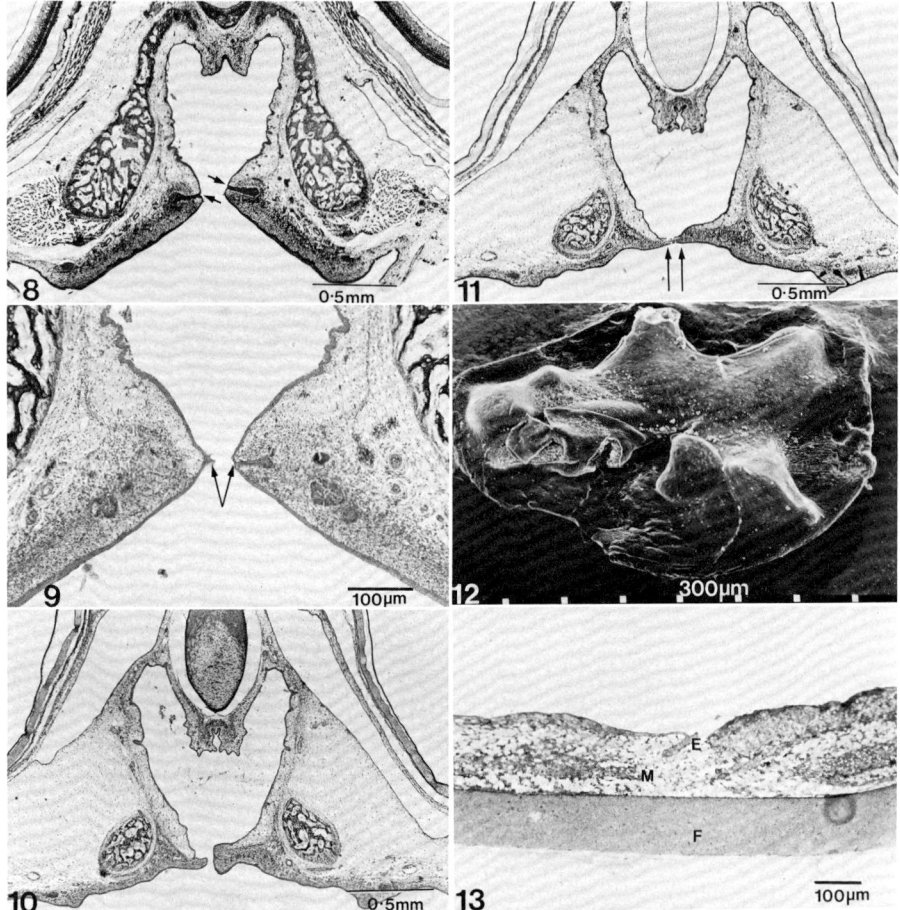

Fig. 8. Transverse section through the palate of a HH stage 38 (day 12) chick embryo that had its palate lacerated at HH stage 32 (day 8). Note the needle track invaginations of the medial edge epithelia (arrowed). Mallory trichrome. Compare with Figures 6 and 7.

Fig. 9. Higher-power view of a more posterior area of the palatal shelf medial edges of the same embryo illustrated in Figure 8. Note the needle track invagination and evidence of epithelial adherence at this zone (arrowed). S = subepithelial connective tissue stroma. Weigert, iron haematoxylin, van Gieson, and alcian blue.

Fig. 10. Transverse section through the head of a HH stage 37 (day 11) chick embryo that had its palatal medial edge epithelia removed at stage 32 (day 8). Note the distorted medial edges of the palatal shelves—compare with Figure 5. H&E and alcian blue.

Fig. 11. Transverse section of a HH stage 37 (day 11) embryonic chick head that had its palatal medial edge epithelia lacerated at stage 33 (day 8). Note the small zone of palatal fusion (arrowed)—compare with Figure 5. Weigert, iron haematoxylin, van Gieson, and alcian blue.

Fig. 12. SEM of a pair of chick palatal shelves explanted at HH stage 32 (day 8) and cultured for 2 days with their lacerated medial edges in contact. Fusion has occurred in the lacerated region.

Fig. 13. Transverse section through a pair of chick palatal shelves explanted at HH stage 35 (day 9) and cultured for 2 days with their lacerated medial edges in contact. Fusion has occurred. E = epithelial seam; F = filter; M = muscle blastemae.

regions where the tungsten needles had lacerated the shelves (Figs. 8,9). These needle tracks consisted of a closed loop of epithelial cells some 4-6 cells thick, resting on a continuous basement membrane (Figs. 8,9). The basal epithelial cells were low columnar/cuboidal but became progressively flatter towards the middle of the loop, where squamous type cells from each side were in contact with each other (Figs. 8,9). The subepithelial connective tissue stroma surrounding such needle tracks appeared normal (compare Figs. 6 and 8), and there were no signs of inflammatory cells or increased vasculature or scar tissue (Fig. 9). Sometimes the mesenchyme and stroma were condensed around the epithelial tracks, as if walling them off (Fig. 9). The remaining medial edge epithelia were normal stratified squamous in type (Figs. 8,9). Occasionally, it appeared as if the epithelia of opposing palatal shelf needle tracks had been adherent (Fig. 9), but there were never any signs of mesenchymal continuity between the two shelves.

In experiments involving either heavy laceration of the palatal shelf medial edges or removal of the medial edge epithelia, a different appearance was observed. The medial edges of such shelves were distorted, being either abnormally bulbous or thinned to small protrusions (Fig. 10). No needle tracks were observed; the medial shelf edges were covered by stratified squamous epithelia with no signs of inflammation, increased vasculature, or scar or scab tissue (Fig. 10). No fusion of opposing shelves was noted.

Only one embryo operated on at stage 33 (day 8) showed evidence of a partially fused palate (Table I, Fig. 11). In this embryo a very small antero-posterior length of the mid-palate had a narrow (oro-nasally) zone of mesenchymal continuity (Fig. 11). The epithelia immediately adjacent to both the oral and nasal sides of this continuity were stratified squamous, indicating that only a portion of the medial shelf edges had fused (Fig. 11). The continuity zone was only approximately five mesenchymal cells thick in the oro-nasal direction (Fig. 11).

Day 9 Operations in Ovo

Operations at HH stage 35 (day 9) resulted in all living embryos at HH stage 39 (day 13) having some sort of fused palate (Table I). These intact fused palates (Figs. 4, 16-19) were abnormal because the palate is normally cleft in chickens (Figs. 5-7). The type of fusion depended upon the type of operation (Table I). Laceration of the entire medial shelf edges and removal of the medial edge epithelia nearly always resulted in fusion of the two shelves throughout their entire length (Table I). Conversely, laceration of restricted lengths of the medial shelf edges resulted in fusion only in these areas (Table I, Figs. 4, 14-16). Fusion did not spread either anteriorly or posteriorly and serial sections through the junctional zones showed the shelves fused (Fig. 16), the epithelia of both shelves in close contact forming a seam-like structure (Fig. 15), and finally the two medial edge epithelia independent of each other (Fig. 14) similar to their normal appearance (eg, Fig. 5). The extent of oro-nasal fusion depended somewhat upon the type of operation. In experiments involving either heavy lacerations or removal of the medial edge epithelia, the areas of mesenchymal continuity were large (Figs. 16,18). The epithelia on the nasal sides of such continuities were pseudostratified ciliated columnar and on the oral sides stratified squamous, indicating that the entire medial shelf edges had fused (Figs. 16,18). Conversely, in experiments involving single light lacerations of both shelves, the extent of oro-nasal fusion was much more limited (Fig. 19). These small areas of continuity had variable epithelial coverings depending upon the oro-nasal location of

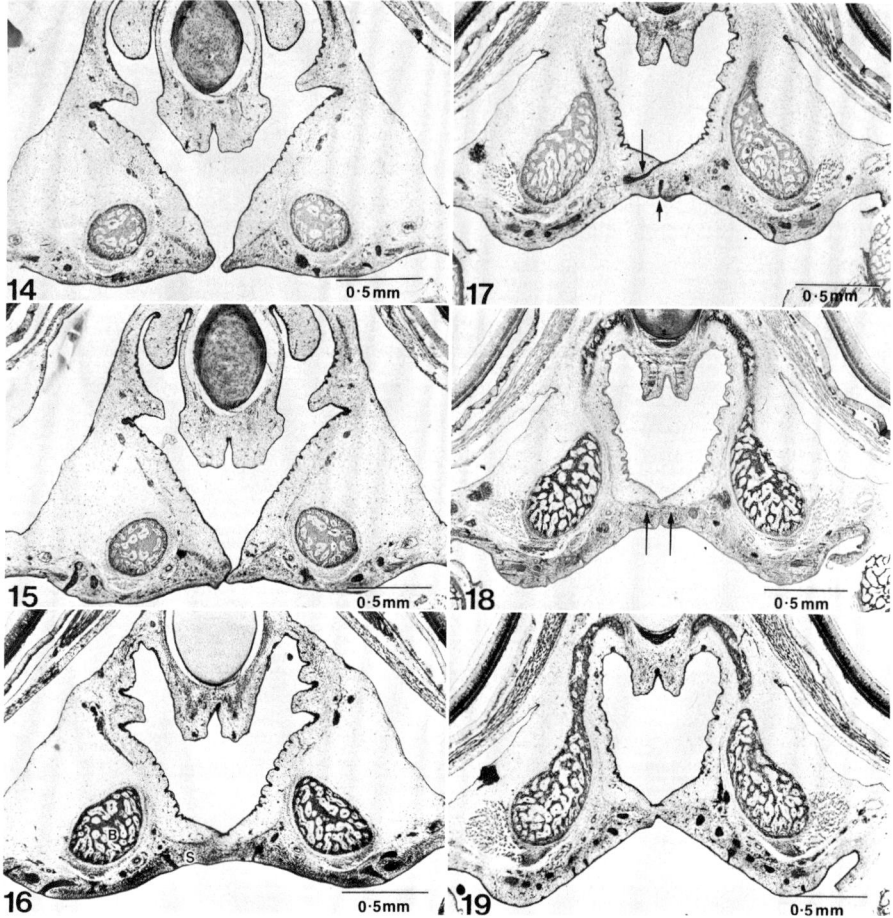

Fig. 14. Transverse section of a HH stage 38 (day 12) embryonic chick head that had its palatal medial edge epithelia partially lacerated at HH stage 35 (day 9). This section is through an anterior unlacerated part of the palate and shows the normal cleft palate (compare with Fig. 5). H&E and alcian blue.

Fig. 15. Transverse section posterior to that in Figure 14 illustrating the junctional area between cleft (Fig. 14) and fused (Fig. 16) palate. Note that the two medial edge epithelia are in contact to form an epithelial seam. H&E and alcian blue.

Fig. 16. Transverse section further posterior to that in Figure 15. Palatal fusion is extensive (compare with Figs. 5 and 14). Note the bony blastemae (B) and subepithelial connective tissue stroma (S) restricted to the oral aspect of the palate. Mallory trichrome.

Fig. 17. Transverse section through a HH stage 38 (day 12) embryonic chick head that had a single light laceration of its palatal medial edge epithelia at HH stage 35 (day 9). Note the extensive palatal fusion and the two epithelial seams (arrowed). Compare with Figures 5 and 6. H&E and alcian blue.

Fig. 18. Transverse section through a HH stage 38 (day 12) embryonic chick head that had its palatal medial edge epithelia removed at HH stage 35 (day 9). Fusion has occurred and bony blastemae (arrowed) are present in the mid-palatal continuity zone. Compare with Figures 6 and 7. Weigert, iron haematoxylin, van Gieson, and alcian blue.

Fig. 19. Transverse section through a HH stage 38 (day 12) embryonic chick head that had a single laceration of its palatal medial edge epithelia at HH stage 35 (day 9). Note the limited extent of palatal fusion. Compare with Figures 6, 7, and 18. Mallory trichrome.

the laceration: most commonly the continuity area was lined by stratified squamous epithelia on both sides, indicating that the medial edges had not fused throughout their entire oro-nasal extents (Fig. 19). Occasionally extensive oro-nasal continuities occurred following such light single lacerations (Fig. 17). In these the mesenchyme from both shelves appeared to consolidate the continuities and cause the remaining medial edge epithelia of both shelves to join together and form incomplete epithelial seams (Fig. 17). These seams (Fig. 17) resembled the needle tracks seen after operations on day 8 (Fig. 8). The epithelial seams were long, often distorted to one side and persisted (perhaps even elongated) throughout later development (Fig. 17). The epithelia were in two layers totaling approximately six cells, ranging from cuboidal basal cells resting on a basement membrane through central squamous cells back to cuboidal basal cells on a basement membrane again. No cell death was evident in the seam, nor were there any signs of reaction in the surrounding connective tissue (Fig. 17). Indeed, none of the fusion zones exhibited any evidence of inflammation or scar tissue, although there were occasionally increased numbers of blood vessels (Figs. 16–19). The dense subepithelial connective tissue stroma was present but localised to the oral aspect of the fused palates, even in the zones of palatal continuity (Fig. 16, compare with Fig. 5). Occasionally differentiating osseous and muscular blastemae were seen crossing the continuity zones of fused palatal shelves (Fig. 18). Such blastemae were highly abnormal because the palate is normally cleft in the chicken. Whether they represent new osseous and muscular elements or merely extensions of existing ones is unknown.

In Vitro Operations at Days 8 and 9

The results of the in vitro experiments were identical regardless of the age of the explanted palatal shelves (Table I). As with the day 9 in ovo experiments, the extent of palatal fusion (antero-posteriorly and oro-nasally) depended upon the type of operation performed (Table I). Fusion occurred only in the areas of laceration or epithelial removal (Table I, Figs. 12,13). Differentiation of the epithelia and mesenchyme were similar to appearances described for day 9 in ovo operations. Occasional epithelial seams were observed in the fusion zones (Fig. 13). Fusion of pairs of palatal shelves in vitro was macroscopically evident following 2 days of culture (Fig. 12). Control shelves explanted with their medial edges in contact, but intact, never fused (Table I); rather, their medial edge epithelia differentiated into the normal stratified squamous phenotype.

DISCUSSION

These experiments document for the first time the ability of chick palatal shelves to fuse in vivo and in vitro to form an intact palate. Such an intact palate is abnormal for chickens, where the palate is naturally cleft. This situation is the reverse of mammals where intact palates are normal and cleft palates abnormal. To some extent the present experiments of making normally cleft palates pathologically intact are the opposite of literally hundreds of mammalian experiments reviewed by Shah [1979], where intact palates have been made pathologically cleft. As such they have some important implications for the pathogenesis of palatal clefting, palatal evolution, embryonic surgery, and embryonic wound healing.

Whether experimental fusion occurs between pairs of chick palatal shelves appears to depend primarily on how close they are to each other at the time of operation. At HH stages 32–33, the shelves are so far apart that the speed of embryonic wound healing is probably such that the shelves are covered by an intact epithelial surface before they contact one another, consequently, fusion does not occur. Conversely, at HH stage 35, when the shelves are already in contact, fusion occurs and precludes re-epithelialisation and wound healing. This hypothesis is supported by the in vitro experiments which demonstrate that operated palatal shelves of any stage will fuse with one another provided that their medial edges are in contact. Importantly, unoperated palatal shelves with their medial edges in contact do not fuse in vitro. The present experiments therefore demonstrate that chick palatal shelves can fuse in ovo and in vitro and that the reason for natural cleft palate in the chick is not related to an unfavourable embryonic environment, eg, excessive shelf movement, small shelf size, or excessive head width.

Instead, the reason may be related to an absence of medial edge epithelial cell death. In previous epithelial mesenchymal recombination experiments, we have shown that chick embryonic palatal epithelium can be induced to die by association with an embryonic mouse palatal mesenchyme [Ferguson and Honig, 1984]. The conclusion from these and other experiments [see Ferguson and Honig, 1984] is that embryonic chick palatal epithelium is capable of responding to mesenchymal instructions to die or migrate, but that such instructions are not received and keratinisation results almost as a default state. The possibilities are that either the chick mesenchyme does not (or cannot) signal medial edge epithelial cell death or that there is some temporal alteration of the sequence of palatal growth and differentiation such that the signal is not received. (There is little possibility that the signal is received at the wrong time, because at no developmental stage do chick medial edge epithelial cells die, ie, there is no asynchrony between cell death and shelf contact). The differentiation of the subepithelial connective tissue stroma on the oral and medial aspects of the chick palatal shelf, also observed by Koch and Smiley [1981], may serve to inhibit such signalling either by a physical barrier or else by the inability of the mesenchymal cells to degrade the latter and so form intimate contacts with either the basement membrane or the epithelial cells themselves. No such subepithelial stroma exists in comparable mammalian palatal shelves, and a similar mechanism has been proposed by Hall and MacSween [1984] to account for the localised signalling of bone differentiation within the embryonic mandible. Such a possibility will be tested in future experiments. In any case the present experiments demonstrate how a subtle alteration in one developmental event, or the synchrony of developmental events, can have profound effects on adult structure and function [Maderson, 1975], ie, cleft or intact palate. Even more intriguing is what the muscular and osseous blastemae crossing the abnormally intact chick palate represent. Are these forerunners of the palatal processes of the maxillae and palatines induced to form by the mere mechanics of palatal closure, or do they represent some abnormal, perhaps ancestral morphology? The answer is of considerable developmental, phylogenetic, and anatomical interest, so that future experimental embryos will be allowed to survive longer to document these structures in detail. It would be interesting to learn how newborn and adult chicks with abnormally intact palates would feed and swallow in view of the extreme physiological adaptations to the normally cleft chicken palate [White, 1968].

Palatal closure did not extend from sites of limited initial experimental fusion in chickens. This is unlike the normal situation in *Alligator mississippiensis* (a close phylogenetic relative) where, after limited medial edge epithelial cell death, extensive epithelial cell migration results in complete palatal closure [Ferguson, 1981a,b, 1982,

1984, 1985]. Of great interest would be a study of palatal development in desmognathous species of birds where the maxillae and/or palatine bones unite in the midline [Bellairs and Jenkins, 1960]. Extrapolation from the present experiments suggests that the medial edge epithelia in the anterior regions of embryonic desmognathous palatal shelves die, resulting in palatal fusion that is unable to progress posteriorly. Comparisons of palatal mesenchymal signalling capabilities in experimental recombinations, the degree of subepithelial stromal development, and the extent of direct mesenchymal/epithelial cell contacts in schizognathous and desmognathous avian species would be most illuminating.

No cell death occurred in the epithelial seams of experimentally fused chick palatal shelves as opposed to that normally seen in mammalian palatal epithelial seams. It would be interesting to compare the ultrastructure and biochemistry of these two seams. It is also unclear how the chick epithelial cells adhere to one another and how they form their basement membranes in both the epithelial seams and the needle tracks. Chick medial edge epithelial cells have a carbohydrate-rich surface coat [Shah and Crawford, 1980], but whether this and/or desmosomes are involved is unknown. If these epithelia can adhere in experimental seams and needle tracks, then why not normally when the two palatal shelves contact each other? Interestingly, despite these extensive persistent epithelial seams, the experimentally fused chick palatal shelves did not pull apart with subsequent development and growth. This casts doubt on the hypothesis of post-fusion rupture as a pathogenetic mechanism in mammalian cleft palate [Goss 1977a,b]. The reason why Goss [1977a,b] did not observe re-fusion of experimentally incised (in utero) day 19½ rat palatal shelves is probably related to the massive tissue distortion and disruption caused by his incisions through the fetal face and nose as well as to the late stage of palatal differentiation. Quite simply, the shelves were not in contact. Even the barely fused experimental chick palatal shelves did not pull apart; rather, they resembled the mammalian condition of submucous cleft palate. Perhaps the pathogenesis of the latter involves limited shelf fusion as well as poor mesenchymal consolidation. The ability of damaged chick palatal shelves to fuse in vitro emphasizes the extreme care needed in handling palatal explants for reliable in vitro experimentation.

The present experiments also document the utility of the developing chicken embryo as a model for studying embryonic (fetal) wound healing and cleft palate surgery. Chick embryos are readily available and inexpensive, surgical access is easier than in mammals, and there are no problems associated with trying to induce cleft palate as the latter is a natural condition. Moreover, comparison of the events of embryonic (fetal) wound healing in the present chick experiments (principally those at day 8) with those of previous monkey [Sopher, 1975] and rat [Sopher, 1975, Goss 1977a,b] experiments reveals many similarities. Thus re-epithelialisation is rapid, and there are no signs of inflammation, infection, or scar or scab tissue formation. These unique features of embryonic (fetal) wound healing probably relate both to the immaturity of the reticulo-endothelial system and the idyllic sterile, aqueous milieu surrounding the embryo. The ingrowths of the chick palatal medial edge epithelia to form needle tracks resemble similar ingrowths down the suture paths and incised wound edges in fetal monkey skin [Sopher, 1975]. Clearly further studies are required to document precisely the sequence of events in embryonic wound healing and cleft palate repair. However, the possibility of embryonic surgery to correct cleft palate in man, with the attendant advantages of scar free healing and prevention of secondary deformities, should be incentive enough to conduct such studies. The naturally cleft chick palate may prove a useful model for the investigation of basic mechanisms in embryonic wound healing and cleft repair.

ACKNOWLEDGMENTS

These experiments were principally conducted in the Laboratory for Developmental Biology, University of Southern California, whose director, Professor H.C. Slavkin, we thank. Collaborative study was made possible by the award of a 1981 Research Travelling Scholarship from the Wellcome Trust to M.W.J.F. This work was supported by grant 8113610CB from the Medical Research Council of Great Britain and grants DE-02848 and DE-03569 from the National Institutes of Health U.S.A. Miss A. Darbyshire kindly typed the manuscript.

REFERENCES

Bellairs A d'A, Jenkin CR: The skeleton of birds. In Marshall AJ (ed): "Biology and Comparative Physiology of Birds, Vol 1." New York: Academic Press, 1960, pp 241–300.

Ferguson MWJ: The value of the American alligator (*Alligator mississippiensis*) as a model for research in craniofacial development. J Craniofacial Genet Dev Biol 1:123–144, 1981a.

Ferguson MWJ: The structure and development of the palate in *Alligator mississippiensis*. Arch Oral Biol 26:427–443, 1981b.

Ferguson MWJ: The structure and development of the palate in *Alligator mississippiensis*. PhD thesis, The Queen's University of Belfast, 1982.

Ferguson MWJ: Craniofacial development in *Alligator mississippiensis*. In (ed): Ferguson MWJ "The Structure, Development and Evolution of Reptiles." London: Academic Press, 1984, pp 233–273.

Ferguson MWJ: The Reproductive Biology and Embryology of Crocodilians. In (eds): Gans C, Billett FS, Maderson P, Biology of the Reptilia, Vol 14: "Development." New York: J Wiley and Sons, (in press), 1985.

Ferguson MWJ, Honig LS: Epithelial-mesenchymal interactions during vertebrate palatogenesis. In: Zimmerman EF (ed) *Current Topics in Developmental Biology,* Vol 19: "Palate development: Normal and Abnormal, Cellular and Molecular Aspects." New York: Academic Press, 1984, pp 137–164.

Ferguson MWJ, Honig LS, Slavkin HC: Differentiation of cultured palatal shelves from alligator, chick and mouse embryos. Anat Rec 209:231–249, 1984.

Goss AN: Intra-uterine healing of fetal rat oral mucosal, skin and cartilage wounds. J Oral Pathol 6:35–43, 1977a.

Goss AN: Post-fusion cleft of the fetal rat palate. Cleft Palate J 14(2):131–139, 1977b.

Greene RM, Pratt RM: Developmental aspects of secondary palate formation. J Embryol Exp Morphol 36:225–245, 1976.

Hall BK, MacSween MC: An SEM analysis of the epithelial-mesenchymal interface in the mandible of the embryonic chick. J Craniofac Genet Dev Biol 4:59–76, 1984.

Hamburger V, Hamilton HL: A series of normal stages in the development of the chick embryo. J Morphol 88:49–92, 1951.

Kock WE, Smiley GR: *In vivo* and *in vitro* studies of the development of the avian secondary palate. Archs Oral Biol 26:181–187, 1981.

Maderson PFA: Embryonic tissue interactions as the basis for morphological change in evolution. Am Zool 15:315–327, 1975.

McLelland J: Digestive system. In King AS, McLelland J (eds): "Form and Function in Birds." London: Academic Press, 1:69–181, 1979.

Poswillo, D.: Causal mechanisms of craniofacial deformity. Br Med Bull 31(2):101–106, 1975.

Shah RM: Current concepts on the mechanisms of normal and abnormal secondary palate formation. In Persaud TVN (ed): "Advances in the Study of Birth Defects, vol 1: Teratogenic Mechanisms." Lancaster: M.T.P. Press Ltd., 1979, pp 69–84.

Shah RM, Crawford BJ: Development of the secondary palate in chick embryo: A light and electron microscopic and histochemical study. Invest Cell Pathol 3:319–328, 1980.

Sopher D: Future prospects for fetal surgery. In Berry CL, Poswillo DE (eds): "Teratology Trends and Applications." Berlin: Springer Verlag, 1975, pp 165–179.

Trasler DG, Fraser FC: Time-position relationships with particular reference to cleft lip and cleft palate. In Wilson JG, Fraser FC (eds): "Handbook of Teratology Vol 2." New York: Plenum Press, 1977, pp 271–292.

White SS: Mechanisms involved in deglutition in *Gallus domesticus*. J Anat 104:177, 1968.

Wouterlood FG, Dullemeijer P: Skull growth after partial prospective lower beak extirpation in chick embryos. Anat Anz 145:1–16, 1979.

Wouterlood FG, Van Pelt W: The influence of the lower beak on the interorbital septum-prenasal process complex in the chick embryo. J Embryol Exp Morphol 49:61–72, 1979.

Experimental Teratological Studies With the Mouse CNS Mutations Cranioschisis and Delayed Splotch

H. Kalter
Children's Hospital Research Foundation and Department of Pediatrics, University of Cincinnati College of Medicine, Cincinnati, Ohio

> Teratological experiments were made with a recessive mouse gene (cranioschisis) causing exencephaly and a semidominant gene (delayed splotch) causing spina bifida. In studies with the cranioschisis gene administration of warfarin and thyroxine resulted in frequencies of exencephaly significantly below that expected of a recessive trait, perhaps indicating selective elimination of abnormal conceptuses. Studies with the delayed splotch gene tested the hypothesis that offspring with a hereditary defect of neural-tube closure have other, unexpressed CNS defects, which may be elicited by teratological impulses. This proposition was decisively upheld by administering 5-bromo-2'-deoxyuridine, cadmium sulfate and retinoic acid, as these treatments all caused significantly greater frequencies of induced exencephaly in offspring with spina bifida than in their genetically normal littermates.

Key words: cranioschisis, delayed splotch, mouse gene, exencephaly, spina bifida

INTRODUCTION

The morphological mutants of the house mouse are an abundant and varied source of teratological research material [Kalter, 1980]. Recognition of the usefulness of this material for numerous types of teratological studies has grown in the last 25 years, but at a snail's pace [eg, Kobozieff et al, 1959; Watney and Miller, 1964; Hamburgh et al, 1970; Seller et al, 1979; Trasler et al, 1984]. Herein are noted several experiments performed with animals carrying two mutant genes, to illustrate some uses of such material.

EXPERIMENTS AND RESULTS

The first of the genes is cranioschisis *(crn)*, a recessive gene with possibly somewhat reduced penetrance, as gauged near term. As its name indicates, it causes exencephaly, usually accompanied by choroid-fissure coloboma of variable extent and other eye defects [Kalter, 1981]. The gene, on a genetically heterogeneous back-

---

Address reprint requests to H. Kalter, Children's Hospital Research Foundation, Elland Avenue, Cincinnati, OH 45229.

© 1985 Alan R. Liss, Inc.

ground, was obtained in March 1977 from Dr. K.S. Brown (NIH); the animals were random bred in my laboratory until they were outbred to a mutant C3H line to improve their vigor, and the random breeding then continued.

The second gene is delayed splotch (Sp^d), a semidominant causing, in homozygotes, lumbosacral spina bifida aperta of variable extent, plus tail, limb, and head abnormalities, and, rarely, exencephaly in offspring with the spinal defect. Affected offspring frequently survive to term, in contrast with those with CNS defects caused by the allele splotch [Auerbach, 1954]. The gene was obtained in April 1977 from the Jackson Laboratory (Bar Harbor, ME), on a C57BL/6J background. Sometime later the animals were outcrossed to a mutant BALB/c line and then random bred. Recently some inbreeding was begun.

The general purpose of the studies to be described was to test the responses of mutant offspring to the effects of various teratogenic chemicals. One series of experiments, made with the cranioschisis stock, attempted to kill exencephalic (ie, crn/crn) embryos and fetuses selectively by maternal injection of warfarin and thyroxine. Previously identified heterozygotes (+/crn) were bred, and the pregnant females given single intraperitoneal (ip) injections of 5–40 mg/kg warfarin (Coumadin, Endo, Garden City, NY) on the 10th or 11th day of gestation, or single or double injections on separate days beginning the 13th day (VP = 1st day). The earlier schedule of treatment had no significant effect on the frequency of exencephaly (expected to be 25%) in near-term offspring, but the later schedule was associated with a greatly reduced frequency of the defect (Table I).

Although it would be tempting to explain the deficiency of affected offspring by their selective elimination, the overall mortality data do not appear to support this interpretation, since the resorption rate in the two groups was similar. A closer analysis of the number affected and number resorbed within each litter is called for.

In the second experiment, with 0.1–0.4 mg/day thyroxine (ICN, Cleveland, OH), given subcutaneously (sc) on two successive days the pattern seemed to be reversed. Comparing an earlier period of treatment (7th–10th) with a later one (10th–14th), the reduced frequency of exencephaly occurred in the former (Table I). Again, however, the overall resorption data do not seem to be helpful in interpreting the results.

Thus in both experiments there was a suggestion that conceptuses with expressed or unexpressed hereditary exencephaly were selectively killed by exposure to a chemical; but the increased prenatal mortality that would be expected to follow such events did not appear to have been present.

TABLE I. Frequency of Hereditary Exencephaly in Offspring of Pregnant Female +/crn Mice (Bred to +/crn Males) Administered Warfarin or Thyroxine at Two Different Periods of Gestation

	Warfarin[1]		Thyroxine[2]		Untreated or saline-injected
	10th, 11th day	13th day	7th–10th day	10th–14th day	
No. litters	16	22	94	21	49
No. offspring	128	193	1027	219	564
% Resorbed	18.5	20.6	10.7	12.1	8.1
% Exencephaly	21.8	5.7	10.9	22.4	21.3

[1]Single injections of 5–40 mg/kg ip on the 10th or 11th day of gestation (VP = 1st day), or single or two successive daily injections beginning the 13th day.
[2]Injections of 0.1–0.4 mg/day sc on two successive days.

An alternative explanation for the reduced frequency in the earlier-treated group in the thyroxine experiment is that in some instances the defect was prevented from occurring, thus in essence further reducing the penetrance of the gene. This possibility could hardly explain the reduced frequency of the defect in the later-treated warfarin group, since these injections were made long after the time of closure of the anterior neuropore [Waterman, 1976].

Another series of experiments, made with the delayed splotch stock, had a different purpose. This was to test the hypothesis that genetic defects of neural tube closure entail additional, albeit ordinarily unexpressed, CNS anomalies. In the specific instance of the delayed splotch gene, it was proposed that in embryos with latent spina bifida the additional anomalous state would be signified by a sensitivity to exencephaly-inducing agents beyond that of their nonbifidous littermates, the latter providing the decided advantage of being an in-built control.

The motive for these studies was to point out a possible bias in the common epidemiological practice of reporting anencephaly and spina bifida as one entity under the heading neural tube defects. This practice has been justified by the several epidemiological similarities of the two defects and their nonrandom concurrence, which have been interpreted as appearing to indicate etiological relatedness.

Several human and experimental observations contradict a common etiology, however. The defects rarely, if ever, occur together in some racial groups [Kurent and Sever, 1973]; although exencephaly is readily induced in laboratory species by numerous chemicals, experimentally induced spina bifida has been reported far more rarely [Kalter, 1968]; the sensitive periods during gestation for the induction of these defects do not coincide [Waterman, 1976].

To test the hypothesis outlined above, chemicals were used that are known to cause exencephaly when given in favorable schedules. Heterozygotes were bred and pregnant females administered 200–500 mg/kg 5-bromo-2'-deoxyuridine (Sigma Chemical Co., St. Louis, MO), ip, on the 8th or 9th day, 3–6 mg/kg cadmium sulfate (Aldrich, Milwaukee, WI), ip, on the 9th day, or 4–30 mg/kg all-trans retinoic acid (Sigma), po, on the 8th or 9th day. All three chemicals gave clear results that supported the proposition (Table II). In all studies, offspring with the hereditary condition spina bifida had a significantly larger frequency of the induced defect, exencephaly, than their littermates without the bifida.

TABLE II. Frequency of Induced Exencephaly in Offspring With and Without Hereditary Spina Bifida Produced by Administration to Pregnant Female $Sp^d/+$ Mice (Bred to $Sp^d/+$ Males) of 5-Bromo-2'-Deoxyuridine (BUDR), Cadmium Sulfate (CdSO$_4$), or All-Trans Retinoic Acid (RA)

	BUDR[1]	CdSO$_4$[2]	RA[3]	Control
No. litters	22	32	20	19
No. offspring	173	234	139	120
% Resorbed	33.5	13.3	18.7	23.1
No. (%) exencephaly/ non-spina bifida	39/143 (27.3)	21/185 (11.4)	13/107 (12.1)	0/95 (0)
No. (%) exencephaly/ spina bifida	19/30 (63.3)	23/49 (46.9)	10/32 (31.2)	3/25 (12.0)

[1]200–500 mg/kg ip, 8th or 9th day.
[2]3–6 mg/kg ip, 9th day.
[3]4–30 mg/kg po, 8th or 9th day.

DISCUSSION

These consistent results, in the face of three very different chemicals, indicate that the cranial neural folds of homozygous delayed splotch embryos are delicately balanced developmentally, possessing a generalized disposition to be deflected from their usual morphogenetic path. This state may be thought of as a step toward the more overt one produced by the gene splotch, another allele at this locus, which frequently causes exencephaly along with spina bifida [Auerbach, 1954; Dempsey and Trasler, 1983].

The developmental instability presented by the delayed splotch gene may have its human counterpart. Thus, the condition of some families, in which both anencephaly and spina bifida occur, in the same individual or not, should perhaps be distinguished from that in which only one or the other of these conditions recurs. Considering these two types of families separately may facilitate analysis of the epidemiological patterns.

ACKNOWLEDGMENTS

This work was supported in part by NIH grant HD15038.

REFERENCES

Auerbach R: Analysis of the developmental effects of a lethal mutation in the house mouse. J Exp Zool 127:305–329, 1954.

Dempsey EE, Trasler DG: Early morphological abnormalities in splotch mouse embryos and predisposition to gene- and retinoic acid-induced neural tube defects. Teratology 28:461–472, 1983.

Hamburgh M, Herz R, Landa G: The effect of trypan blue on expressivity of the brachyury gene "T," in mice. Teratology 3:111–113, 1970.

Kalter H: Teratology of the central nervous system. Induced and spontaneous malformations of laboratory, agricultural, and domestic mammals. University of Chicago, Chicago, 1968.

Kalter H: A compendium of the genetically induced congenital malformations of the house mouse. Teratology 21:397–429, 1980.

Kalter H: Eye defects associated with a gene for exencephaly in mice. Teratology 23:44A, 1981.

Kobozieff N, Tuchmann-Duplessis H, Mercier-Parot L, Domriaskinsky-Kobozieff NA: Influence de bleu trypan sur la frequence d'apparition et la gravite des malformations chez des souris presentant une polydactylie hereditaire. Rec Med Vet 135:317–324, 1959.

Kurent JE, Sever JL: Perinatal infections and epidemiology of anencephaly and spina bifida. Teratology 8:359–361, 1973.

Seller MJ, Embury S, Polani PE, Adinolfi M: Neural tube defects in curly tail mice. II. Effect of maternal administration of vitamin A. Proc R. Soc Lond B 206:95–107.

Trasler DG, Kemp D, Trasler TA: Increased susceptibility to 6-aminonicotinamide-induced cleft lip of heterozygote dancer mice. Teratology 29:101–104, 1984.

Waterman RE: Topographical changes along the neural fold associated with neurulation in the hamster and mouse. Am J Anat 146:151–172, 1976.

Watney MJ, Miller JR: Prevention of a genetically determined congenital eye anomaly in the mouse by the administration of cortisone during pregnancy. Nature 202:1029–1031, 1964.

Index

Abnormal growth syndromes. *See* Craniofacial dysmorphology in abnormal growth syndromes, roentgencephalometry; specific syndromes
Achondroplasia, craniofacial morphometry and roentgencephalometry, 139–163
    basion-anterior nasal spine distance, 151
    calvaria, 152, 159–161
        hydrocephalus, 160–161
        hypotonia and slow motor development, 160
        megalocephaly, 160
    cephalometric measurements, 144–149
        area measurements, 148, 155
        with defined points, listed, 144–145
        linear and angular, 146, 149, 154, 155
        linear, perpendicular to sellar vertical, 147
        morphologic disarticulation, 148
        ratios, 149
    computer morphometric model, 142–143, 145
        Calcomp plot, 143, 152
        model, 2-dimensional, 142–143
    cranial base and angle, 156–159
        cribiform and sphenoid bones, 157
        early closure of spheno-occipital synchondrosis, 158
        endochondral bone formation, 156
        foramen magnum, 158–159
        functional matrix theory, 156–157
        occipital bony protuberance, 159
        trunk length and vertebral column, 157, 160
    data analysis, 149–150
        IBM system 360 and MIDAS statistical package, 149
        multivariate, 150
    face, 161–163
    females cf. normal females, 150, 152
    frontal sinus area, 151, 152
    histograms, 150
    males cf. females, 150, 153, 162
    males cf. normal males, 150, 151
    mandibular alveolar prognathism, 151, 162
    normals, males cf. females, 153
    profile patterns, standard deviation, 154, 161, 163
    subjects (Little People of America), 141
    cf. controls, 142
    sample bias, 141–142
Adenoids. *See under* Velopharyngeal inadequacy without overt cleft palate
Age
    cleft palate surgical closure, 71–73, 83
    determination, bone, 43–44
Agent Orange and dioxin, teratogenic/mutagenic effects, 259–264

cf. animals and plants, 259, 262–263
birth defects, 259, 260, 263–264
    listed, 260
chromosomal damage, 259–264
epidemiologic evidence, 263–264
    Italy, 263
    Oregon and Australia, 264
formulations, 259, 262
G-banded karyotyping, 260–261
lipophilicity, 264
peripheral neuropathy, 260
SCE, 259, 261–263
Vietnam veterans, 260, 264
Aglossia and agnathia, 241, 243, 246
Agnathia without holoprosencephaly, developmental field complex, 241–248
    aglossia, 241, 243, 246
    cleft lip and palate, 242, 243, 246, 247
    cloudy corneas, 243
    cyclopia, 241
    down-slanting palpebral fissures, 242, 243, 246, 247
    ear position, 241–246
    cf. guinea pig and mouse, 242, 247
    cf. with holoprosencephaly, 246–247
    maternal alcohol abuse, 242
    microstomia, 241–246
    neural crest, 247–248
    patent ductus arteriosus, 244
    polyhydramnios, 242, 245, 246
    prechordal mesoderm, 247–248
    PROM, 243
    race and sex, 242, 243, 245, 246
    respiratory distress and cardiac anomalies, 244
    review of reported cases, 246–247
Airway, Beckwith-Wiedemann syndrome, 180, 181; *see also* Hallerman-Streiff syndrome with cardiorespiratory insufficiency
A/J mice, clefting, 306, 314, 319–322; *see also* Cleft palate, corticosterone-induced, A/J mice
Alcohol abuse, maternal, agnathia without holoprosencephaly, 242
Amblyopia, Duane retraction syndrome, 274
Ameloblast-specific gene expression, and pattern formation during craniofacial development, 59, 61–65
Amelogenin, 63, 64
Anisometropia, Duane retraction syndrome, 274
Apert syndrome, 19–20, 37, 45, 49
Aphasia, 110
Apnea, sleep, 106, 192–197
Apraxia, VPI, 110–111
Ascertainment bias, 53–54
Astigmatism, Duane retraction syndrome, 274

Index

Asymmetric dysmorphism, 50; *see also* Hemifacial microsomia *entries;* Mandibular condyle in facial asymmetry, longitudinal roentgencephalometry; Plagiocephaly, longitudinal roentgencephalometry
Australia, Agent Orange and dioxin, 264
Autoimmunity and laterality, 85

BALB/c mice, 340
Beckwith-Wiedemann syndrome, longitudinal roentgencephalometric study (single case), 179–187
   airway, 180–181
   anterior cross-bite, 180, 183, 186
   dentoalveolar protrusion, 184, 186
   difficulty swallowing, 180, 181
   EMG syndrome (exomphalos, macroglossia, gigantism), 179
   hernia, 180–182
   mandibular prognathism, 180, 184, 186
   macroglossia, 179–181, 183, 185–187
     cf. cleft lip, 184, 185
   midface hypoplasia, 180
   speech, 181–182
Bias, ascertainment, 53–54
Blastemae, 332, 333
Blastula, cell-specific gene expression, 58
Blebs. *See* Cleft lip/palate, nasomaxillary blebs and hematomas, mice
Blepharophimosis
   diphenylhydantoin-induced cf. spontaneous anomalies, 307
   Dubowitz syndrome, 286
Blindness, Hallerman-Streiff syndrome, 189–190, 194
Bloom syndrome cf. Dubowitz syndrome, 283
Brachycephaly, Hallerman-Streiff syndrome, 190, 192, 194
Branchio-oto-renal syndrome. *See* Hemifacial microsomia with branchio-oto-renal syndrome
BrdU and delayed splotch (sp^d) gene, mouse spina bifida, 341
Buccopharyngeal membrane, persistent, and VPI, 104

Cadmium sulfate and delayed splotch (sp^d) gene, mouse spina bifida, 341
Calcomp plot, 143, 152
Calvaria, achondroplasia, 152, 159–161
Cardiac anomalies
   agnathia without holoprosencephaly, 244
   velocardiofacial syndrome, 113
Cardiorespiratory insufficiency. *See* Hallermann-Streiff syndrome with cardiorespiratory insufficiency
C57BL/6J mice
   cleft palate, corticosterone-induced, 301, 303
   and delayed splotch (sp^d) gene, mouse spina bifida, 340
Cell death, 334–335
Cell-specific gene expression. *See* Gene expression, cell-specific, and pattern formation during craniofacial development
Cephalometric roentgenology. *See* Roentgencephalometric *entries*
Cerebral gigantism, 212, 222, 224
Ceruloplasmin, diphenylhydantoin-induced cf. spontaneous anomalies, 311
Chick. *See* Cleft palate, natural, experimental fusion in embryonic chick
C3H mice and cranioschisis gene, mouse exencephaly, 340
Chromosomal damage, Agent Orange and dioxin, 259–264; *see also* Trisomy
Cleft lip
   cf. Beckwith-Wiedemann syndrome, 184, 185
   and mandibular condyle in facial asymmetry, 228
   right-sided, excess of parental non-righthandedness, 85–87
     with or without cleft palate, 86, 87
     cf. left-sided or bilateral, 86
Cleft lip/palate
   agnathia without holoprosencephaly, 242, 243, 246, 247
   diphenylhydantoin-induced cf. spontaneous anomalies, 305–309
   Duane retraction syndrome, 277
   hemifacial microsomia with branchio-oto-renal syndrome, 291, 292
Cleft lip/palate, nasomaxillary blebs and hematomas, mice, 313–322
   A/J mice, 314, 319–322
   CL/Fr mice, 314–319, 321, 322
   diphenylhydantoin, 313
   left cf. right, 314
   mesenchyme-epithelial adhesion, 313, 319–322
     cf. human collagen diseases, 322
   pedigree of events, 321
   phenotypic frequencies of various abnormalities, 314
Cleft lip/palate, unilateral, measurements cf. normals, 89–95
   and lip repair, 94
   maxillary arch size, 89–94
     arch height, 92, 93
     at birth, 91, 93
     at 5 years of age, 91–92, 94
     intercanine width, 91–94
     intermolar width, 91–93
     linear arch dimensions at 5 years, 92
   model, 90
   occlusion, 94
   palatal mucosa, 89, 93–94
     at birth, 90–91, 93, 94
     and development of maxillary arch, 94–95
   speech, 95
Cleft, median facial, Duane retraction syndrome, 280
Cleft palate
   Dubowitz syndrome, 284–286
   spontaneous closure, 73–74, 76
   see also Velopharyngeal inadequacy without overt cleft palate
Cleft palate, corticosterone-induced, A/J mice, 299–304
   cf. C57BL/6J (resistant) fetuses, 301, 303

diurnal corticosterone patterns in pregnancy, 299–302
    cf. chronic stress, 302
    and fetal growth, 303
    P450 enzymes, 303
    receptor physiology, 301, 303
        EGF and insulin, 301
Cleft palate, natural, experimental fusion in embryonic chick, 323–336
    cf. alligators, 324, 326, 334
    collagen, 328
    embryonic wound healing, 333–336
    epithelial-mesenchyme interactions, 324, 328, 331, 334
    evolution, 324, 326, 333–335
    experimental mortality, 328
    explants, 324–327, 333
        schema, 325, 334
    GAGs, 328
    in ovo surgery, 324–334
        schema, 35
    cf. mammals, 324, 333, 335
        monkeys, 335
    palatal shelf movements, 324, 326, 328, 331
        blastemae, 322, 323
            cell death, 334–335
            medial edge epithelia, 324–326, 328, 331–332, 334
Cleft palate, surgical closure, timing, 71–83
    aesthetics, 72, 82
    age, 71–73, 83
    case illustrations, 75–79
    dentition, 73
    feeding, 72, 81
    Island Flap, 73, 79
    isolated cleft palate, 79
    late, after prosthetic obturation, 71–72, 77, 79
    lip repair, two-stage 80–81
    nonphysiological surgery, 72, 78, 79
    palate and facial development, 72, 79, 80, 82
        palatal compression technique, 73
    palatopharyngeal action, 82
    Pierre Robin syndrome, 81
    size of cleft space, 72
        customizing surgery, results, 72–74
    speech, 71, 72, 82
        and neonatal orthopedics, 79
            phenomic development of articulation, 72
    spontaneous closure, 73–74, 76
    stimulation of cleft space to close faster, 78
CL/Fr mice, clefting
    diphenylhydantoin-induced cf. spontaneous anomalies, 306–310
    nasomaxillary blebs and hematomas, mice, 314–319, 321, 322
Cockayne syndrome, 219
Collagen, 328
    diseases, human, 322
Coloboma, Duane retraction syndrome, 274, 276–280
Computer morphometric model, achondroplasia, 142–143, 149
    Calcomp plot, 143, 152

see also Record, craniofacial patient, computerized multi-use
Condyle. *See* Mandibular condyle *entries*
Copper, serum, diphenylhydantoin-induced, 311
Cornea, cloudy, agnathia without holoprosencephaly, 243
Cornelia de Lange syndrome. *See* de Lange syndrome
Coronal synostosis, unilateral, plagiocephaly, 199–202, 209
    neurosurgical release, 204, 209–210
Coronoid process
    achondroplasia, 162
    and mandibular condyle in facial asymmetry, 228
Cor pulmonale, Hallerman-Streiff syndrome, 196, 197
Corticosterone. *See* Cleft palate, corticosterone-induced, A/J mice
Craniofacial dysmorphology in abnormal growth syndromes, roentgencephalometry, 211–225
    data analysis, 215–218
        cross-sectional, 215–217
        longitudinal, 217–218
    growth increment ratios of facial components, 224
    hexagon, 213, 214, 218, 222, 225
    landmarks and planes, 213
    maxilla cf. mandible, 213, 214, 219, 220, 222
    neurocranium, 213, 214, 219, 220, 222, 223
    splanchnocranium, 214–215
    University of Illinois CCFA, 213
    see also specific syndromes
Craniofacial Profile Pattern Analysis, dimension used, 46, 47
Cranioschisis *(crn)* gene, mouse exencephaly, 339–342
    C3H mice, 340
    eye defects, 339
    warfarin and thyroxine administration, 340–341
Cribiform bone, achondroplasia, 157
crn gene. *See* Cranioschisis *(crn)* gene, mouse exencephaly
Crouzon syndrome, 19–20, 37, 49, 53
Cryptorchidism, Dubowitz syndrome, 284, 286
Cyclopia, 241

Data bank, University of Illinois, 35–36
Database management, 253, 254, 257
Deafness/hearing loss
    Duane retraction syndrome, 275–277, 280
    Dubowitz syndrome, 285
    hemifacial microsomia with branchio-oto-renal syndrome, 287, 288, 290, 292–294
    see also Ear; Microtia
de Lange syndrome, 49–50, 54
    craniofacial dysmorphology, 212, 217–218, 220–222, 224
Delayed splotch (sp^d) gene, mouse spina bifida, 340–341
    BrdU, cadmium sulfate, and retinoic acid, 341
    C57BL/6J and BALB/c mice, 340
Dentition

and cleft palate surgical closure, 73
Dubowitz syndrome, 284-286
and neural crest, cell-specific gene expression, 59
see also Hemifacial microsomia, teeth maturation; Gene expression, cell-specific, and pattern formation during craniofacial development
Dento-alveolar process
  and mandibular condyle in facial asymmetry, 236-237
  protrusion and Beckwith-Wiedemann syndrome, 184-186
Dermoids, Duane retraction syndrome, 274, 277-279, 280
Developmental fields. *See* Agnathia without holoprosencephaly, developmental field defect
Diagnostic homogeneity, problems with, Robin sequence example, 50-53
Dioxin. *See* Agent Orange and dioxin, teratogenic/mutagenic effects
Diphenylhydantoin-induced cf. spontaneous craniofacial anomalies, 305-311
  A/J mice, 306
  cleft lip/palate, 305-309
  CL/Fr mice, 306-310
  failure of eyelid closure, 307
  genetics, 306-310
    autosomal recessive, 308, 309
    fertility, 308
    model proposed, 310
  hydantoin syndrome, 306
  increased serum copper and ceruloplasmin, 311
  primary and secondary epithelial closure defects, 306-311
  Star mice, 306-309
Diphenylhydantoin-induced cleft lip/palate, nasomaxillary blebs and hematomas, mice, 313, 313
cDNA clones, ameloblast enamel genes, 61-64
DNA sequence identification, cell-specific gene expression, 59-61
Down syndrome, craniofacial dysmorphology, 212, 219-221, 224
Duane retraction syndrome (restrictive strabismus), craniofacial malformations, 273-281
  amblyopia, 274
  anisometropia, 274
  astigmatism, 274
  cleft lip/palate, 277
  coloboma, 274, 276-277, 279, 280
  dermoids, 274, 277-280
  ear abnormalities and deafness, 275-277, 280
  EMG data, 274
  Goldenhar syndrome, 276-281
  hemifacial microsomia, 277-279, 281
  Klippel-Feil anomaly, 275, 277, 280
  lacrimal gland and tearing, 279
  macrostomia, 277-279
  median facial cleft, 280
  microstomia, 277

  paradoxical innervation, 279-280
  Wildervanck syndrome, 277, 280
Dubowitz syndrome, 283-286
  cf. Bloom syndrome, 283
Dwarfism. *See* Achondroplasia, craniofacial morphometry and roentgencephalometry
Dysarthria, dyspraxia, and VPI, 110-113; *see also* Speech

Ear
  Duane retraction syndrome, 275-277, 280
  otitis, VPI, 106-108, 110
  position, agnathia without holoprosencephaly, 241-246
  see also Deafness/hearing loss; Microtia
Edema, pedal, Hallerman-Streiff syndrome with cardiorespiratory insufficiency, 191
EGF, 301
Ehlers Danlos syndrome, 322
Electromyography
  Duane retraction syndrome, 274
  plagiocephaly, 201, 202, 206-209
  and VPI, 102
Embryonic surgery and wound healing. *See* Cleft palate, natural, experimental fusion in embryonic chick
EMG syndrome (exomphalos, macroglossia, gigantism), 179
Enamel genes. *See under* Gene expression, cell-specific, and pattern formation during craniofacial development
Endochondral bone formation, achondroplasia, 156
Epilepsy, 306
Epithelium/epithelial
  closure defects, diphenylhydantoin-induced cf. spontaneous anomalies, 306-311
  -mesenchyme adhesion, cleft lip/palate, nasomaxillary blebs and hematomas, mice, 313, 319-322
  cf. human collagen diseases, 322
  see also Cleft palate, natural, experimental fusion in embryonic chick
Evolution, natural cleft palate, chick, 324, 326, 333-335
Exencephaly, cranioschisis *(crn)* gene, mouse, 339-342
Exomphalos, Beckwith-Wiedemann syndrome, 179
Experimental surgery, *See* Cleft palate, natural, experimental fusion in embryonic chick
Eye defects and cranioschisis gene, mouse exencephaly, 339; *see also* Duane retraction syndrome (restrictive strabismus), craniofacial malformations; Oculo-*entries*

Facial paresis, hemifacial microsomia with branchio-oto-renal syndrome, 288, 293
Faucial pillar abnormalites, VPI, 103-104
Feeding and cleft palate surgical closure, 72, 81
Fertility, diphenylhydantoin, 308
Fistula, congenital palatal, and VPI, 99, 102
  cf. overt clefts, 102
Foramen magnum, achondroplasia, 158-159

Index

Forebrain. *See* Agnathia without holoprosencephaly, developmental field complex
Forth (computer language), 254, 257
Frontal sinus, achondroplasia, 151, 152
Functional matrix theory, 156–157, 227

Gatlinburg Conference (1959) 5, 23–24, 58
G-banded karyotyping, Agent Orange and dioxin, chromosomal effects, 260–261
Gene expression, cell-specific, and pattern formation during craniofacial development, 57–65
   control, 58–59
      blastula, 58
      craniofacial paradigm, 60–61
   DNA sequence identification, 59–61
   enamel genes, ameloblast, 59, 61–65
      amelogenin, 63, 64
         de novo expression during mouse molar formation, 64–65
         inductive signals, 65
         mouse cDNA clones, 61–64
         restriction endonuclease cleavage, 63
   generalized schema, 60
   investigative strategies, 59–60
   neural crest and dentition, 59
   recombinant DNA technology, 58
Genetic counseling, hemifacial microsomia with branchio-oto-renal syndrome, 295
Gigantism
   cerebral, craniofacial dysmorphology, 212, 222, 224
   EMG syndrome, 179
Glucocorticoids. *See* Cleft palate, corticosterone-induced, A/J mice
Glycosaminoglycans, 328
Goldenhar syndrome, 167, 168, 172, 173, 176, 177
   with Duane retraction syndrome, 276–281
   hemifacial microsomia with branchio-oto-renal syndrome, 288
   tooth maturation, 268
Growth deficiency/failure
   Dubowitz syndrome, 283, 285, 286
   syndromes, prenatal-onset, 44–45, 49–50
   see also Craniofacial dysmorphology in abnormal growth syndromes, roentgencephalometry

Hallerman-Streiff syndrome, teeth, 191, 268
Hallerman-Streiff syndrome with cardiorespiratory insufficiency, 189–197
   brachycephaly, 190, 192, 194
   cor pulmonale, 196, 197
   dental defects, 191
   hypoplastic mandible, 190, 192–194
      surgical correction, 197
      TMJ, 192–194
   micrognathia, 190, 194, 196
      cf. Treacher-Collins syndrome and progeria, 190, 194, 197
   obstructive sleep apnea, 192–197
   oculomandibulodyscephaly with hypotrichosis, 189–190, 194
   ophthalmologic abnormalities, 190, 194
   pedal edema, 191
   platybasia, 193
   respiratory obstruction, chronic, 190, 193–196
   roentgenocephalometric findings, summarized, 195
   spina bifida, 191
   treatment, 192, 197
Hand-foot-uterus syndrome, 45–47
Hearing loss/deafness
   Duane retraction syndrome, 275–277, 280
   Dubowitz syndrome, 285
   hemifacial microsomia with branchio-oto-renal syndrome, 287, 288, 290, 292–294
   see also Ear; Microtia
Hematoma formation theory, hemifacial microsomia, 176, 270, 279; *see also* Cleft lip/palate, nasomaxillary blebs and hematomas, mice
Hemifacial microsomia
   accessory vertebra, 171, 173, 175
   cranial base malformations, 168–176
      angle (kyphosis), 168, 169, 173
      basilar invagination, 169–170
      occipitalization of atlas, 169–171, 173, 175
      platybasia, 168, 169, 173
   craniovertebral malformations, roentgencephalometry, 167–177
   and Duane retraction syndrome, 277–279, 281
   first and second branchial syndrome, 175
   frequency, 172–173, 176
   hematoma formation theory, 176, 270, 279
   heterogeneity, 270, 271
   with Klippel-Feil anomaly, 173, 175–176
   mandible, grades I-III deformities, 267–268
   maxilla, 267
   microtia, 167, 168, 170, 172–177, 267, 270
      foramen magnum and odontoid process, 174
   oculoauriculovertebral dysplasia, 167, 168, 173, 175–177, 288
   scoliosis, 171, 172, 175, 176
   spina bifida, 170, 172, 175, 176
   tooth maturation, 267–271
      cf. other syndromes, 268
      unequal patterns, 269–271
   University of Illinois, CCFA, 168
   vertebral fusion, 170, 171, 173, 175
   see also Goldenhar syndrome; Mandibular condyle in facial asymmetry, longitudinal roentgencephalometry
Hemifacial microsomia with branchio-oto-renal syndrome, 287–295
   autosomal dominant, 287, 294–295
   bifid uvula, 292
   branchial cleft cartilage, 287, 290, 292–294
   branchial cleft sinuses/fistulas, 287, 289, 293, 294
   cephalometry, 291
   cleft lip/palate, 291, 292
   facial paresis, 288, 293
   genetic counseling, 295

kidney, 288, 291, 292, 294
lacrimal duct aplasia, 288
mandibular hypoplasia, 288–294
microtia and hearing loss, 287, 288, 290, 292–294
preauricular pits/sinuses/tags, 287–290, 292–294
Hernia, Beckwith-Wiedemann syndrome, 180–182
Holoprosencephaly, 246–247; see also Agnathia without holoprosencephaly, developmental field complex
Hurler syndrome, 45
Hydantoin syndrome, 306; see also Diphenylhydantoin-induced cf. spontaneous craniofacial anomalies
Hydrocephalus, achondroplasia, 160–161
Hypertelorbitism, 19
Hypospadias, Dubowitz syndrome, 284, 286
Hypotonia, achondroplasia, 160
Hypotrichosis, Hallerman-Streiff syndrome, 189–190, 194

IBM
    PC-XT, 254
    System, 360, 149
Immune defects, Dubowitz syndrome, 286
Implants, 35, 38; see also Mandible, backward rotation, metallic implant, roentgencephalometry
In ovo surgery. See Cleft palate, natural, experimental fusion in embryonic chick
Insulin, 301
Intelligence
    Dubowitz syndrome, 283–286
    and laterality, 85
Intercanine and intermolar width, unilateral clefts, 91–94
Intracranial pressure, increased, plagiocephaly, 202
Italy, Agent Orange and dioxin, 263

Johanson-Blizzard syndrome, 212, 216, 219–220, 224
Juvenile rheumatoid polyarteritis, 131–134

Kidney. See Hemifacial microsomia with branchio-oto-renal syndrome
Klippel-Feil anomaly, 173, 175–176, 275, 277, 280
Kyphosis, 168, 169, 173

Lacrimal gland
    Duane retraction syndrome, 279
    duct aplasia, hemifacial microsomia with branchio-oto-renal syndrome, 288
Laterality
    cleft lip, right sided, excess of parental non-rightedness, 85–87
    intelligence, autoimmunity, schizophrenia, and NTDs, 85
    preferential, 50
    twins, 85, 87

Levator palatini, VPI, 101
Lip repair, 80–81, 94
Little People of America, 141–142
Long face syndrome, 129–131
    symphysis, 129, 131

Macroglossia, Beckwith-Wiedemann syndrome, 179–181, 183, 185–187
    cf. cleft lip, 184, 185
Macrostomia, Duane retraction syndrome, 277–279
Malignancy, Dubowitz syndrome, 286
Mandible/mandibular
    hemifacial microsomia, 267–268
    hypoplasia, branchio-oto-renal syndrome, 288–294
    hypoplastic, Hallerman-Streiff syndrome, 190, 192–194
        surgical correction, 197
        TMJ, 192–194
    plagiocephaly, 200–202, 204–206, 209
    prognathism
        alveolar, achondroplasia, 151, 162
        Beckwith-Wiedemann syndrome, 180, 184, 186
        see also Agnathia without holoprosencephaly, developmental field complex
Mandible, backward rotation, metallic implant, roentgencephalometry, 127–138
    craniofacial tracings, 130, 133, 136
    intramatrix rotation, 127–129, 131, 132, 135, 137
    juvenile rheumatoid polyarteritis, 131–134
        maxillary growth, 132, 134
        molars, 132
        resorption at condylar head, 131
        Still's disease, 131
    long face syndrome, 129–131
        symphysis, 129, 131
    mandibulofacial dysostosis, 134–137
        molars, 137
    matrix rotation, 128, 131
    total rotation, 131
Mandibular condyle
    cartilage in mandibulofacial dysostosis, 134
    head resorption, juvenile rheumatoid polyarteritis, 131
Mandibular condyle in facial asymmetry, longitudinal roentgencephalometry, 227–237
    cleft lip, 228
    congenital agenesis, 228–230
    coronoid process, 228
    degeneration, 227, 234–236
    dento-alveolar process, 236–237
    fracture, condylar, 230–234
        functional appliance, 232
    functional matrix theory, 227
    implications for development, 227
    importance of early recognition, 234–236
    and maxilla, 236
    microtia, 228–230
    orthodontics, 229–231, 234, 236
        bite block, 236

and ramus, 228, 230–231, 234
regeneration, 227
zygoma, 229
Mandibulofacial dysostosis, 134–137
March of Dimes Birth Defects Information System, 254, 258
Marfan syndrome, 212, 222–224
Maxilla/maxillary
　achondroplasia, 161
　arch measurements, unilateral clefts, 89–95
　growth, juvenile rheumatoid polyarteritis, 132, 134
　hemifacial microsomia, 267
　and mandibular condyle in facial asymmetry, 236
　plagiocephaly, 199–202, 205, 209
Megaloencephaly, achondroplasia, 160
Mesenchyme-epithelial adhesion, cleft lip/palate
　chick, 324, 328, 331, 334
　cf. human collagen diseases, 322
　mice, 313, 319–322
Mesoderm, prechordal, agnathia without holoprosencephaly, 247–248
Mice. *See* Cleft palate, corticosterone-induced, A/J mice; Cleft lip/palate, nasomaxillary blebs and hematomas, mice; Cranioschisis *(crn)* gene, mouse exencephaly; Delayed splotch *(sp^d^)* gene, mouse spina bifida; Diphenylhydantoin-induced cf. spontaneous craniofacial anomalies, mice; specific strains
Microcephaly, Dubowitz syndrome, 283, 285, 286
Micrognathia, Dubowitz syndrome, 284–286
Microstomia
　agnathia without holoprosencephaly, 241–246
　Duane retraction syndrome, 277
Microtia
　hemifacial microsomia, 167, 168, 170, 172–177, 267, 270
　　with branchio-oto-renal syndrome, 287, 288, 290, 292–294
　and mandibular condyle in facial asymmetry, 228–230
　see also Ear; Deafness/hearing loss
MIDAS statistical package, 149
Molars
　juvenile rheumatoid polyarteritis, 132
　mandibulofacial dysostosis, 137
Motor development, slow, achondroplasia, 160
Musculus uvulae, and VPI, 102
Myoclonus, palatal, and VPI, 111

Nasal bone, achondroplasia, 161
Nasal respiration, reduced, and VPI, 106
Nasomaxillary blebs and hematomas. *See* Cleft lip/palate, nasomaxillary blebs and hematomas, mice
Nasopharyngeal constriction, achondroplasia, 161–162
Nasopharyngoscopy, and VPI, 101
National Institute for Dental Research, 5, 23
Neural crest
　agnathia without holoprosencephaly, 247–248
　and dentition, cell-specific gene expression, 59

Neural tube defects, laterality, 85; *see also* Spina bifida
Neurocranium, abnormal growth syndromes, 213, 214, 219, 220, 222, 223
Neuromotor deficits. *See under* Velopharyngeal inadequacy without overt cleft palate
Neuropathy, peripheral, Agent Orange and dioxin, teratogenic/mutagenic effects, 260
Nystagmus, palatal, and VPI, 111

Obesity, 196
Obturator, 71–72, 77, 79
Occipital bony protuberance, achondroplasia, 159
Oculoauriculovertebral dysplasia and hemifacial microsomia, 167, 168, 173, 175–177
　with branchio-oto-renal syndrome, 288
Oculomandibulodyscephaly with hypotrichosis, Hallerman-Streiff syndrome, 189–190, 194
Oculo-motor. *See* Duane retraction syndrome, craniofacial malformations
Oligohydramnics, Robin sequence, 51, 52
Oregon, Agent Orange and dioxin, 264
Orthodontics, mandibular condyle in facial asymmetry, 229–231, 234, 236
Osteogenesis imperfecta, 322
Otitis and VPI, 106–108, 110
Oto-palato-digital syndrome, MZ twins, 47, 48

Palate/palatal
　fistula, congenital, and VPI, 99, 102
　　cf. overt clefts, 102
　myoclonus, and VPI, 111
　shelf movements, 324, 326, 328, 331
　see also Cleft *entries*
Palatopharyngeal disproportion, and VPI, 104–105
Paresis, facial, hemifacial microsomia with branchio-oto-renal syndrome, 288, 293
Patent ductus arteriosus, agnathia without holoprosencephaly, 244
Patient record. *See* Record, craniofacial patient, computerized multi-use
Pattern formation. *See* Gene expression, cell-specific, and pattern formation during craniofacial development
P450 enzymes, cleft palate, corticosterone-induced, 303
Pierre Robin syndrome. *See* Robin sequence
Plagiocephaly, longitudinal roentgencephalometry, 199–210
　asymmetry, craniofacial
　　cranial base, 199–202, 204, 206, 208, 209
　　development in early infancy, 201, 208
　　mandibular, 200–202, 204–206, 209
　　maxillary, 199–201, 205, 209
　　progressive facial, 203
　　ramus, 200, 201
　coronal synostosis, unilateral, 199–202, 209
　　neurosurgical release, 204, 209–210
　electromyography, temporal and masseter muscles, 201, 202, 206–209
　　cf. visual torticollis in strabismus, 209
　increased intracranial pressure, 202
　sphenofrontal synostosis, 199, 200, 209
　supraorbital depression, 202, 204

Platybasia
  Hallerman-Streiff syndrome with cardiorespiratory insufficiency, 193
  and hemifacial microsomia, 168, 169, 173
Polyarteritis, juvenile rheumatoid, 131–134
Polyhydramnios, agnathia without holoprosencephaly, 242, 245, 246
Preauricular pits/sinuses/tags, hemifacial microsomia with branchio-oto-renal syndrome, 287–290
Preferential laterality, 50
Premature rupture of membranes (PROM), agnathia without holoprosencephaly, 243
Prenatal-onset growth deficiency syndromes, 44–45, 49–50
Progeria
  craniofacial dysmorphology, 212, 215, 218, 224
  cf. Hallerman-Streiff syndrome with cardiorespiratory insufficiency, 190, 194, 197
Progeroid cranoifacial dysmorphology, 212, 219, 224
Prognathism, mandibular
  alveolar, achondroplasia, 151, 162
  and Beckwith-Wiedemann syndrome, 180, 184, 186
Pruzansky, Samuel, 5–9, 19–21
  bibliography, 10–16
  encouragement of younger colleagues, 8
  Gatlinburg Conference (1959), 5, 23–24, 58
  interdisciplinary approach, 57–58
  National Institute for Dental Research, 5, 23
  professional focus, three issues, 7
  professional memoir, 19–21
  and roentgencephalometry, 33, 35–38
  as speaker and writer, 7–8
  wife (Donna), 6, 9
  University of Illinois–Chicago, 7, 25–29; see also Univeristy of Illinois–Chicago
  youth and education, 5
Psychological factors, VPI, 113

Race, agnathia without holoprosencephaly, 242, 243, 245, 246
Ramus
  in facial asymmetry, 228, 230–231, 234
  mandibulofacial dysostosis, 137
  plagiocephaly, 200, 201
Recombinant DNA technology, cell-specific gene expression, 58
Record, craniofacial patient, computerized multi-use, 251–258
  classification system, 251, 253–254, 258
    listed, 255–257
  computer user access, 253
  core record, 251–252
  cost, 252
  database management, 253, 254, 257
  hard copy, 252
  IBM PC-XT, 254
  linking research information with treatment, 251
  March of Dimes Birth Defects Information System, 254, 258
  software design, 252–254
    MMS Forth, 254, 257
    word processing, 253, 254
Respiration, nasal, reduced, and VPI, 106
Respiratory distress, agnathia without holoprosencephaly, 244; see also Hallermann-Streiff syndrome with cardiorespiratory insufficiency
Restriction endonuclease cleavage, ameloblast enamel genes, 63
Retinoic acid, and delayed splotch (sp^d) gene, mouse spina bifida, 341
Rheumatoid polyarteritis, juvenile, 131–134
Robin sequence, 47–49
  and cleft palate surgical closure, 81
  etiologic implies phenotypic heterogeneity, 52
  oligohydramnios, 51–53
  partial trisomy 11q, 51, 52
  problems in diagnostic homogeneity, 50–53
Roentgencephalometric principles of syndromic dysmorphic growth and development, 43–54
  Apert syndrome, 37, 45, 49
  ascertainment bias problems, 53–54
    diagram of phenotypic spectrum for a syndrome, 52
    Rubenstein-Taybi syndrome, 54
  asymmetric dysmorphism and preferential laterality, 50
  bone age determination, 43–44
  Crouzon syndrome, 37, 49, 53
  de Lange syndrome, 49–50, 54
  dysharmonic maturation and patterned dysmorphism, 45–49
    Craniofacial Profile Pattern Analysis, 46, 47
    hand-foot-uterus syndrome, 45–47
    Hurler syndrome, 45
    oto-palato-digital syndrome, MZ twins, 47, 48
    Robin sequence, 47–49
    trisomy 18, 45, 49
  limitations of radiologic assessment in syndromic dysmorphism, 44–45
  prenatal-onset primary growth deficiency syndromes, 44–45, 49–50
  problems in diagnostic homogeneity, Robin sequence example, 50–53
  see also specific applications
Roentgencephalometric techniques, 26, 31–38
  analytic techniques, 34–35
    multivariate, 35, 38
  craniofacial anomalies, 35–37
    data bank, University of Illinois, 35–36
    qualitative and quantitative analysis, 36
  development of technique, 32–33
  improving resolution, 37
  infant cephalometry, 33–34, 37
    lateral, frontal, axial projections 33–34
  longitudinal studies, 38
  metallic implant technique, 35, 38
  Pruzansky, S.J., and, 33, 35–38

Rubinstein-Taybi syndrome, 54
Russel-Silver syndrome, 212, 217, 220, 224

Schizophrenia and laterality, 85
Scoliosis, hemifacial microsomia, 171, 172, 175, 176
Sedlackova syndrome, 113
Sex, agnathia without holoprosencephaly, 242, 243, 245, 246; *see also under*
    Achondroplasia, craniofacial morphometry and roentgencephalometry
Sinus, frontal, achondroplasia, 151, 152
Sister chromatid exchange, Agent Orange and dioxin, 259, 261–263
Sleep apnea, 106, 192–197
sp^d (delayed splotch) gene, mouse spina bifida, 340–341
Speech
    Beckwith-Wiedemann syndrome, 181–182
    cleft palate, 71, 72, 82
        neonatal orthopedics, 79
        phonemic development of articulation, 72
        unilateral, 95
    Dubowitz syndrome, 284–286
    and VPI, 106–108, 110
    dysarthria (neuromotor deficit), 110–113
    hypernasal, 98–100, 103, 105, 108–110, 113, 114
    hyponasal, 98, 108
Speech pathologist and VPI, 109
Sphenofrontal synostosis, plagiocephaly, 199, 200, 209
Sphenoid bone, achondroplasia, 157
Spheno-occipital-synchondrosis, achondroplasia, 158
Spina bifida
    delayed splotch (sp^d) gene, mouse, 340–341
    Hallerman-Streiff syndrome with cardiorespiratory insufficiency, 191
    and hemifacial microsomia, 170, 172, 175, 176
Splanchnocranium, abnormal growth syndromes, 214–215
Star mice, diphenylhydantoin-induced cf. spontaneous anomalies, 306–309
Stickler syndrome, problems in diagnostic homogeneity, 51, 52
Still's disease, juvenile rheumatoid polyarteritis, 131
Strabismus, 209; *see also* Duane retraction syndrome, craniofacial malformations
Supraorbital depression, plagiocephaly, 202, 204
Surgery. *See* Cleft palate, natural, experimental fusion in embryonic chick; Cleft palate, surgical closure timing
Swallowing difficulty, Beckwith-Wiedemann syndrome, 180–181
Symphysis
    long face syndrome, 129, 131
    mandibulofacial dysostosis, 137
Synostosis, plagiocephaly
    sphenofrontal, 199, 200, 209
    unilateral coronal, 199–202, 209
        neurosurgical release, 204, 209–210
Tear glands, 279, 288

Teeth. *See* Dentition
Temperomandibular joint, Hallerman-Streiff syndrome, 192–194
Thumb, supernumerary, 228
Thyroxine and cranioschisis gene, mouse exencephaly, 340–341
Treacher-Collins syndrome
    cf. Hallerman-Streiff syndrome, 190, 194, 197
    Pruzansky and, 19–20
    tooth maturation, 268
Trisomy
    11q, partial, Robin sequence, 51, 52
    18, 45, 49
    21 (Down syndrome), 212, 219–221, 224
Trunk length, achondroplasia, 157, 160
Turner syndrome, craniofacial dysmorphology, 212, 218, 220, 224
Twins
    and laterality, 85, 87
    MZ, oto-palato-digital syndrome, 47, 48

University of Illinois-Chicago, 7, 25–29
    Center for Craniofacial Anomalies, 25, 27–29
        abnormal growth syndromes, 213
        Data Bank, 27, 28, 35–36
        establishment (1967), 28
        hemifacial microsomia, 168
        Maxillofacial Prosthetics Clinic, 27
    Cleft Palate Center, 26–28
    team approach, 25–26
        academic vs. service, 28–29
        role of dentist, 29
Uvula, bifid
    Dubowitz syndrome, 285, 286
    hemifacial microsomia with branchio-oto-renal syndrome, 292
    and VPI, 98–101, 104

Velocardiofacial syndrome and VPI, 113
Velopharyngeal inadequacy (VPI) without overt cleft palate, 97–115
    adenoids and VP function, 104–110
        adenoidectomy for otitis and compromised speech, 106–108, 110
        auditory tube, 106–107
        embryology, 105–106
        incidence, 109
        reduced nasal respiration, effects, 106
        speech pathologist, 109
        velum-adenoid closure in childhood, 106
    bifid uvula, 98–101, 104
    congenital palatal fistula, 99, 102
    cf. overt clefts, 102
    electromyography, 102
    faucial pillar abnormalities, 103–104
        persistent buccopharyngeal membrane, 104
    hypernasal speech, 98–100, 103, 105, 108–110, 113, 114
        cf. hyponasal, 98, 108
    levator palatini, 101
    nasopharyngoscopy, 101
    neuromotor deficits, 110–113
        cf. aphasia, 110
        apraxia and dyspraxia, 110–111

categorization, 112
dysarthria, 110–113
general neurologic defect, 113
link with psychological factors, 113
palatal myoclonus or nystagmus, 111
palatopharyngeal disproportion, 104–105
discovery at adenoidectomy, 104–105
phoneme-specific, 98–99, 114–115
stress, in wind instrument playing, 113–114
submucous anatomic defects of secondary palate, 98–102, 104
classic, 100–101
musculus uvulae, 102
occult muscular deficiencies, 101
tonsils, 109–110
cf. VP incompetence, 98
Vertebrae. See Spina bifida; under Hemifacial microsomia

Vietnam veterans. See Agent Orange and dioxin, teratogenic/mutagenic effects
Visual torticollis, 209
Voice, high-pitched, Dubowitz syndrome, 284–286

Waldeyer's ring, 105
Warfarin and cranioschisis gene, mouse exencephaly, 340–341
Wildervanck syndrome, 277, 280
Wind instruments, VPI, 113–114
Word processing, 253, 254
Wound healing, embryonic, experimental cleft palate fusion, chick, 333–336

Zygoma in facial asymmetry, 229